病毒感染与人类肿瘤
从基础科学到临床预防

Viruses and Human Cancer
From Basic Science to Clinical Prevention

〔美〕Mei Hwei Chang
      Kuan-Teh Jeang 编著

卢建红 等 编译

本书受以下基金项目资助：
国家自然科学基金（81372139，81171931，81471959，81501746，31470263）
国家重点基础研究发展计划（973计划，2015CB554301）
科技部科技基础性工作专项（2013FY113300）
湖南省自然科学基金（2015JJ2149）
云南省应用基础研究计划（2013FZ143）
中国医学科学院医学生物学研究所重点项目（2014IMB03ZD）

科学出版社
北　京

图字：01-2016-1755

内 容 简 介

本书来自2014年Springer出版的肿瘤研究最新进展Recent Results in Cancer Research丛书，原书作者都是相关领域的专家，对当前的研究进展内容描述比较详尽，体现了最新进展。本书阐述了已发现的几种常见肿瘤病毒感染的致瘤机制及其预防，领域涉及病毒学和肿瘤学研究，内容涉及外泌体、非编码RNA、炎症与肿瘤、肿瘤微环境等当前在肿瘤研究领域的热点概念。

本书适合于从事肿瘤相关基础研究与临床预防的科研人员和临床医生，也适合于从事肿瘤病毒或病毒学相关学习和研究的本科生及硕士、博士研究生参考。

Translation from English language edition:
Viruses and Human Cancer
From Basic Science to Clinical Prevention
edited by Mei Hwei Chang and Kuan-Teh Jeang
Copyright©Springer Berlin Heidelberg 2014
Springer Berlin Heidelberg is a part of Springer Science+Business Media
All Rights Reserved

图书在版编目(CIP)数据

病毒感染与人类肿瘤：从基础科学到临床预防/张美惠等编著；卢建红等编译. —北京：科学出版社，2016.3
书名原文：Viruses and Human Cancer: From Basic Science to Clinical Prevention
ISBN 978-7-03-047942-6

Ⅰ. ①病… Ⅱ. ①张… ②卢… Ⅲ. ①致肿瘤病毒–研究 Ⅳ. ①R730.231

中国版本图书馆CIP数据核字（2016）第060284号

责任编辑：罗 静 刘 晶/责任校对：郑金红
责任印制：徐晓晨/封面设计：刘新新

科学出版社出版
北京东黄城根北街16号
邮政编码：100717
http://www.sciencep.com
北京凌奇印刷有限责任公司 印刷
科学出版社发行 各地新华书店经销
*
2016年3月第 一 版　　开本：720×1000 B5
2018年4月第四次印刷　　印张：21
字数：406 000
定价：120.00元
（如有印装质量问题，我社负责调换）

《病毒感染与人类肿瘤：从基础科学到临床预防》编译人员名单

主 编 译　　卢建红（中南大学基础医学院肿瘤研究所）

　　　　　　　李义平（中山大学中山医学院、人类病毒学研究所）

　　　　　　　瞿小旺（南华大学转化医学研究所）

副主编译　　刘红旗（中国医学科学院医学生物学研究所）

其他参加人员（按姓名拼音排序）

　　　　　　　刘灵芝　刘文培　刘玉良　邵卫星

　　　　　　　陶玉芬　徐占雪　杨　静　尹　典

　　　　　　　郑福祥　周　诠　周中林　左垿莲

　　　　　　　Wu Hongzhuan

编 译 者 序

目前已知大约有 12%的人类肿瘤与病毒有关，病毒是治疗和预防相关性肿瘤的重要切入点。与一般的病毒性疾病一样，对于病毒相关性肿瘤，人类需要了解病毒的致病机制、获取流行病学数据；目标是开发有效的疫苗和治疗手段，最终控制或消灭致病性病毒。肿瘤病毒研究的发展在肿瘤研究中具有不可磨灭的历史，从 20 世纪初第一个肿瘤病毒即鸡 Rous 肉瘤病毒的发现到第一个原癌基因 *src* 的发现、著名的抑瘤基因 *p53* 的发现，以及从 1964 年第一个人类肿瘤病毒即 EB 病毒到当前多种人类肿瘤病毒的发现，无不体现了这点。到目前为止，至少有 5 个诺贝尔生理学或医学奖与肿瘤病毒的研究或发现有关。需要指出的是，上述的有些发现来自于动物肿瘤病毒，不包含在本书中。

无疑，病毒学与肿瘤学已相互交叉，互为渗透。虽然目前获取信息的途径很多，对于从事肿瘤病毒学的研究人员和临床医生来说，有几本好的工具书仍然是必要的。编译这本书，源自偶然。2014 年我留学回国时获得刚出版的原版书，发现书的内容新颖，编写详细，内容涉及基础科学与临床预防，便萌发了翻译出版的想法。由于有一系列从事病毒学和肿瘤学科研工作的专业人员及资深翻译人员的尽心参与，这本编译版的书终于得以面世。本书的主要内容忠实于原著，只对部分章节进行了编辑。关于 EB 病毒的致瘤作用和预防（原书第 10 章），原作者在移植后淋巴细胞增生性疾病描述较多，我们结合自己和当前的研究进展进行了编译，补充了 EB 病毒通过编码和诱导 microRNA 发挥作用等内容（编译版第 5 章和第 6 章）；第 4 章也是增加的内容。

在本书出版之际，特别感谢付出辛勤劳动的所有参编参译人员和科学出版社。

科学技术和研究的发展日新月异，相信还会有更多的病毒被发现与肿瘤发生相关或者更多的肿瘤与病毒感染有关。尽管我们很努力，书中错误也在所难免，而且书籍逐渐会有些赶不上时代的步伐。我们一方面希望读者对书中错误不吝指正，另一方面相信很多内容会是经典。如果这本书能给读者带来较大的收获，即是达成了我们的心愿。

卢建红

2016 年 3 月于长沙

目　　录

编译者序
第1章　概论：病毒感染与人类肿瘤 1
  1　引起人类肿瘤的病毒 3
  2　致瘤机制 4
    2.1　病毒感染与肿瘤的因果联系 5
    2.2　确认一种病毒的病因学的基础和临床意义 5
    2.3　发现新的致瘤病毒 7
  参考文献 7

第2章　病毒感染与人类肿瘤的流行病学 11
  1　引言 12
  2　全球范围内致瘤病毒感染率 13
  3　全球范围内的一些病毒引起的癌症发病率 18
  4　肿瘤病毒的致瘤机制 20
  5　一些病毒引起的癌症的终生累积发病率 21
  6　一些病毒引起的癌症的共同作用因子 21
  7　HBV 引起的肝细胞癌的风险计算 23
  8　通过疫苗和抗病毒治疗减少癌症发生率 25
  9　未来展望 26
  参考文献 26

第3章　病毒感染、炎症与肿瘤的预防 32
  1　引起肿瘤的慢性病毒感染 33
  2　炎症与肿瘤 34
    2.1　炎症与肿瘤生长的内在联系 34
    2.2　肿瘤相关性炎症过程中细胞因子信号机制和分子途径 35
    2.3　炎症过程中的肿瘤微环境 36
    2.4　肿瘤生长过程中的炎症、缺氧和血管生成 37
    2.5　慢性病毒感染和恶性肿瘤中的 T 细胞耗竭 38
  3　炎症与转移 39
  4　炎症相关性肿瘤的预防 40
    4.1　抗病毒疫苗和治疗 41

4.2　抗纤维化治疗 42
　　　4.3　抗炎治疗 44
　5　展望：肿瘤免疫治疗的前景 46
　参考文献 47

第 4 章　病毒感染与肿瘤微环境 59
　1　引言 59
　2　病毒感染与肿瘤微环境的形成及其相互影响 59
　　　2.1　炎症、癌变与肿瘤微环境 60
　　　2.2　免疫细胞与肿瘤微环境 61
　　　2.3　microRNA 与肿瘤微环境 62
　　　2.4　肿瘤细胞代谢与肿瘤微环境 62
　3　几种病毒的感染与肿瘤微环境 63
　　　3.1　EBV 与肿瘤微环境 63
　　　3.2　HBV 与肿瘤微环境 64
　　　3.3　HCV 与肿瘤微环境 65
　　　3.4　HPV 与肿瘤微环境 66
　　　3.5　HIV 与肿瘤微环境 66
　4　针对肿瘤微环境的靶向治疗及展望 67
　参考文献 68

第 5 章　EB 病毒的致瘤作用 73
　1　引言 73
　2　EB 病毒的感染与复制 74
　　　2.1　EB 病毒的感染与进入细胞 74
　　　2.2　EB 病毒的主要编码产物 77
　　　2.3　EB 病毒的复制 79
　3　EBV 相关性肿瘤和疾病 80
　　　3.1　EBV 与上皮性肿瘤 80
　　　3.2　EBV 与淋巴瘤 82
　　　3.3　EBV 与移植后淋巴组织增生性疾病 84
　4　EBV 通过 microRNA 发挥致瘤作用 84
　　　4.1　EBV 编码的 miRNA 85
　　　4.2　EBV 诱导宿主 miRNA 的异常表达 87
　　　4.3　EBV 相关的 miRNA 调控共同的靶基因 88
　　　4.4　EBV 相关的 miRNA 与免疫逃逸 89
　　　4.5　EBV 相关的 miRNA 与炎症和肿瘤微环境 90

  4.6　EBV 相关的 miRNA 与临床应用 ·· 91
 5　小结 ·· 91
 参考文献 ·· 91

第 6 章　EB 病毒感染及相关性疾病的预防 ·· 102
 1　引言 ·· 102
 2　EBV 感染的血清学检测 ·· 102
 3　EBV 疫苗 ·· 103
 4　PTLD 的治疗 ·· 104
 5　小结 ·· 106
 参考文献 ·· 107

第 7 章　乙型肝炎病毒的致癌作用 ·· 110
 1　引言 ·· 110
 2　HBV 基因组及复制 ·· 111
 3　HBx——一个具有复杂结构和功能的反式激活因子 ······················ 113
 4　HBx 与 E3 泛素连接酶：不仅仅是蛋白稳定性的一种联系？ ········ 114
 5　HBx 与肝细胞恶性转化 ·· 117
 6　HCC 中 HBV DNA 整合及突变的 X 基因 ·· 118
 7　结论与展望 ·· 118
 参考文献 ·· 120

第 8 章　乙型肝炎病毒感染与肝癌的预防 ·· 126
 1　引言 ·· 126
 2　HCC 造成的疾病负担 ·· 127
 3　HBV 感染的传播途径 ·· 127
 4　慢性 HBV 感染与 HCC ·· 128
  4.1　发生 HCC 的病毒（HBV）风险因素 ······································ 129
  4.2　HCC 宿主因素 ·· 130
  4.3　母体影响 ·· 131
  4.4　环境或生活方式因素 ·· 131
 5　HCC 预防 ·· 131
  5.1　一级预防：通过免疫接种预防 HBV 感染 ···························· 133
  5.2　接种 HBV 疫苗有效地减少 HBV 感染及相关并发症 ·········· 133
 6　通过免疫接种阻止 HBV 感染和预防 HCC 的效果 ························ 134
 7　肝癌预防中亟待解决的问题 ·· 136
  7.1　覆盖率低 ·· 136
  7.2　疫苗接种后的突破性感染（免疫失败） ······························ 137

8　有效控制 HBV 相关性 HCC 的策略······138
　　　　8.1　预防 HBV 突破性感染······138
　　　　8.2　高危人群筛查和 HBV 相关 HCC 的二级预防······139
　　9　其他癌症预防的未来前景和意义······140
　　参考文献······140

第 9 章　丙型肝炎病毒的致癌作用······146
　　1　引言······146
　　2　HCV 和病毒蛋白······147
　　3　HCV 在肝癌发生中的可能作用······148
　　4　HCV 在小鼠体内表现致癌作用······148
　　5　HCV 增强产生氧化应激作用和调节胞内信号······150
　　6　HCV 感染中的 ROS 来自线粒体······151
　　7　HCV 在诱导 ROS 的同时减弱某种抗氧化系统······152
　　8　HCV 感染的代谢改变：肝病发展的共同因素······153
　　9　小结······154
　　参考文献······155

第 10 章　HCV 感染与肝癌的预防······161
　　1　引言······161
　　2　HCV 感染······162
　　3　丙型肝炎和发生 HCC 的风险因子······163
　　4　预防丙肝导致的肝硬化患者发生 HCC······164
　　5　预防慢性丙肝患者发生肝硬化和 HCC······165
　　6　丙型肝炎的抗病毒治疗······166
　　　　6.1　标准治疗方法······166
　　　　6.2　聚乙二醇化 IFN/利巴韦林抗病毒应答的预测因子······167
　　　　6.3　直接作用抗病毒药物······167
　　　　6.4　靶向宿主的药物······171
　　　　6.5　治疗性疫苗······171
　　7　HCV 高发人群的预防······172
　　　　7.1　预防性疫苗······172
　　　　7.2　公共卫生措施······172
　　8　小结······173
　　参考文献······173

第 11 章　人类乳头状瘤病毒在肿瘤发生中的作用······182
　　1　引言······182

1.1　HPV 的生命周期 ··184

　　1.2　HPV 基因组 ··185

　　1.3　癌蛋白：E5、E6 和 E7 ···186

　2　小结 ···190

　参考文献 ···190

第 12 章　通过疫苗接种控制 HPV 感染及其相关性肿瘤 ·····························196

　1　引言 ···197

　2　目前市售的预防性疫苗 ··198

　3　第二代预防性疫苗的开发 ···201

　4　治疗性疫苗的临床开发策略 ···203

　　4.1　治疗性疫苗的概念和目标 ···203

　　4.2　基于活载体的治疗性 HPV 疫苗 ··204

　　4.3　基于多肽的治疗性 HPV 疫苗 ···205

　　4.4　基于蛋白质的疫苗 ···206

　　4.5　基于树突状细胞的疫苗 ··207

　　4.6　基于 DNA 的疫苗 ···208

　　4.7　联合策略 ··209

　5　小结 ···210

　参考文献 ···210

第 13 章　HTLV-1 与白血病：成人 T 细胞白血病发生中的病毒-细胞相互作用 ··219

　1　引言 ···219

　2　HTLV-1 的感染 ···220

　　2.1　流行病学 ··220

　　2.2　嗜性和受体 ··220

　　2.3　病毒增殖 ··221

　　2.4　病毒的基因表达 ··223

　3　Tax 的表达决定 HTLV-1 感染细胞的命运 ··224

　　3.1　Tax 促进 HTLV-1 感染细胞的存活和增殖 ·································224

　　3.2　Tax 表达细胞中 DNA 损伤的累积 ··227

　4　ATL ···228

　　4.1　Tax 表达的缺失与对宿主免疫监测的逃避 ··································228

　　4.2　HBZ 的表达 ···229

　5　小结 ···230

　参考文献 ···230

第 14 章　人类嗜 T 淋巴细胞病毒 1 型感染与成人 T 细胞白血病/淋巴瘤的预防 ······241

1　引言 ······242
2　HTLV-1 感染的流行病学 ······242
　2.1　全球概况 ······242
　2.2　日本 ······242
3　传播模式和临床转归 ······242
4　成人 T 细胞白血病/淋巴瘤的流行病学 ······243
5　HTLV-1 的传播机制 ······243
6　HTLV-1 传播的预防 ······244
　6.1　垂直传播的预防 ······244
　6.2　水平传播的预防 ······244
　6.3　输血和性传播的预防 ······245
7　成人 T 细胞白血病/淋巴瘤的病程 ······245
　7.1　成人 T 细胞白血病/淋巴瘤的致病性 ······245
　7.2　从无症状带毒发展到 ATLL 的决定因素 ······246
8　成人 T 细胞白血病/淋巴瘤患者的预后 ······246
　8.1　急性和淋巴瘤亚型 ······246
　8.2　慢性和郁积亚型 ······247
9　当前的治疗措施 ······247
　9.1　传统化疗方法 ······247
　9.2　异体造血干细胞移植 ······247
　9.3　α干扰素（IFN-α）和叠氮脱氧胸苷 ······248
　9.4　ATLL 的预防 ······248
　9.5　ATLL 预防的未来展望 ······248
10　小结 ······249
参考文献 ······250

第 15 章　人疱疹病毒 8 型分子生物学：病毒致病性和复制相关的新功能及病毒-宿主相互作用 ······255

1　引言 ······256
2　HHV-8 潜伏期产物与自分泌调节紊乱 ······257
　2.1　潜伏相关核抗原（LANA）······257
　2.2　病毒 FLICE 抑制蛋白（vFLIP）······259
　2.3　kaposins ······260
　2.4　PEL 中的病毒白细胞介素-6（vIL-6）······261

    2.5　PEL 中病毒干扰素调节因子 3（vIRF-3）……………………………264
    2.6　MicroRNA（miRNA）……………………………………………264
3　通过裂解活性的新型病毒-宿主相互作用……………………………………268
    3.1　病毒白细胞介素-6（vIL-6）……………………………………………268
    3.2　病毒 CC 趋化因子配体（vCCL）………………………………………268
    3.3　病毒 G 蛋白偶联受体（vGPCR）………………………………………269
    3.4　病毒干扰素调节因子（vIRF）…………………………………………270
    3.5　K7 编码的病毒凋亡抑制蛋白（vIAP）…………………………………272
4　末端膜蛋白…………………………………………………………………273
    4.1　K1/可变包含 ITAM 的蛋白（VIP）……………………………………273
    4.2　K15 编码的膜蛋白………………………………………………………274
5　小结…………………………………………………………………………276
参考文献…………………………………………………………………………279

第 16 章　抗病毒治疗与癌症控制………………………………………………300
1　引言…………………………………………………………………………300
2　乙肝病毒（HBV）和丙肝病毒（HCV）………………………………………301
    2.1　抗乙肝病毒治疗…………………………………………………………302
    2.2　抗 HCV 治疗……………………………………………………………305
3　HBV-HCV 共感染……………………………………………………………305
4　HBV-HIV 共感染和 HCV-HIV 共感染………………………………………306
5　卡波西肉瘤相关疱疹病毒……………………………………………………307
6　人类嗜 T 淋巴细胞病毒 1 型（HTLV-1）……………………………………308
7　EB 病毒（EBV）……………………………………………………………309
8　人乳头瘤病毒（HPV）………………………………………………………310
9　梅克尔细胞多瘤病毒…………………………………………………………311
10　结论与展望…………………………………………………………………311
参考文献…………………………………………………………………………312

第1章 概论：病毒感染与人类肿瘤

John T.Schiller 和 Douglas R. Lowy

摘　要　据估计，目前全世界大约10%的癌症由病毒感染引起，其中绝大部分（>85%）出现在发展中国家。致癌病毒包括很多种类的 DNA 和 RNA 病毒，诱发癌症的机制也多种多样。总体上，肿瘤发生在少数被感染的个体，并且要经过多年的慢性感染。与癌症病例相关最多的病毒有人乳头状瘤病毒（HPV），以及肝炎病毒 HBV 和 HCV。HPV 会引起宫颈癌及其他几种上皮恶性肿瘤，而大多数的肝细胞肝癌由后两者引起。其他致瘤病毒包括 Epstein-Barr 病毒（EBV）、卡波西肉瘤相关疱疹病毒（KSHV）、人类 T 淋巴细胞白血病病毒（HTLV-I），以及梅克尔细胞多瘤病毒（MCPyV）。对感染病原的鉴定使人类找到了一些可以降低肿瘤发生风险的干预手段，这些手段包括：HBV 和 HPV 疫苗、基于 HPV 检测的宫颈癌筛查、针对慢性 HBV 和 HCV 感染的抗病毒治疗，以及筛查血液制品中可能存在的 HBV 和 HCV 病毒。更多致瘤病毒的成功鉴定，将加深对病因和发病机制的认识，同时也可提供新的治疗和预防手段。

特定的某些人类病毒的感染，是相当一部分人类恶性肿瘤的主因，这种认识的确立是癌症病因学最显著的成就之一。根据最近的估计，全球每年1300万的人类肿瘤病例中，有超过10%是由以下人类病毒引起的：人乳头状瘤病毒（HPV）、乙型肝炎病毒（HBV）、丙型肝炎病毒（HCV）、EB 病毒（EBV）、卡波西肉瘤相关性疱疹病毒（KSHV）（又称人类疱疹病毒8型）、人类 T 淋巴细胞白血病病毒（HTLV-I），以及梅克尔细胞多瘤病毒（MCPyV）（de Martel et al. 2012）。此外，全球范围内还有5%的癌症（主要是胃癌）是由幽门螺杆菌引起的。这个结论是基于过去50年间大量的实验室结果及流行病学研究得出的。在第2章我们会更加详细地讨论，不同病毒引发的新发病例数相差甚远，从 HPV 导致的60

J. T. Schiller (✉) _ D. R. Lowy
Laboratory of Cellular Oncology, Center for Cancer Research, National Cancer Institute,
Bethesda, MD, USA
e-mail: schillej@mail.nih.gov

D. R. Lowy
e-mail: dl60z@nih.gov

万人，到 HTLV 导致的 2100 人（表 1-1）。超过 85%的由病毒引发的癌症患者来自发展中国家，这就意味着，病毒引发的癌症问题可以解读为公共卫生预防问题。

表 1-1 不同发展状况地区中由特定病毒感染新引发的癌症病例数量（de Martel et al. 2012）

病毒	全球	发展中国家	发达国家
HPV	600 000	520 000	80 000
HBV	380 000	330 000	44 000
HCV	220 000	190 000	37 000
EBV	110 000	96 000	16 000
KSHV	43 000	39 000	4 000
HTLV	2 100	660	1 500

由不同病毒引起的癌症类型及比例都大不相同，这是因为病毒感染情况差异很大（de Martel et al. 2012）（表 1-2）。此外，肿瘤病例间的病毒流行情况也因地理位置不同而有差别。HPV 通常感染复层鳞状上皮，与一些生殖器癌症相关。宫颈癌几乎 100%与之相关，外阴癌则不足 50%。最近，HPV 病毒也更多地与口咽部癌联系在一起，不同地区间的感染率估值也大不相同（Gillison 2008）。HPV 相关的口咽部癌比例似乎大大增加，目前，美国及其他几个（Arora et al. 2012）工业化国家（Chaturvedi et al. 2011；Chaturvedi et al. 2012）的感染率达 50%。HBV 和 HCV 对肝细胞有严格的嗜性，它们是肝癌的主要病因（El-Serag 2012）。EBV 通常感染上皮细胞和淋巴细胞，特别是 B 细胞，它是绝大多数霍奇金淋巴瘤及伯基特淋巴瘤的病因（Saha and Robertson 2011），同时也是上皮来源的肿瘤如大多数鼻咽癌的致病因子（Kutok and Wang 2006）。几乎所有的卡波西肉瘤中都可以检测到 KSHV，它同时也与两种比较稀少的 B 细胞淋巴瘤（多中心性巨大淋巴结增生症和原发性渗出性淋巴瘤）的形成密切关联。HTLV-1 也以淋巴细胞作为靶细胞，它是成人 T 细胞白血病和淋巴瘤的主因（Gallo 2011）。MCPyV 似乎是皮肤正常菌群的一部分，也因此与接近 3/4 的梅克尔细胞癌（一种少见的皮肤癌）相关（Aror et al. 2012）。

表 1-2 病毒相关癌症中的病毒感染率（de Martel et al. 2012）

病毒	癌症	地理区域	病例中感染率/%
HPV	宫颈	全球	100
HPV	阴茎	全球	50

续表

病毒	癌症	地理区域	病例中感染率/%
HPV	肛门	全球	88
HPV	外阴	全球	43
HPV	阴道	全球	70
HPV	口咽部	北美	56
HPV	口咽部	南欧	17
HPV	口咽部	日本	52
HBV	肝	发展中国家	59
HBV	肝	发达国家	23
HCV	肝	发展中国家	33
HCV	肝	发达国家	20
EBV	霍奇金淋巴瘤	发展中国家-儿童	90
EBV	霍奇金淋巴瘤	发展中国家-成人	60
EBV	霍奇金淋巴瘤	发达国家	40
EBV	伯基特淋巴瘤	撒哈拉以南非洲	100
EBV	伯基特淋巴瘤	其他地区	20~30
EBV	鼻咽癌	高发地区	100
EBV	鼻咽癌	低发地区	80
KSHV	卡波西肉瘤	全球	100
HTLV-1	成人T细胞白血病	全球	100
MCPyV	梅克尔细胞癌	全球	74

1 引起人类肿瘤的病毒

人类肿瘤病毒包含几种显著不同的病毒组，包括小基因组（HPV、HBV 和 MCPyV）、大基因组（EBV 和 KSHV）、正链 RNA 基因组（HCV）和逆转录病毒组（HTLV-1）（表 1-3）（Butel and Fan 2012），它们各自的致瘤机制也大不一样。但是，人类肿瘤病毒的一个共同特征是，肿瘤的形成是病毒生命周期的一种失常，也是感染的一种异常形式。对于有的病毒，如 HPV 和 MCPyV，癌细胞内的病毒基因组发生了突变，并且/或者整合至宿主 DNA，因而它们不再产生传染性病毒子（Vinokurova et al. 2008；Arora et al. 2012）。通常在很多年后，病毒相关的癌症几乎都会由慢性感染升级为单克隆增殖过程，这说明感染只是致癌过程中众多步骤的一部分。一个明显的例外是 KSHV 引起的卡波西肉瘤，它在感染的几个月内就可以在免疫抑制的个体中升级为多克隆肿瘤（Mesri et al. 2010）（也可见第 15 章）。

表 1-3 人类致癌病毒的基本特征

病毒	基因组	病毒粒子结构	正常嗜性	分离年份（参考文献）
HPV16	7.9kb 双链环状 DNA	55nm，裸露二十面体	复层鳞状上皮	1983（Dürst et al.1983）
HBV	3.2kb 部分双链环状 DNA	42nm，有包膜	肝细胞	1970（Dane et al. 1970）
HCV	9.6k nt 线性正链 RNA	有包膜	肝细胞	1989（Choo et al. 1989）
EBV	172kb 线性双链 DNA	有包膜	上皮细胞和 B 细胞	1964（Epstein et al. 1964）
KSHV	165kb 线性双链 DNA	有包膜	口咽部上皮细胞	1994（Chang et al. 1994）
HTLV-1	9.0k nt 线性正链 RNA	有包膜	T 细胞和 B 细胞	1980（Poiesz et al. 1980）
MCPyV	5.4kb 双链环状 DNA	40nm，裸露二十面体	皮肤	2008（Feng et al. 2008）

2　致瘤机制

在下文中将会谈到，大部分肿瘤病毒的致瘤机制包括特定病毒基因（致癌基因）产物的持续表达，这些基因产物通过与细胞基因产物的相互作用来控制增殖或抗凋亡。癌基因蛋白的例子包括 HPV 的 E6 和 E7、EBV 的 LMP1，还有 HTLV-1 的 Tax（分别见第 5、6、11 和第 13 章）。病毒（如 EBV）编码微小 RNA（miRNA），会通过抑制细胞生长负调控因子的表达，产生致瘤作用（Raab-Traub 2012）。KSHV 则主要通过改变复杂的细胞因子/趋化因子网络起作用（Mesri et al. 2010）（见第 15 章）。相反地，一些肿瘤，如 HCV 和 HBV，可能会通过持续损害组织及其再生，以及宿主对持续感染的慢性炎症反应，以这种更加间接的方式诱发癌症（Alsion et al. 2011）（见第 3、8 和第 9 章）。

一些病毒，特别是逆转录病毒，可以在动物模型中以插入突变的方式诱发癌症（Fan and Johnson 2011）。但是，这种机制并没有在人类有令人信服的记录，只有一些患者在实验性的基因导入试验中的记录，这些实验都涉及使用高剂量的重组逆转录病毒载体（Romano et al. 2009）。HIV 也可被认为是一种肿瘤病毒，因为 HIV 感染是几种癌症的极高风险因素，不过，这些癌症绝大部分还与其他病毒相关（Parkin 2006）。HIV 感染对肿瘤形成的影响被认为是间接的，它抑制正常的人类免疫功能，使其不能控制或者清除致瘤病毒感染，并且/或者不能对初期肿瘤进行免疫监视（Clifford and Franceschi 2009）。与这个推测一致的是，在其他形式的免疫抑制患者中，这些癌症的比率也会提高。

2.1 病毒感染与肿瘤的因果联系

以上 7 种病毒及特定癌症间的因果联系的确立是较完善的，即使不完全，也大体上符合 A. Bradford Hill 爵士在 20 世纪 70 年代初期提出的因果关系标准（Hill 1971）。感染与癌症关联的强烈性和一致性是高度建立在不同背景下的多种流行病学研究基础上的。例如，对于 HPV 和 KSHV 感染分别对宫颈癌和卡波西肉瘤发生的相对风险，有超过 100 个研究。在一些情况下，鉴定特定致瘤型对其强相关性分析尤为重要，需要鉴定特定的肿瘤亚型，如黏膜高危型 HPV 中的 HPV16 型和 18 型、头颈之间的口咽部癌。感染可以发展成癌症，并且通常是经过很多年，这满足了时间性标准。某些病例中，确认了在癌症前期病变中可以持续检测到病毒，HPV 及其他高级别宫颈上皮内瘤变就是如此（见第 11 章）。大部分情况下，病毒感染率高的人群，相关肿瘤的比率也更高，如 HBV 与肝癌，这满足了剂量-反应关系（El-Serag 2012）（见第 8 章）。但是，当普通人群也有致瘤病毒高感染率，以及其他风险因素引起感染率变化时，这些相关性有时候会混淆。典型的例子是普通人群中 EBV 的高感染率，以及在 EBV 阳性伯基特淋巴瘤的诱发中与疟疾感染密切相关的共同作用因子（Magrath 2012）（见第 5 和第 6 章）。在无数实验室研究中，确认了携有增殖、凋亡关键调控因子的病毒蛋白之间的相互作用，它们在体外永生化的转化作用，以及它们在动物模型中的致瘤作用，满足了致瘤因子的生物学合理性标准（见第 5、6、7、9、11、13 和第 15 章）。这些研究也支持了一个标准：相关性须与目前对发病机制的理解一致。在这个病例中，该理解是指肿瘤发生的过程。最后一个标准——减少暴露于病原可以预防疾病，这是最有说服力的标准，它已被 HBV 证实，在下文以及第 8 章中将会谈到。

2.2 确认一种病毒的病因学的基础和临床意义

确认一种病毒是某种特定癌症的主要原因，这可能是一项重要发现，原因如下。

第一，它可以加深对致癌过程的基础认识，因此可以为干预治疗确认潜在的靶细胞，这些干预通常对病毒性肿瘤和非病毒性肿瘤都有意义。例如，抑癌基因 p53 和 pRb 最先在实验系统中都被认为是小 DNA 肿瘤病毒的结合伴侣，后来都被证明其实是人类致瘤病毒的标靶。它们在非病毒肿瘤中也是最活跃的突变基因（Howley and Livingston 2009）（见第 11 章）。

第二，病毒的存在可以用于癌症的诊断或风险评估。HPV DNA 用于宫颈癌筛查已经很好地说明了这一点（Schiffman et al. 2011）。HPV DNA 测试对于高级别癌前病变和宫颈癌来说，要比标准巴氏试验更灵敏，所以宫颈检测中，HPV DNA 为阴性的妇女，两次检测的间隔时间可以更长（Saslow et al. 2012）。另外一个例子是给肝硬化和肝癌的高风险个体做 HCV 筛查确认。美国最近推荐 1945~1965

年间出生的人做 HCV 筛查（Smith et al. 2012）。

第三，病毒基因产物为通过治疗药物或疫苗对癌症、癌前期病变，或者是有患癌高风险的慢性感染患者的治疗，提供了潜在目标。这个潜力无限的领域曾有过实证研究，虽然没有形成恶性肿瘤或癌前病变的基于病毒的治疗手段，但是也在慢性 HBV 和 HCV 感染的抗病毒治疗方面取得了一些临床实践的成功（见第 16 章）。聚乙二醇化干扰素 α，或者核苷/核苷酸模拟物，现在都被用于抑制 HBV 复制（见第 8 章），由此抑制肝硬化以及降低肝细胞癌的风险。HCV 感染也可用类似的方法治疗。然而，持续的病毒学反应是有限的。幸运的是，一些直接作用于病毒基因产物的潜在备选药物现在正在开发中，它们似乎更有效，耐受性也更好（Poordad and Dieterich 2012）（见第 10 章）。类似的是，对 AIDS 携带者 KSHV 感染的治疗降低了卡波西肉瘤发生的风险（Uldrick and Whitby 2011）。另外，在使用高效抗逆转录病毒治疗（HAART）后，卡波西肉瘤病变在 HIV 感染个体中通常会减退，但这主要是重构免疫系统的间接结果，而不是药物直接针对 KSHV 的效果（Uldrick and Whitby 2011）。另外，HIV 感染个体的 HAART 治疗与部分（但并不是所有）病毒诱发肿瘤发生风险的降低呈相关性（Shiels et al. 2011）。

第四，对病毒病因学的认识可以为癌症预防手段服务。其中一种方法是：降低感染易感性的行为干预，例如，对于 HBV 和 HCV，限制与血液制品的接触（见第 8 和第 10 章）；对于 HPV，限制性伴侣人数；或者劝阻已感染的母亲哺乳，以防止 HTLV-1 传播（Ruff 1994）（见第 14 章）。另外，人类致瘤病毒的识别可以用来开发有效的疫苗，防止致瘤病毒感染。这个方法已经卓有成效地应用于 HBV 和 HPV。HBV 预防性疫苗已经使用了 20 余年（综述见第 8 章）。在肝癌高发的中国台湾地区，儿童肝癌病例大大地减少了 2/3（Chang et al. 2009）。被有效阻止接触 HBV 的婴儿达到肝癌高发年龄时，可以预见成人肝癌病例也会大大减少。针对 HPV16 型和 18 型的 HPV 疫苗拿到许可仅仅 6 年（Schiller and Lowy 2012）（见第 12 章）。在未来至少 10 年中，并不能期望 HPV 相关癌症会显著减少。然而，在澳大利亚，疫苗覆盖率高，筛查项目包括了比较年轻的妇女，癌前宫颈疾病正大大减少，群体免疫力大有提高（Brotherton et al. 2011）。在开发针对 EBV 和 HCV 的预防药物以及/或者治疗疫苗方面，有很多人正在付出巨大的努力（Wu et al. 2010；Feinstone et al. 2012）（见第 5 和第 6 章）。然而，它们特定的生物学特征使得开发有效疫苗极具挑战性。例如，HBV 有潜伏期，HCV 有基因不稳定性。针对这些病毒的疫苗产品可能具有商业价值。KSHV 和 HTLV-1 的疫苗开发比较少，因为它们在全球范围内引发的癌症更少，而且与 HBV 和 HCV 比较而言，它们似乎并不常引起医学上很重要的良性疾病（Schiller and Lowy 2010）。它们也被证明易受其他干预手段影响。具体而言，治疗 HIV 感染减少了 KSHV 引发的卡波西肉瘤，劝阻被感染的母亲哺乳减少了 HTLV-1 的传播（见第

14 章）。

2.3 发现新的致瘤病毒

是否还有其他人类致瘤病毒没有被发现？对整个细胞基因组进行测序的高通量核酸测序技术，现在被广泛应用于各种人类肿瘤，为相关研究提供了无比宝贵的原始数据（Lizardi et al. 2011）。MCPyV 的发现证明了这个技术可以用于识别新的人类致瘤病毒（Feng et al. 2008）。然而，这种研究可能会遗漏携有 RNA 基因组的致瘤病毒。此外，对肿瘤中病毒的核酸序列识别仅仅是第一步。确认一种病毒的感染与癌症发生有因果联系而不是被动寄生于肿瘤，需要更多实验、临床和流行病学研究。如果病毒是一种普通人群中的常见感染，那么建立因果联系就变得尤为困难。同样，在病毒仅仅参与了肿瘤的发生，而没有参与维持的情况下，因果联系的建立也会很困难。这种情况是合理的，但是作为一种人类致瘤机制还没有被证明，常被称为"打了就跑"的游击战（Schiller and Buck 2011）。有人认为，病毒感染可能与其他几种癌症有关。例如，免疫抑制后，非黑色素瘤皮肤癌患病概率会急剧增加（Schiller and Buck 2011），并且，一些流行病学研究将前列腺癌风险与性行为变量联系在一起，认为通过性传播的感染原参与其中（Sutcliffe 2010）。还有一种有趣的观点，认为结直肠癌和儿童白血病可能是由尚未确认的病毒感染引起的。

毋庸置疑，在过去数十年中，致瘤病毒的研究一直处于生物医学研究的前沿。这些研究提供了对于基础细胞学和致病机制的重要认识，并促生了重要的控制人类主要癌症的公共卫生干预手段。本文重点总结了当前在这个动态领域的发展状况。我们期待这片领域的进一步研究将会促进对癌症起因的新认识，并促生新的防治干预手段。

（卢建红，尹典 译）

参 考 文 献

Alison MR, Nicholson LJ, Lin WR (2011) Chronic inflammation and hepatocellular carcinoma. Recent Results Cancer Res 185:135–148

Arora R, Chang Y, More PS (2012) MCV and Merkel cell carcinoma: a molecular success story. Curr Opin Virol 2(4):489–498

Brotherton JM, Fridman M, May CL et al (2011) Early effect of the HPV vaccination programme on cervical abnormalities in Victoria, Australia: an ecological study. Lancet 377(9783):2085–2092

Butel JS, Fan H (2012) The diversity of human cancer viruses. Curr Opin Virol 2(4):449–452

Chang MH, You SL, Chen CJ et al (2009) Decreased incidence of hepatocellular carcinoma in hepatitis B vaccinees: a 20-year follow-up study. J Natl Cancer Inst 101(19):1348–1355

Chang Y, Cesarman E, Pessin MS et al (1994) Identification of herpesvirus-like DNA sequences in AIDS-associated Kaposi's sarcoma. Science 266(5192):1865–1869

Chaturvedi AK (2012) Epidemiology and clinical aspects of HPV in head and neck cancers. Head Neck Pathol 6(Suppl 1):S16–S24

Chaturvedi AK, Engels EA, Pfeiffer RM et al (2011) Human papillomavirus and rising oropharyngeal cancer incidence in the United States. J Clin Oncol 29(32):4294–4301

Choo QL, Kuo G, Weiner AJ et al (1989) Isolation of a cDNA clone derived from a blood-borne non-A, non-B viral hepatitis genome. Science 244(4902):359–362

Clifford GM, Franceschi S (2009) Cancer risk in HIV-infected persons: influence of CD4(+) count. Future Oncol 5(5):669–678

Dane DS, Cameron CH, Briggs M et al (1970) Virus-like particles in serum of patients with Australia-antigen-associated hepatitis. Lancet 1(7649):695–698

de Martel C, Ferlay J, Franceschi S et al (2012) Global burden of cancers attributable to infections in 2008: a review and synthetic analysis. Lancet Oncol 13(6):607–615

Dürst M, Gissmann L, Ikenberg H et al (1983) A papillomavirus DNA from a cervical carcinoma and its prevalence in cancer biopsy samples from different geographic regions. Proc Natl Acad Sci USA 80:3812–3815

El-Serag HB (2012) Epidemiology of viral hepatitis and hepatocellular carcinoma. Gastroen-terology 142(6):1264–1273 e1261

Epstein MA, Achong BG, Barr YM et al (1964) Virus particles in cultured lymphoblasts from Burkitt's lymphoma. Lancet 1(7335):702–703

Fan H, Johnson C (2011) Insertional oncogenesis by non-acute retroviruses: implications for gene therapy. Viruses 3(4):398–422

Feinstone SM, Hu DJ, Major ME (2012) Prospects for prophylactic and therapeutic vaccines against hepatitis C virus. Clin Infect Dis 55(Suppl 1):S25–S32

Feng H, Shuda M, Chang Y et al (2008) Clonal integration of a polyomavirus in human Merkel cell carcinoma. Science 319(5866):1096–1100

Gallo RC (2011) Research and discovery of the first human cancer virus, HTLV-1. Best Pract Res Clin Haematol 24(4):559–565

Gantt S, Casper C (2011) Human herpesvirus 8-associated neoplasms: the roles of viral replication and antiviral treatment. Curr Opin Infect Dis 24(4):295–301

Gillison ML (2008) Human papillomavirus-related diseases: oropharynx cancers and potential implications for adolescent HPV vaccination. J Adolesc Health 43(4 Suppl):S52–S60

Hill A (1971) Statistical evidence and inference. Principles of medical statistics, 9th edn. Oxford University Press, New York, pp 309–323

Howley PM, Livingston DM (2009) Small DNA tumor viruses: large contributors to biomedical sciences. Virology 384(2):256–259

Kutok JL, Wang F (2006) Spectrum of Epstein-Barr virus-associated diseases. Annu Rev Pathol 1:375–404

Lizardi PM, Forloni M, Wajapeyee N (2011) Genome-wide approaches for cancer gene discovery. Trends Biotechnol 29(11):558–568

Magrath I (2012) Epidemiology: clues to the pathogenesis of Burkitt lymphoma. Br J Haematol 156(6):744–756

Mesri E, Cesarman E, Boshoff C (2010) Kaposi's sarcoma and its associated herpesvirus. Nat Rev Cancer 10(10):707–719

Parkin DM (2006) The global health burden of infection-associated cancers in the year 2002. Int J Cancer 118(12):3030–3044

Poiesz BJ, Ruscetti FW, Mier JW et al (1980) Detection and isolation of type C retrovirus particles from fresh and cultured lymphocytes of a patient with cutaneous T-cell lymphoma. Proc Natl Acad Sci U S A 77(12):7415–7419

Poordad F, Dieterich D (2012) Treating hepatitis C: current standard of care and emerging direct-acting antiviral agents. J Viral Hepat 19(7):449–464

Raab-Traub N (2012) Novel mechanisms of EBV-induced oncogenesis. Curr Opin Virol 2(4):453–458

Rama I, Grinyo JM (2010) Malignancy after renal transplantation: the role of immunosuppres- sion. Nat Rev Nephrol 6(9):511–519

Romano G, Marino IR, Pentimalli F et al (2009) Insertional mutagenesis and development of malignancies induced by integrating gene delivery systems: implications for the design of safer gene-based interventions in patients. Drug News Perspect 22(4):185–196

Ruff AJ (1994) Breastmilk, breastfeeding, and transmission of viruses to the neonate. Semin Perinatol 18(6):510–516

Saha A, Robertson ES (2011) Epstein-Barr virus-associated B-cell lymphomas: pathogenesis and clinical outcomes. Clin Cancer Res 17(10):3056–3063

Saslow D, Solomon D, Lawson HW et al (2012) American Cancer Society, American Society for Colposcopy and Cervical Pathology, and American Society for Clinical Pathology screening guidelines for the prevention and early detection of cervical cancer. CA Cancer J Clin 62(3):147–172

Schiffman M, Wentzensen N, Wacholder S et al (2011) Human papillomavirus testing in the prevention of cervical cancer. J Natl Cancer Inst 103(5):368–383

Schiller JT, Buck CB (2011) Cutaneous squamous cell carcinoma: a smoking gun but still no suspects. J Invest Dermatol 131(8):1595–1596

Schiller JT, Lowy DR (2010) Vaccines to prevent infections by oncoviruses. Annu Rev Microbiol

64:23–41

Schiller JT, Lowy DR (2012) Understanding and learning from the success of prophylactic human papillomavirus vaccines. Nat Rev Microbiol 10(10):681–692

Shiels MS, Pfeiffer RM, Gail MH et al (2011) Cancer burden in the HIV-infected population in the United States. J Natl Cancer Inst 103(9):753–762

Smith BD, Jorgensen C, Zibbell JE et al (2012) Centers for Disease Control and Prevention initiatives to prevent hepatitis C virus infection: a selective update. Clin Infect Dis 55(Suppl 1):S49–S53

Sutcliffe S (2010) Sexually transmitted infections and risk of prostate cancer: review of historical and emerging hypotheses. Future Oncol 6(8):1289–1311

Uldrick TS, Whitby D (2011) Update on KSHV epidemiology, Kaposi Sarcoma pathogenesis, and treatment of Kaposi Sarcoma. Cancer Lett 305(2):150–162

Vinokurova S, Wentzensen N, Kraus I et al (2008) Type-dependent integration frequency of human papillomavirus genomes in cervical lesions. Cancer Res 68(1):307–313

Wu TT, Blackman MA, Sun R (2010) Prospects of a novel vaccination strategy for human gamma-herpesviruses. Immunol Res 48(1–3):122–146

zur Hausen H (2009) Childhood leukemia's and other hematopoietic malignancies: interdepen- dence between an infectious event and chromosomal modifications. Int J Cancer 125(8):1764–1770

zur Hausen H (2012) Red meat consumption and cancer: reasons to suspect involvement of bovine infectious factors in colorectal cancer. Int J Cancer 130(11):2475–2483

第 2 章 病毒感染与人类肿瘤的流行病学

Chien-Jen Chen，Wan-Lun Hsu，Hwai-I Yang，Mei-Hsuan Lee，
Hui-Chi Chen，Yin-Chu Chien 和 San-Lin You

摘　要　国际癌症研究机构（IARC）全面地评估了生物因子对人体的致癌性，包括 Epstein–Barr 病毒（EBV）、乙型肝炎病毒（HBV）、丙型肝炎病毒（HCV）、卡波西肉瘤相关疱疹病毒（KSHV）（又称人类疱疹病毒 8 型）、人类免疫缺陷病毒 1 型（HIV-1）、人类 T 淋巴细胞白血病病毒 1 型（HTLV-1）和人乳头状瘤病毒（HPV）在内的 7 种病毒已被 IARC 归为 1 类人体致癌物，这是基于流行病学和致病机制研究的成果得出的结论。EBV、HPV、HTLV-1 和 KSHV 均为直接致癌物；HBV 和 HCV 是通过慢性炎症间接致癌；HIV-1 是通过抑制免疫间接致癌。有些病毒可以引起不止一种癌症，有些癌症则由一种以上病毒引起。然而，只有感染了这些致癌病毒的部分人群会产生特定癌症。现已有一系列研究来评估某些癌症的病毒、宿主和环境辅因子，这些癌症包括 EBV 相关的鼻咽癌、HBV/HCV 相关的肝细胞癌和 HPV 相关的宫颈癌。持续感染和高病毒量是对这些病毒引发的癌症进行风险预测的重要因素。现已建立了考虑宿主和病毒因素的计算肝细胞癌长期风险的方法。这些方法对于被感染患者的分类与临床管理十分有用。无论是临床试验，还是国家免疫计划或抗病毒治疗项目，都证实 HBV、HCV 和 HPV 引发的癌症显著降低。我们迫切需要对致瘤病毒与人类宿主的基因-基因、

C.-J. Chen (✉) _ W.-L. Hsu _ H.-C. Chen _ S.-L. You

Genomics Research Center, Academia Sinica, 128 Academia Road, Section 2,

Taipei 115, Taiwan

e-mail: chencj@gate.sinica.edu.tw

C.-J. Chen

Graduate Institute of Epidemiology and Preventative Medicine, National Taiwan University,

Taipei, Taiwan

H.-I. Yang _ Y.-C. Chien

Molecular and Genomic Epidemiology Center, China Medical University Hospital

and Graduate Institute of Clinical Medical Science, China Medical University,

Taichung, Taiwan

M.-H. Lee

Institute of Clinical Medicine, National Yang-Ming University, Taipei, Taiwan

基因-环境相互作用做进一步研究。

关键词 肿瘤，EBV，流行病学，HBV，HCV，HIV，HPV，HTLV-I，KSHV

1 引言

国际癌症研究机构（IARC）基于流行病学和致病机制数据，全面地评估了生物因子对人体的致癌性（IARC 2009）。包括 Epstein–Barr 病毒（EBV）、乙型肝炎病毒（HBV）、丙型肝炎病毒（HCV）、卡波西肉瘤相关疱疹病毒（KSHV）（又称人类疱疹病毒 8 型）、人类免疫缺陷病毒 1 型（HIV-1）、人类 T 淋巴细胞白血病病毒（HTLV-1）、人乳头状瘤病毒（HPV）在内的 7 种病毒已被 IARC 归为 1 类人类致癌物，见表 2-1。

表 2-1 根据 IARC 标准的充分和有限证据划分的 1 类致瘤病毒引起的癌症

病毒	证据充分的肿瘤	证据有限的肿瘤
EB 病毒（EBV）	鼻咽癌、伯基特淋巴瘤、免疫抑制相关的非霍奇金淋巴瘤、结外 NK/T 细胞淋巴瘤（鼻型）、霍奇金淋巴瘤	胃癌、淋巴上皮瘤样癌
乙型肝炎病毒（HBV）	肝细胞癌	胆管癌、非霍奇金淋巴瘤
丙型肝炎病毒（HCV）	肝细胞癌、非霍奇金淋巴瘤	胆管癌
人类免疫缺陷病毒 1 型（HIV-1）	卡波西肉瘤、非霍奇金淋巴瘤、霍奇金淋巴瘤、宫颈癌、肛门癌、结膜癌	外阴癌、阴道癌、阴茎癌、非黑色素瘤皮肤癌、肝细胞癌
人乳头状瘤病毒 16 型（HPV-16）	宫颈癌、外阴癌、阴道癌、阴茎癌、肛门癌、口腔癌、口咽癌、扁桃体癌	喉癌
人乳头状瘤病毒 18、31、33、35、39、45、51、52、56、58、59 型	宫颈癌	
人乳头状瘤病毒 26、30、34、53、66、67、68、69、70、73、82、85、97 型		宫颈癌
人类 T 淋巴细胞白血病病毒 1 型（HTLV-1）	成人 T 细胞白血病和淋巴瘤	
卡波西肉瘤疱疹病毒（KSHV）	卡波西肉瘤、原发性渗出性淋巴瘤	多中心卡斯尔曼病

EBV 引起人类鼻咽癌、伯基特淋巴瘤、免疫抑制相关的非霍奇金淋巴瘤、结外 NK/T 细胞淋巴瘤（鼻型）和霍奇金淋巴瘤，证据充分；EBV 引起胃癌和淋巴上皮瘤样癌的证据则不足。HBV 和 HCV 引起肝细胞癌，证据充分。HCV 引起非霍奇金淋巴瘤，特别是 B 细胞淋巴瘤，证据充分，不过，HBV 和 HCV 引起胆管

癌的证据不足。HIV-1 引起卡波西肉瘤、非霍奇金淋巴瘤、霍奇金淋巴瘤，以及宫颈癌、肛门癌、结膜癌，证据充分；但是 HIV-1 引起外阴癌、阴道癌、阴茎癌、非黑色素瘤皮肤癌和肝细胞癌的证据不足。

HPV-16 引起宫颈癌、外阴癌、阴道癌、阴茎癌、肛门癌、口腔癌、口咽癌、扁桃体癌，证据充分；但是 HPV-16 引起喉癌的证据不足。宫颈癌由几种 HPV 引起，包括 HPV-18、31、33、35、39、45、51、52、56、58、59。HPV-26、30、34、53、66、67、68、69、70、73、82、85、97 引起宫颈癌的证据不足。HTLV-1 引起成人 T 细胞白血病和淋巴瘤，证据充分。KSHV 引起卡波西肉瘤和原发性渗出性淋巴瘤，证据充分；但是，KSHV 引起多中心性巨大淋巴结增生症的证据不足。

感染原引起癌症的比例估计最近超过 20%（IARC 2009）。鉴定更多这些感染原引起的癌症部位，意味着可能有更多癌症可以被预防。本章将主要回顾致瘤病毒的流行病学以及它们引起的癌症。

2 全球范围内致瘤病毒感染率

EBV 在全球有相当高的感染率，在偏远地区，甚至达 90%的成人感染了 EBV （IARC 2009）。感染 EBV 的人数估计已超过 55 亿。EBV 初次感染的年龄在全球范围内差异很大。在人口过于稠密、卫生条件差的居住环境中，初次感染的年龄比环境好的更小。EBV 的两种主要类型均已被鉴别，它们的区域分布并不相同，EBV-2 在非洲和同性恋中更为常见。特定的 EBV 类型在不同癌症中发挥何种作用仍有待阐明。EBV 感染普遍存在，而 EBV 相关恶性肿瘤（包括地方性伯基特氏淋巴瘤和鼻咽癌）的区域分布情况更有可能归因于其他可刺激 EBV 复制的共同作用因子的分布差异。

图 2-1 展示了致瘤病毒感染率在全球范围内的区域差异。全球范围内，HBV 感染人群超过 20 亿，其中超过 3 亿人是慢性 HBV 携带者（IARC 2009）。如图 2-1A 显示，全球 HBV 慢性感染的差异很大[①]。HBV 慢性感染率高（乙肝表面抗原血清阳性率>8%）、中（2%~7%）、低（<2%）地区人口，分别占全球人口的 45%、43%、12%。撒哈拉以南非洲、亚马孙盆地、中国大陆、韩国、中国台湾，以及东南亚一些国家的感染率最高。在高发区，HBV 感染的终生风险高于 60%，大部分感染来自产期和儿童间传播，在此时期，转为慢性感染的风险最高。在中国大陆、韩国、中国台湾，孕妇的乙肝 e 抗原的血清阳性率高，产期（垂直）传播占主要地位；而在撒哈拉以南的非洲，孕妇的乙肝 e 抗原的血清阳性率低，儿

---

① CDC http://wwwnc.cdc.gov/travel/yellowbook/2012/chapter-3-infectious-diseases-related-totravel/hepatitis-b.htm

童间（横向）传播更为普遍。在感染率中等的地区，则呈现出婴儿期、幼童期、青春期、成人期等多种 HBV 传播混合的模式。在低发区，大部分 HBV 感染发生在青少年之间，传播途径有毒品注射、男性同性恋行为、医疗保健和常规输血或血液透析。

乙肝病毒表面抗原的血清阳性率在全球范围内有显著的区域差异，8 种基因型的 HBV 在不同国家的分布也明显不同（IARC 2009）。A 基因型在欧洲、非洲和北美洲地区流行；B、C 基因型在东亚及东南亚地区流行；D 基因型在南亚、中东和地中海地区占主要地位；E 基因型仅限于西非；F、G 基因型在中美洲和南美洲发现；H 基因型则发现于中美洲。

HCV 感染了全球大约 1.5 亿人口，感染率估计为 2.2%（IARC 2009），如图 2-1B 所示，在不同地区差异显著。在英国和斯堪的纳维亚半岛 HCV 感染（HCV 抗体血清阳性率）估计小于 0.1%，而在埃及则高达 15%~20%（Alter 2007）。在蒙古国、北非、巴基斯坦、中国、南意大利和日本局部地区，均观察到较高的 HCV 感染率。至少有 6 种主要的 HCV 基因型已被鉴定。全球范围内，HCV 基因型的区域分布差别极大。不同的 HCV 基因型对抗病毒治疗的反应不同。感染 2、3 基因型的患者，治疗效果比 1、4 基因型要好。

HCV 有两种主要的传播途径，即毒品注射，以及输血、移植、不安全的注射治疗等医源性暴露。1990 年后，日本、意大利等发达国家的 HCV 医源性传播有所减少，然而在资源匮乏的国家，一次性针头可能反复使用，医源性传播仍然常见。在发达国家，毒品注射是新的获得性 HCV 感染最重要的传播途径。与医源性暴露和毒品注射相比，通过产期传播、性传播和针头意外暴露传播的效率较低。

据估计，截止到 2010 年末，全球有 3400 万人感染了 HIV（IARC 2009）[①]。全球 15~49 岁的成年人中，大约有 0.8%携带有 HIV，如图 2-1C 所示，这种状况在不同国家和地区间也有显著差异。撒哈拉以南的非洲地区情况一直最严重，感染率达 4.9%。尽管撒哈拉以南非洲的 HIV 感染率要高于亚洲 25 倍，南亚、东南亚、东亚的 HIV 携带者人数总共也有近 500 万。感染严重程度仅次于撒哈拉以南非洲的是加勒比地区、东欧和中亚，2011 年，这些地方有 1.0%的成年人携带有 HIV。2011 年，HIV 感染者新增 250 万人，其中包括 39 万儿童。2001 年以来，在 33 个国家中，HIV 年度新增病例有所减少，其中 22 个国家位于撒哈拉以南的非洲。然而，尽管在 21 世纪初，东亚和中亚的新增病例曾有所减缓，目前却再次加速增长，并且中东和北非的新增感染也在增加。

---

① UNAIDS http://data.unaids.org/pub/epislides/2012/2012_epiupdate_en.pdf

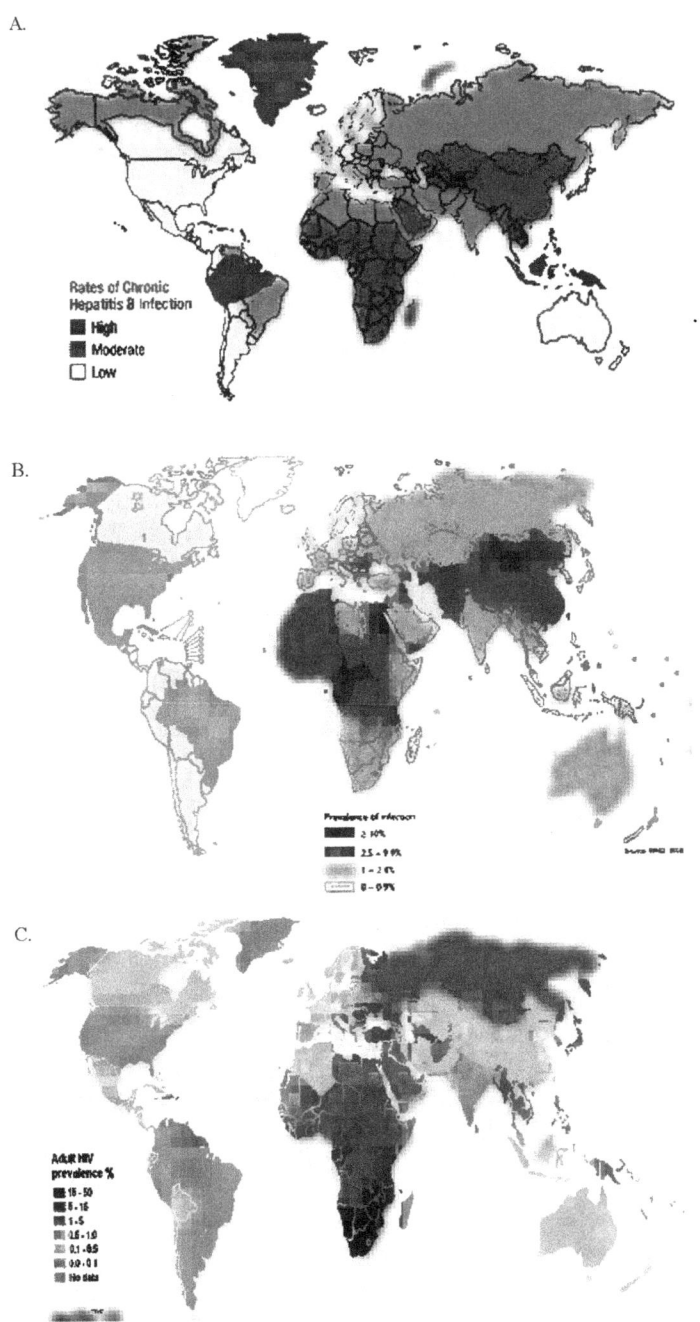

图 2-1　1 类致瘤病毒在全球的感染率估值（每 100 人）。A. HBV；B. HCV；C. HIV-1；D. HPV；E. HTLV-1；F. KSHV。

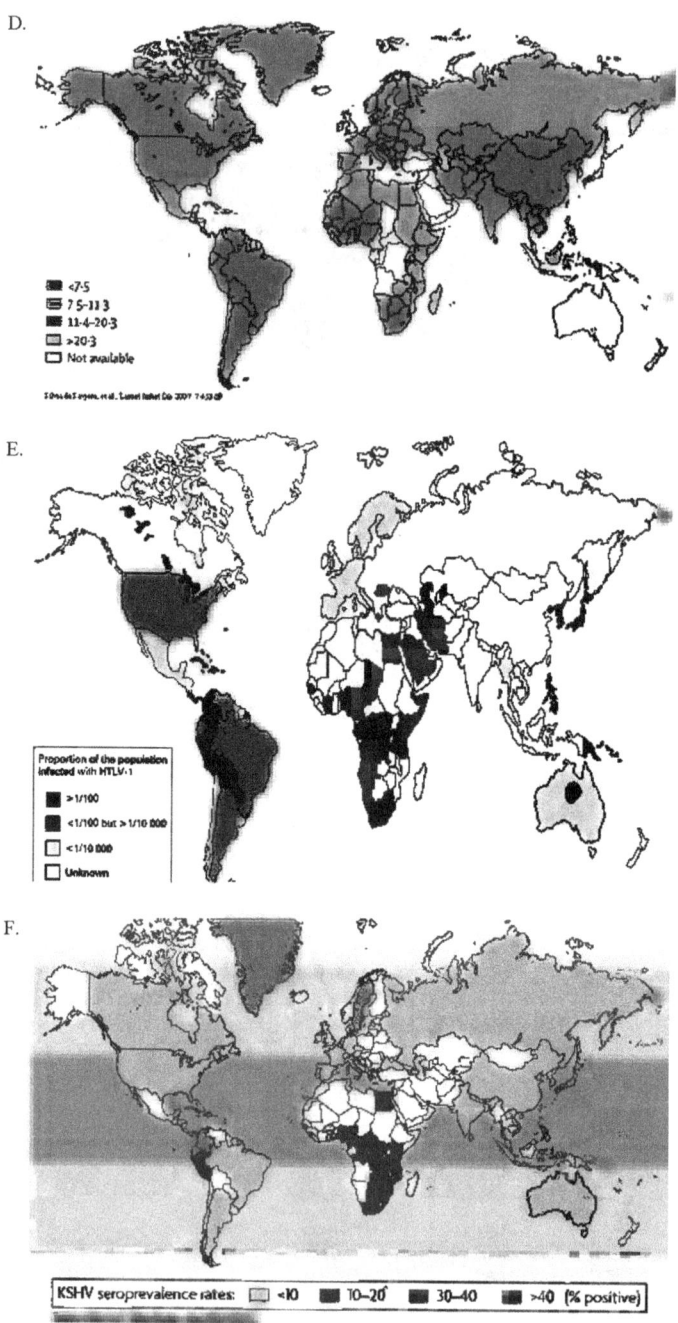

图 2-1 （续）

HIV-1 感染有三种主要传播途径：性行为、血液接触及母婴传播。HIV-1 的传染性由病原、宿主和环境三个因素的相互作用决定。输血传播 HIV-1 的可能性最高，其次是母婴传播、共用注射针头、男性同性恋行为传播。女性通过性行为传播给男性的可能性最低。

在性行为最活跃的人群中，HPV 感染率非常高，他们在一生中会染上至少一种基因型的 HPV（IARC 2009）。在对 157 879 位细胞学检验正常的妇女的荟萃分析中，HPV 致瘤 DNA 的时点患病率（point prevalence）估值高达 10%，这意味着大约 6 亿人被感染（de Sanjose et al. 2007）。时点患病率在非洲、东欧和拉丁美洲最高（20%~30%）；在南欧、西欧和东南亚最低（6%~7%），验证了图 2-1D 中显著的区域差异。时点患病率估值动态变化很大，因为发病率和清除率都很高。

13 种致瘤 HPV 基因型中，流行最普遍的包括 16、18、31、33、35、45、52、58 型。HPV 16 型在所有地区最常见，感染率为 2.3%~3.5%。HPV 感染通过直接皮肤接触或者皮肤-黏膜接触传播。肛殖型 HPV 主要通过青少年和年轻成人的性行为传播。非性行为途径则包括产褥期和医源性传播，这只占 HPV 感染的一小部分。

全球大约 1500 万~2000 万人感染了 HTLV-1（IARC 2009）。如图 2-1E 所示，HTLV-1 感染的特点是小流行热点区，周围为低发地区（Proietti et al. 2005）。中国大陆、韩国和中国台湾的 HTLV-1 感染率低于 0.1%，日本九州、冲绳高达 20%。高发地区包括日本西南部、撒哈拉以南非洲部分地区、加勒比地区和南非。HTLV-1 有三种主要的传播途径：垂直传播、性传播和非肠道传播。通过哺乳的垂直传播很容易导致母婴感染。然而，子宫内垂直传播率很低，因为被 HTLV-1 感染的淋巴细胞能穿越胎盘的数量有限。HTLV-1 的性传播效率受前病毒载量和安全套使用的影响。通过血液制品的敏感的血清学检查，非肠道注射传播的数量大大减少。毒品注射相关的共用针头是 HTLV-1 传播的另外一种非肠道途径。

如图 2-1F 所示，血清学检查确认的 KSHV 感染率在全球范围内有着很大差异（Dukers and Rezza 2003），从北欧的 2%~3%到刚果的 82%（IARC 2009）。在北欧、美国和亚洲，感染率普遍较低（<10%），在地中海地区稍高（10%~30%），在撒哈拉以南非洲很高（>50%）。KSHV 最初通过唾液传播。在 KSHV 感染率高的国家，通常在童年时期感染，随着年龄增长加重。男同性恋之间的 KSHV 传播同样是通过唾液。KSHV 也有可能通过长期毒品注射、输血和器官移植途径低效率传播。

3 全球范围内的一些病毒引起的癌症发病率

图 2-2 显示了一些致瘤病毒相关癌症的年龄标化发病率在全世界范围的分布。如图 2-2A 所示，鼻咽癌的年龄标化发病率范围在每 100 000 人小于 0.1 人与 8.05 人患病之间。在中国南部、东南亚和撒哈拉以南非洲，患病率最高，而在欧洲、西非和中美洲，患病率最低。不同的记录均显示，中国人患鼻咽癌的概率最高。EBV 感染在人类中分布较均匀，而中国人鼻咽癌患病率特别高，这意味着中国人的生活方式或者遗传易感性可能在鼻咽癌的发生中起到重要作用。

图 2-2B 显示了伯基特淋巴瘤的年龄标化发病率。中美洲、赤道附近的南美洲、巴布亚新几内亚和加勒比地区的国家都是伯基特淋巴瘤的高发区。但是，在其他

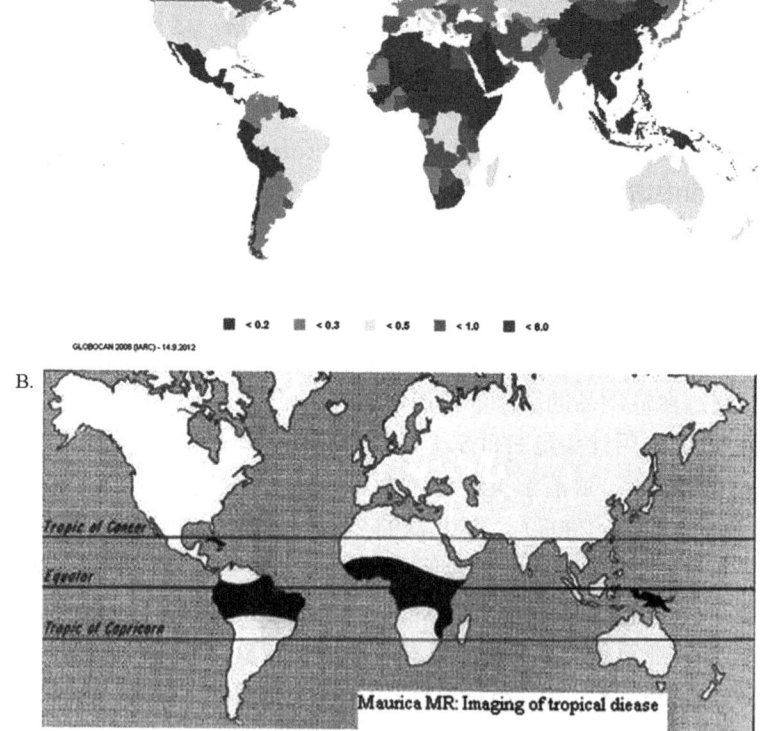

图 2-2 病毒引起的癌症在全球的年龄标准发生率（每 100 000 人）。A. 鼻咽癌；B.伯基特淋巴瘤；C.肝癌；D.宫颈癌；E.卡波西肉瘤。

第2章　病毒感染与人类肿瘤的流行病学

C. Estimated age-standardised incidence rate per 100,000
Liver: both sexes, all ages

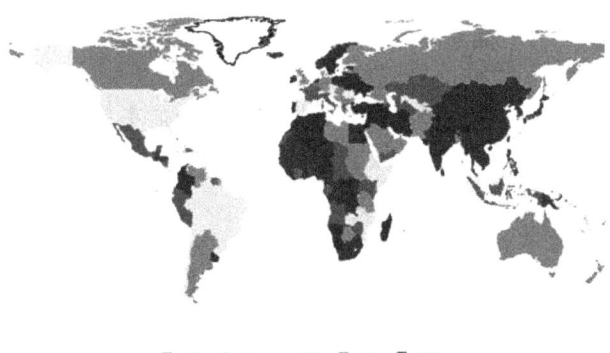

D. Estimated age-standardised incidence rate per 100,000
Cervix uteri, all ages

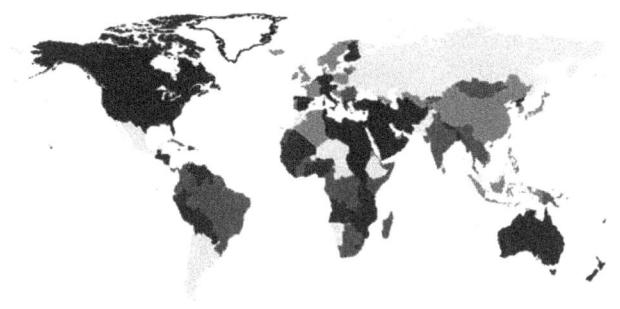

E.

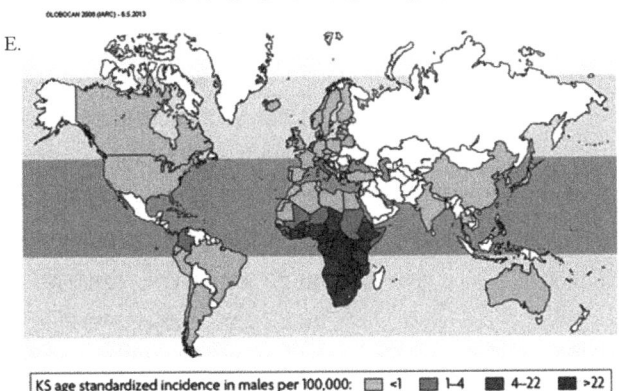

图 2-2　（续）

国家，伯基特淋巴瘤的发病率比较低。EBV 感染在人类中分布较均匀，但是非洲的伯基特淋巴瘤发病率格外高，这意味着地域环境或者遗传易感性在地方性伯基特淋巴瘤的发生中起到重要作用。

如图 2-2C 所示，肝癌的年龄标化发病率从每 100 000 人中 0.70 人到 94.4 人不等。东亚、东南亚、埃及和撒哈拉以南非洲的发病率最高，欧洲、中东、澳大利亚、新西兰、加拿大的发病率最低。肝癌发病率的地域差异与 HBV 和 HCV 血清阳性率的地域差异是一致的。

如图 2-2D 所示，宫颈癌的年龄标化发病率从每 100 000 人中 2.14 人到 56.29 人不等。拉丁美洲、南亚和撒哈拉以南非洲的发病率最高，欧洲、北美、澳大利亚、新西兰和中东地区的发病率最低。宫颈癌发病率的地域差异与致瘤 HPV 血清阳性率的地域差异是一致的。

如图 2-2E 所示，卡波西肉瘤的年龄标化发病率从每 100 000 人中低于 1.0 人到 30 人不等。撒哈拉以南非洲的发病率最高，欧洲、澳大利亚、北美和东亚的发病率最低。卡波西肉瘤发病率的地域差异与 KSHV 血清阳性率的地域差异是一致的。

4　肿瘤病毒的致瘤机制

如表 2-2 所示，7 种 1 类致瘤病毒的致瘤机制主要有 3 种，即直接作用、慢性炎症间接作用和免疫抑制间接作用（IARC 2009）。直接致瘤病毒包括 EBV、HPV、HTLV-1 和 KSHV；慢性炎症间接致瘤病毒包括 HBV 和 HCV；免疫抑制间接致瘤病毒包括 HIV-1。

表 2-2　已确定的致瘤病毒的致瘤机制

机制	1 类病毒（致瘤属性）
直接作用	EBV（细胞增殖、细胞凋亡抑制、基因组不稳定性、细胞移行）
	HPV（永生化、基因组不稳定性、DNA 损伤应答抑制、抗凋亡活动）
	HTLV-1（永生化和 T 细胞转化）
	KSHV（细胞增殖、细胞凋亡抑制、基因组不稳定性、细胞移行）
通过慢性炎症的间接作用	HBV（炎症、肝硬化、慢性肝炎）
	HCV（炎症、肝硬化、肝纤维化）
通过免疫抑制的间接作用	HIV-1（免疫抑制）

直接致瘤病毒有以下特点：①每个癌细胞中，通常都能找到全部或部分病毒基因组；②在体外，病毒可以在靶细胞发育后永生化；③病毒表达的致瘤基因与细胞蛋白相互作用，破坏细胞周期的检测点、抑制凋亡和 DNA 损伤应答，引起

基因组不稳定，诱发细胞的永生化、转化和转移。

HBV 和 HCV 都是通过慢性炎症引起受感染细胞和/或炎症细胞分泌趋化因子、细胞因子和前列腺素，从而引起肝细胞癌。慢性炎症也会通过直接诱变效应产生反应性氧化产物，从而解除对免疫系统的控制，促进血管生成，这对于新血管形成和肿瘤的生存十分关键。

感染 HIV-1 的患者有很高的风险患上由另一种感染原引起的癌症。HIV-1 感染，主要是通过免疫抑制，会促进 EBV、KSHV 等致瘤因子的复制。虽然抗逆转录病毒治疗可以降低很多 HIV-1 相关癌症的风险，但是，在全球范围内，该风险仍然很高。

5 一些病毒引起的癌症的终生累积发病率

一些病毒可能引起一种以上癌症，而有些癌症可能是由多种病毒共同引起。然而，感染这些致瘤病毒的患者中，只有部分会发展成特定癌症。表 2-3 显示了一些病毒引起的癌症的终生累积发病率。EBV VCA IgA 抗体或 EBV DNase 抗体血清反应阳性的人中，鼻咽癌的终生累积（30~75 岁）风险是 2.2%，而这两个抗体血清反应均为阴性的人，该风险是 0.48%。

只有 1/4 的 HBV 慢性感染患者会发展成肝细胞癌，并且性别差异很大，男性为 27.4%，女性为 8.0%（Huang et al. 2011）。HBV 引起的肝细胞癌发生被认为是多级的，有多原病因，包括 HBV、化学致瘤物、宿主特征和遗传易感性的相互作用（Che et al. 1997；Chen and Chen 2002；Chen and Yang 2011；IARC 2009）。

HCV 抗体血清反应阳性的患者中，大约 1/5 会发展成肝细胞癌，性别差异稍小，男性为 23.7%，女性为 16.7%（Huang et al. 2011）。丙肝抗体血清反应阳性的患者中，血清 HCV RNA 水平可测的，肝细胞癌的终生累积风险为 3.53%，不可测的为 24.2%。他们的肝细胞癌的发展包括很多共同作用因子（Lee et al. 2010；IARC 2009）。

感染 HPV16、HPV52、HPV58 和任何 1 类致瘤 HPV 的女性，宫颈癌的终生累积（30~75 岁）风险分别为 34.3%、23.3%、33.4% 和 20.3%。持续感染致瘤 HPV 的女性比短期感染的女性，宫颈癌的终生累积风险要高很多（Chen et al. 2011b）。

6 一些病毒引起的癌症的共同作用因子

感染致瘤病毒的人中，只有一部分会发展成特定癌症。事实充分说明，致瘤过程包括了其他共同作用因子。如表 2-3 所示，致瘤作用可能由多种风险因素共同作用，包括病毒、宿主和环境因素。病毒因素包括多种感染标志物，如病毒载量、基因型、变体、突变体、抗体、血清滴定量。宿主因素包括年龄、性别、种族、人体测量特征、免疫系统状况、激素水平、个人病史和家族肿瘤病史。环境因素包括化学致瘤物、营养状况、电离辐射、免疫抑制药物和其他感染原的混合感染。若干额外的因素促进了病毒相关癌症发育，这种作用似乎十分重要，但尚未具体阐明。

表 2-3 病毒引起的癌症的终生累积发病率和风险共同作用因子

病毒（癌症）	终生发病率	病毒因素	宿主因素	环境因素
EBV（鼻咽癌）	男性，2.0%	EBV 抗体血清滴定量、EBV 病毒载量高	男性、家族病史、遗传多态性（异型生物质新陈代谢、DNA 修复、人白细胞抗原）	广式咸鱼、饮食亚硝胺、木屑、甲醛、烟草
HBV（肝细胞癌）	男性，27.4% 女性，8.0%	持续感染、病毒载量、基因型、突变体、血清乙肝表面抗原水平	老年、男性、肥胖、糖尿病、血清雄激素和 ALT 水平、家族病史、遗传多态性（DNA 修复、人白细胞抗原、雄激素和异型生物质新陈代谢）	黄曲霉素、酒精、烟草、类胡萝卜素、硒、HCV 感染
HCV（肝细胞癌）	男性，23.7% 女性，16.7%	持续感染、病毒载量、基因型、突变体	老年、男性、肥胖、糖尿病、血清 ALT 水平、家族病史、遗传多态性	酒精、烟草、槟榔、HBV 或 HTLV-1 感染、辐射
HPV（宫颈癌）	HPV-16，34.3% HPV-52，23.3% HPV-58，33.4% 任何致瘤 HPV，20.3%	持续感染、病毒载量、基因型	老年、怀孕次数、家族病史、血清雌激素水平、遗传多态性（DNA 修复、人白细胞抗原）	烟草、免疫抑制、HIV-1 感染、避孕药、营养素

鼻咽癌的若干共同作用因素之前已被讨论过（Chien and Chen 2003）。与 EBV 引起的鼻咽癌相关的病毒因素包括 EBV 抗体（抗 EBV VCA IgA、抗 EBV DNase 和抗 EBNA1）血清效价高（Chien et al. 2001；Hsu et al. 2009），以及血清 EBV DNA 水平（病毒载量）高。宿主因素包括男性性别、鼻咽癌家族史（Hsu et al. 2011）和异型代谢酶的遗传多态性（Hildesheim et al. 1997）、DNA 修复酶（Cho et al. 2003）和人白细胞抗原（Hildesheim et al. 2002；Hsu et al. 2012b）。环境因素包括食用广东咸鱼、饮食含有过高的亚硝酸盐和亚硝胺（Ward et al. 2000）、对木屑和甲醛的职业暴露（Hildesheim et al. 2001）、长期吸烟（Hsu et al. 2009），以及饮食摄入植物维生素、鲜鱼、绿茶和咖啡较少（Hsu et al. 2012a）。

与 HBV 引起的肝细胞癌相关的病毒因素有血清乙肝 e 抗原水平高（Yang et al. 2002）、血清 HBV DNA 水平（Yang et al. 2002；Chen et al. 2006；Chen et al. 2009）、HBV 基因型和突变体类型（Yang et al. 2008）、血清乙肝表面抗原水平高（Lee et al. 2013）。宿主因素包括老年、男性、血清丙氨酸转氨酶（ALT）水平高、肝细胞癌家族病史（Chen et al. 1991；Yu et al. 2002a；Yang et al. 2010）、肥胖和糖尿病的病况（Chen et al. 2008）、血清雄激素水平高、雄性激素相关的遗传多态性（Yu and Chen 1993；Yu et al. 2000b）、异生代谢酶和 DNA 修复酶的遗传多态性（Chen et al. 1996a；Yu et al. 1995a，1999a，2003）。环境因素包括黄曲霉毒素暴露（Chen et al. 1996b；Wang et al. 1996）、烟酒习惯（Chen et al. 1991；Wang et al. 2003）、类胡萝卜素和硒摄取不足（Yu et al. 1995b，1999a，b）、HCV 共同感染（Huang et al. 2011）。

与 HCV 引起的肝细胞癌相关的病毒因素包括血清 HCV RNA 和基因 1 型 HCV 水平高（Lee et al. 2010；Huang et al. 2011）。宿主因素包括老年、男性、肥胖、糖尿病、血清 ALT 水平高和遗传多态性（Sun et al. 2003；Chen et al. 2008；Lee et al. 2010；IARC 2009）。环境因素包括饮酒、吸烟、嚼槟榔、辐射暴露、HBV 或 HTLV-1 的共同感染（Sun et al. 2003；Huang et al. 2011；IARC 2009）。

与致瘤 HPV 引起的宫颈癌相关的病毒因素包括长期感染、高病毒载量、HPV 基因型和变异（Chen et al. 2011a，b；Chang et al. 2011；IARC 2009）。宿主因素包括老年、怀孕次数、宫颈癌家族病史、血清雌激素水平、DNA 修复酶的遗传多态性和人白细胞抗原（Chen et al. 2011a；Chuang et al. 2012；IARC 2009）。环境因素包括吸烟、免疫抑制、HIV-1 共同感染、口服避孕药的使用、微量元素摄入不足（IARC 2009）。

7 HBV 引起的肝细胞癌的风险计算

每种病毒引起的癌症都有很多风险因子，整合这些因子，做出一个预测癌症累积患病率的风险模型或风险计算器，是十分有用的。这些风险计算器可以给临床医生提供重要信息，用以识别谁是强化治疗患者，谁只需常规随诊。已有一些风险模型/计算器被用于预测慢性丙肝患者的肝细胞癌患病率（Yang et al. 2010），而只有 REACH-B 评分通过了外部验证（Yang et al. 2010）。近来，REACH-B 评分被用于检查抗病毒治疗的效果，以减少慢性丙肝患者的肝癌风险。

表 2-4 显示最新的慢性乙肝患者的 HCC 风险计算器（Lee et al. 2013）。计算器中包括的因子有年龄、性别、家族肝细胞癌病史、血清 ALT 水平、乙肝 e 抗原血清状况、血清 HBV DNA 和乙肝表面抗原水平，以及 HBV 基因型。风险评分受多种类型的风险因子影响。例如，一位 60 岁（风险评分=6）的男性（风险评分=2）丙肝患者，有家族肝细胞癌病史（风险评分=2），ALT 血清水平为 90 IU/L（风险评分=2），乙肝 e 抗原血清反应阳性，血清 HBV DNA 水平为 10^7 拷贝/毫升，血清乙肝表面抗原水平为 104 IU/mL，感染了 HBV 基因型 C（风险评分=7），

风险评分总分为 19。图 2-3 的诺模图显示了由风险评分计算出的 5 年、10 年、15 年的肝细胞癌累积风险。风险评分高达 19 的患者，其 5 年、10 年、15 年的肝细胞癌累积风险分别为 35%、80% 和 90%。相反，一个 34 岁的女性，没有家族肝细胞癌病史，血清 ALT 水平为 10 IU/L，乙肝 e 抗原阴性，血清 HBV DNA 水平为 10^3 拷贝/mL，血清乙肝表面抗原水平为 50 IU/mL（风险评分总分=0），其 5 年、10 年、15 年的肝细胞癌风险分别为 0.0075%、0.025% 和 0.065%。

表 2-4　HBV 引起的肝细胞癌的风险因子评分

风险因子	风险评分
年龄/岁	
30~34	0
35~39	1
40~44	2
45~49	3
50~54	4
55~59	5
60~64	6
性别	
女	0
男	2
家族肝细胞癌病史	
无	0
有	2
血清 ALT 水平/（IU/L）	
<15	0
15~44	1
≥45	2
乙肝 e 抗原/HBV DNA（拷贝/mL）/乙肝表面抗原（IU/mL）/基因型	
阴性/<10^4/<100/任何类型	0
阴性/<10^4/100~999/任何类型	2
阴性/<10^4/≥1000/任何类型	2
阴性/10^4~10^6/<100/任何类型	3
阴性/10^4~10^6/100-999/任何类型	3
阴性/10^4~10^6/≥1000/任何类型	4
阴性/≥10^6/任何水平/乙肝或乙肝+丙肝	5

风险因子	风险评分
阴性/≥10^6/任何水平/丙肝	7
阳性/任何水平/任何水平/乙肝或乙肝+丙肝	6
阳性/任何水平/任何水平/丙肝	7

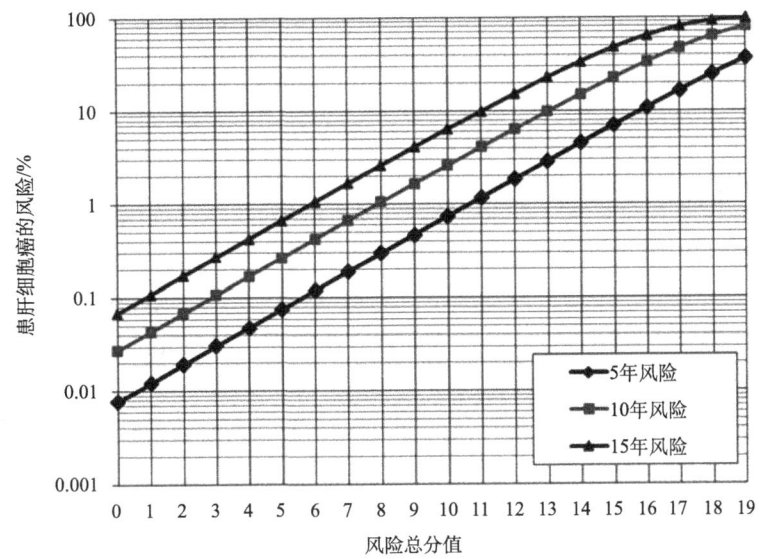

图 2-3 根据风险评分肝细胞癌 5 年、10 年、15 年的风险预测线图

鼻咽癌和宫颈癌等其他病毒引起的癌症的风险计算也会有利于分类和对有其他致瘤病毒感染患者的临床管理。风险计算器的开发需要大规模的预期群体,需要对他们进行长期的风险因子的精确跟踪测量。人口特征、病毒感染生物标记、家族病史和遗传易感性的多态性均需要整合,以建立有效、实用的癌症风险计算器。

8 通过疫苗和抗病毒治疗减少癌症发生率

防止病毒引起的癌症的最有效策略,是通过疫苗防止病毒感染,或者通过抗病毒治疗来清除人类宿主中的致瘤病毒。表 2-5 显示的是目前正在使用的预防致瘤病毒感染的疫苗或抗病毒策略。疫苗可用于预防 HBV 引起的肝细胞癌和 HPV 引起的宫颈癌,抗病毒治疗可用于 HBV、HCV 和 HIV 慢性感染的治疗。

表 2-5　通过疫苗和抗病毒治疗的预防策略减少病毒引起的癌症发生率

病毒	癌症	预防策略
HBV	肝细胞癌	疫苗和抗病毒治疗
HCV	肝细胞癌	抗病毒治疗
HIV-1	卡波西肉瘤	抗病毒治疗
HPV	宫颈癌	疫苗

很多临床试验都验证了 HPV 疫苗可以有效预防宫颈肿瘤、宫颈癌的前期病变，用于肝硬化患者的抗病毒治疗，也可以有效预防肝细胞癌（Liaw et al. 2004）。中国台湾在 1984 年实施了 HBV 免疫规划，出生时接种了疫苗的世代，6~19 岁时的肝细胞癌发生率大大降低（Chang et al. 1997，2009；Chien et al. 2006）。澳大利亚因为实施 HPV 免疫规划，在青少年群体中进行疫苗接种，宫颈肿瘤发生率被有效地降低。2003 年，中国台湾实施了抗病毒治疗计划，用以控制乙肝病毒或丙肝病毒的慢性感染，以期减少肝癌在成年患者中的发病率和死亡率。然而，它对预防肝细胞癌的有效性仍然有待评估。

9　未来展望

随着蛋白质组学和基因组学的发展，越来越多的与病毒引起的癌症发育相关的生物标志物得到鉴定。它们可以应用于癌症的风险预测或早期检测。例如，多种微 RNA 已被组合用于肝细胞癌的诊断。但是，肝细胞癌早期诊断的有效性和成本效益需要进一步评估，并与其他方式进行比较，如腹部超声检查（Chen and Lee 2011）。更重要的是，对生物标志物的重复测量可能进一步改善对于病毒引起的癌症的风险预测或早期检测（Chen 2005）。例如，血清 HBV DNA 水平的轨迹已可以用来有效地预测肝细胞癌的长远风险（Chen et al. 2011c）。我们亟需更多纵向的研究，对多种生物标志物进行常规跟踪检验，以鉴定优质的分子靶标，推进研发预防药物、诊断，或多种病毒引起的癌症的治疗。对这些生物药品的卫生经济学评估可能有利于它们的临床应用。

（卢建红，尹典，周诠 译）

参 考 文 献

Alter MJ (2007) Epidemiology of hepatitis C virus infection. World J Gastroenterol 13:2436–2441

Chang MH, Chen CJ, Lai MS, Kong MS, Wu TC, Liang DC, Hsu HM, Shau WY, Chen DS (1997) Taiwan Childhood Hepatoma Study Group. Universal hepatitis B vaccination in Taiwan and the incidence of hepatocellular carcinoma in children. New Engl J Med 336:1855–1859

Chang MH, You SL, Chen CJ, Liu CJ, Lee CM, Lin SM, Chu HC, Wu TC, Yang SS, Kuo HS, Chen DS (2009) The Taiwan hepatoma study group. decreased incidence of hepatocellular carcinoma in hepatitis B vaccinees: a 20-year follow-up study. J Natl Cancer Inst 101:1348–1355

Chang YJ, Chen HC, Lee BH, You SL, Lin CY, Pan MH, Chou YC, Hsieh CY, Chen YM, Chen YJ, Chen CJ (2011) Unique variants of human papillomavirus genotypes 52 and 58 and risk of cervical neoplasia. Int J Cancer 129:965–973

Chen CJ (2005) Time-dependent events in natural history of occult hepatitis B virus infection: Importance of population-based long-term follow-up study with repeated measurements (Editorial). J Hepatology 42:438–440

Chen CJ, Chen DS (2002) Interaction of hepatitis B virus, chemical carcinogen and genetic susceptibility: multistage hepatocarcinogenesis with multifactorial etiology (editorial). Hepatology 36:1046–1049

Chen CJ, Lee MH (2011) Early diagnosis of hepatocellular carcinoma by multiple microRNAs: validity, efficacy and cost-effectiveness (editorial). J Clin Oncol 29:4745–4747

Chen CJ, Yang HI (2011) Natural history of chronic hepatitis B REVEALed. J Gastroenterol Hepatol 26:628–638

Chen CJ, Liang KY, Chang AS, Chang YC, Lu SN, Liaw YF, Chang WY, Sheen MC, Lin TM (1991) Effects of hepatitis B virus, alcohol drinking, cigarette smoking and familial tendency on hepatocellular carcinoma. Hepatology 13:398–406

Chen CJ, Yu MW, Liaw YF, Wang LW, Chiamprasert S, Matin F, Hirvonen A, Bell AB, Santella RM (1996a) Chronic hepatitis B carriers with null genotypes of glutathione S-transferase M1 and T1 polymorphisms who are exposed to aflatoxins are at increased risk of hepatocellular carcinoma. Am J Hum Genet, 59:128–134

Chen CJ, Wang LY, Lu SN, Wu MH, You SL, Li HP, Zhang YJ, Wang LW, Santella RM (1996b) Elevated aflatoxin exposure and increased risk of hepatocellular carcinoma. Hepatology 24:38–42

Chen CJ, Yu MW, Liaw YF (1997) Epidemiological characteristics and risk factors of hepatocellular carcinoma. J Gastroen Hepatol 12:S294–S308

Chen CJ, Yang HI, Su J, Jen CL, You SL, Lu SN, Huang GT, Iloeje UH (2006) Risk of hepatocellular carcinoma across a biological gradient of serum hepatitis B virus DNA level. JAMA 2006(295):65–73

Chen CL, Yang HI, Yang WS, Liu CJ, Chen PJ, You SL, Wang LY, Sun CA, Lu SN, Chen DS, Chen CJ (2008) Metabolic factors and risk of hepatocellular carcinoma by chronic hepatitis B/ C virus infection: a follow-up study in Taiwan. Gastroenterology 135:111–121

Chen CJ, Yang HI, Iloeje UH (2009) REVEAL-HBV Study Group. Hepatitis B virus DNA levels and outcomes in chronic hepatitis B. Hepatology 49:S72–S84

Chen CF, Lee WC, Yang HI, Chang HC, Jen CL, Iloeje UH, Su J, Hsiao KC, Wang LY, You SL, Lu SN, Chen CJ (2011a) Changes in serum levels of HBV DNA and alanine aminotransferase determine risk for hepatocellular carcinoma risk. Gastroenterology 141:1240–1248

Chen HC, You SL, Hsieh CY, Lin CY, Pan MH, Chou YC, Liaw KL, Schiffman M, Hsing AW, Chen CJ (2011b) For CBCSP-HPV Study Group. Prevalence of genotype- specific human papillomavirus infection and cervical neoplasia in Taiwan: a community-based survey of 10,602 women. Int J Cancer 128:1192–1203

Chen HC, Schiffman M, Lin CY, Pan MH, You SL, Chuang LC, Hsieh CY, Liaw KL, Hsing AW, Chen CJ (2011c) CBCSP-HPV study group. persistence of type-specific human papilloma- virus infection and increased long-term risk of cervical cancer. J Natl Cancer Inst 103:1387–1396

Chien YC, Chen CJ (2003) Epidemiology and etiology of nasopharyngeal carcinoma: gene-environment interaction. Cancer Rev Asia-Pacific 1:1–19

Chien YC, Chen JY, Liu MY, Yang HI, Hsu MM, Chen CJ, Yang CS (2001) Serologic markers of Epstein-Barr virus infection and nasopharyngeal carcinoma in Taiwanese men. New Engl J Med 345:1877–1882

Chien YC, Jan CF, Kuo HS, Chen CJ (2006) Nationwide hepatitis B vaccination program in Taiwan: Effectiveness in 20 years after it was launched. Epidemiol Rev 28:126–135

Cho EY, Hildesheim A, Chen CJ, Hsu MM, Chen IH, Mittl BF, Levine PH., Liu MY, Chen JY, Brinton LA, Cheng YJ, Yang CS (2003) Nasopharyngeal carcinoma and genetic polymorphisms of DNA repair enzymes XRCC1 and hOGG1. Cancer Epidemiol Biomarker Prev, 12:1100–1104

Chuang LC, Hu CY, Chen HC, Lin PJ, Lee B, Lin CY, Pan MH, Chou YC, You SL, Hsieh CY, Chen CJ (2012) Associations of human leukocyte antigen class II genotypes with human papillomavirus 18 infection and cervical intraepithelial neoplasia risk. Cancer 118:223–231

de Sanjose S, Diaz M, Castellsague X, Clifford G, Bruni L, Munoz N, Bosch FX (2007) Worldwide prevalence and genotype distribution of cervical human papillomavirus DNA in women with normal cytology: a meta-analysis. Lancet Infect Dis 7:453–459

Dukers NH, Rezza G (2003) Human herpesvirus 8 epidemiology: what we do and do not know. AIDS 17:1717–1730

Hildesheim A, Anderson LM, Chen CJ, Cheng YJ, Brinton LA, Daly AK, Reed CD, Chen IH, Caporaso NE, Hsu MM, Chen JY, Idle JR, Hoover RN, Yang CS, Chabra SK (1997) CYP2E1 genetic polymorphisms and risk of nasopharyngeal carcinoma in Taiwan. J Natl Cancer Inst 89:1207–1212

Hildesheim A, Dosemeci M, Chan CC, Chen CJ, Cheng YC, Hsu MM, Chen IH, Mittl BF, Sun B, Levine PH, Chen JY, Brinton LA, Yang CS (2001) Occupational exposure to wood, formaldehyde, and solvents and risk of nasopharyngeal carcinoma. Cancer Epidemiol Biomarker Prev 2001(10):1145–1153

Hildesheim A, Apple RJ, Chen CJ, Wang SS, Cheng YC, Klitz W, Mack SJ, Chen IH, Hsu MM, Yang CS, Brinton LA, Levine PH, Erlich HA (2002) Association of HLA class I and II alleles and extended haplotypes with nasopharyngeal carcinoma in Taiwan. J Natl Cancer Inst 94:1780–1789

Hsu WL, Chen JY, Chien YC, Liu MY, You SL, Hsu MM, Yang CS, Chen CJ (2009) Independent effects of EBV and cigarette smoking on nasopharyngeal carcinoma: a 20-year follow-up study on 9,622 males without family history in Taiwan. Cancer Epidemiol Biomarkers Prev 18:1218–1226

Hsu WL, Yu KJ, Chien YC, Chiang JY, Cheng YJ, Chen JY, Liu MY, Chou SP, You SL, Hsu MM, Lou PJ, Wang CP, Hong JH, Leu YS, Tsai MH, Su MC, Tsai ST, Chao WY, Ger LP, Chen PR, Yang CS, Hildesheim A, Diehl SR, Chen CJ (2011) Familial tendency and risk of nasopharyngeal carcinoma in Taiwan: effects of covariates on risk. Am J Epidemiol 173:292–299

Hsu WL, Pan WH, Chien YC, Yu KJ, Cheng YJ, Chen JY, Liu MY, Hsu MM, Lou PJ, Chen IH, Yang CS, Hildesheim A, Chen CJ (2012a) Lowered risk of nasopharyngeal carcinoma and intake of plant vitamin, fresh fish, green tea and coffee: a case-control study in Taiwan. PLoS ONE 7:e41779

Hsu WL, Tse KP, Liang S, Chien YC, Su WH, Yu KJ, Cheng YJ, Tsang NM, Hsu MM, Chang KP, Chen IH, Chen TI, Yang CS, Golstein AM, Chen CJ, Chang YS, Hildesheim A (2012b) Evaluation of human leukocyte antigen-A (HLA-A), other non-HLA markers on chromosome 6p21 and risk of nasopharyngeal carcinoma. PLoS ONE 7:e42767

Huang YT, Jen CL, Yang HI, Lee MH, Lu SN, Iloeje UH, Chen CJ (2011) REVEAL-HBV/HCV Study Group. Lifetime risk and gender difference of hepatocellular carcinoma among patients affected with chronic hepatitis B and C. J Clin Oncol 29:3643–3650

IARC (2009)(International Agency for Research on Cancer) *A review of human carcinogens. Part B: biological agent*. IARC, Lyon, IARC

Lee MH, Yang HI, Lu SN, Jen CL, Yeh SH, Liu CJ, Chen PJ, You SL, Wang LY, Chen WJ, Chen CJ (2010) Hepatitis C virus seromarkers and subsequent risk of hepatocellular carcinoma: long-term predictors from a community-based cohort study. J Clin Oncol 28:4587–4593

Lee MH, Yang HI, Liu J, Batrla-Utermann R, Jen CL, Iloeje UH, Jun J, Lu SN, You SL, Wang LY, Chen CJ (2013) For the R.E.V.E.A.L.-HBV Study Group. Models predicting long-term risk of liver cirrhosis and hepatocellular carcinoma in chronic hepatitis B patients: risk scores integrating characteristics of host and hepatitis B virus. Hepatology (in press)

Liaw YF, Sung JJ, Chow WC, Farrell G, Lee CZ, Yuen H, Tanwandee T, Tao QM, Shue K, Keene

ON, Dixon JS, Gray DF, Sabbat J (2004) Lamivudine for patients with chronic hepatitis B and advanced liver disease. N Engl J Med 351:1521–31

Proietti FA, Carneiro-Proietti AB, Catalan-Soares BC, Murphy EL (2005) Global epidemiology of HTLV-1 infection and associated diseases. Oncogene 24:6058–6068

Sun CA, Wu DM, Lin CC, Lu SN, You SL, Wang LY, Wu MH, Chen CJ (2003) Incidence and co-factors of hepatitis C virus-related hepatocellular carcinoma: a prospective study of 12,008 men in Taiwan. Am J Epidemiol 157:674–682

Wang LY, Hatch M, Chen CJ, Levin B, You SL, Lu SN, Wu MH, Wu WP, Wang LW, Wang Q, Huang GT, Yang PM, Lee HS, Santella RM (1996) Aflatoxin exposure and the risk of hepatocellular carcinoma in Taiwan. Int J Cancer 67:620–625

Wang LY, You SL, Lu SN, Ho HC, Wu MH, Sun CA, Yang HI, Chen CJ (2003) Risk of hepatocellular carcinoma and habits of alcohol drinking, betel quid chewing, and cigarette smoking: a cohort of 2416 HBsAg-seropositive and 9421 HBsAg-seronegative male residents in Taiwan. Cancer Cause Control 14:241–250

Ward MH, Pan WH, Cheng YJ, Li FH, Brinton LA, Chen CJ, Hsu MM, Chen IH, Levine PH, Yang CS, Hildesheim A (2000) Dietary exposure to nitrite and nitrosamines and risk of nasopharyngeal cancer in Taiwan. Int J Cancer 2000(86):603–609

GLOBOCAN http://globocan.iarc.fr/factsheets/populations/factsheet.asp?uno=900

Yang HI, Lu SN, You SL, Sun CA, Wang LY, Hsiao K, Chen PJ, Chen DS, Liaw YF, Chen CJ (2002) Hepatitis B e antigen and the risk of hepatocellular carcinoma. New Engl J Med 347:168–174

Yang HI, Yeh SH, Chen PJ, Iloeje UH, Jen CL, Wang LY, Lu SN, You SL, Chen DS, Liaw YF, Chen CJ, REVEAL-HBV Group (2008) Association between Hepatitis B virus genotype and mutants and the risk of hepatocellular carcinoma. J Natl Cancer Inst, 100: 1134–1143

Yang HI, Sherman M, Su J, Chen PJ, Liaw YF, Iloeje UH, Chen CJ (2010) Nomograms for risk of hepatocellular carcinoma in patients with chronic hepatitis B virus infection. J Clin Oncol 28:2437–2444

Yang HI, Yuen MF, Chan HL, Han KH, Chen PJ, Kim DY, Ahn SH, Chen CJ, Wong VW, Seto WK (2011) Risk estimation for hepatocellular carcinoma in chronic hepatitis B (REACH-B): development and validation of a predictive score. Lancet Oncol 12:568–574

Yu MW, Chen CJ (1993) Elevated serum testosterone levels and risk of hepatocellular carcinoma. Cancer Res 53:790–794

Yu MW, Gladek-Yarborough A, Chiamprasert S, Santella RM, Liaw YF, Chen CJ (1995a) Cytochrome P-450 2E1 and glutathione S-transferase M1 polymorphisms and susceptibility to hepatocellular carcinoma. Gastroenterology 109:1266–1273

Yu MW, Hsieh HH, Pan WH, Yang CS, Chen CJ (1995b) Vegetable consumption, serum retinol level and risk of hepatocellular carcinoma. Cancer Res 55:1301–1305

Yu MW, Chiu YH, Chiang YC, Chen CH, Lee TH, Santella RM, Chen HD, Liaw YF, Chen CJ (1999a) Plasma carotenoids, glutathione S-transferases M1 and T1 genetic polymorphisms, and risk of hepatocellular carcinoma: Independent and interactive effects. Am J Epidemiol 149:621–629

Yu MW, Horng IS, Hsu KH, Chiang YC, Liaw YF, Chen CJ (1999b) Plasma selenium levels and risk of hepatocellular carcinoma among men with chronic hepatitis B virus infection. Am J Epidemiol 150:367–374

Yu MW, Chang HC, Liaw YF, Lin SM, Lee SD, Chen PJ, Hsiao TJ, Lee PH, Chen CJ (2000a) Familial risk of hepatocellular carcinoma among chronic hepatitis B carriers and their relatives. J Natl Cancer Inst 92:1159–1164

Yu MW, Cheng SW, Lin MW, Yang SY, Liaw YF, Chang HC, Hsiao TJ, Lin SM, Lee SD, Chen PJ, Liu CJ, Chen CJ (2000b) Androgen-receptor CAG repeat, plasma testosterone levels, and risk of hepatitis B-related hepatocellular carcinoma. J Natl Cancer Inst 92:2023–2028

Yu MW, Yang SY, Pan IJ, Lin CL, Liu CJ, Liaw YF, Lin SM, Chen PJ, Lee SD, Chen CJ (2003) Polymorphisms in XRCC1 and glutathione S-transferase genes and hepatitis B-related hepatocellular carcinoma. J Natl Cancer Inst 95:1485–1488

第3章 病毒感染、炎症与肿瘤的预防

Norman Woller 和 Florian Kühnel

摘 要 在过去的20年中,我们从分子水平对肿瘤生物学的了解取得了实质性进展。近年的研究结果表明,炎症在肿瘤发生过程中是一个主要的驱动力,这是由于慢性病毒感染和肿瘤生成是密切相关的。这个视角让我们深刻认识到,持续性病毒感染和慢性炎症在肿瘤发生、生长和转移中起决定性作用。研究成果解释了肿瘤细胞如何与邻近的上皮细胞和浸润免疫细胞相互作用及联系,从而形成所谓的"肿瘤微环境"并建立肿瘤特异的耐受性。这种对恶性肿瘤的进一步认识使得我们可以设计出合理的干预治疗措施,将目标瞄准炎症和潜在的信号通路,从而预防和治疗炎症相关性肿瘤。本章概括了肿瘤发生过程中病毒介导炎症的角色,进而阐明了肿瘤相关的炎症机制和肿瘤微环境的特征。其中,肿瘤微环境近些年被认为在肿瘤维持和进展中起关键作用。最后,本章还讨论了预防炎症相关性肿瘤的最新进展,并简要展望肿瘤免疫治疗的前景。

在19世纪,Rudolph Virchow猜测组织损伤先于该部位的肿瘤发生。他根据在肿瘤组织中观察到的白细胞浸润现象推测,伤口愈合中的炎症过程可能与肿瘤发生有关(Balkwill and Mantovani 2001)。根据这些观点,肿瘤在后来被描述为是"可能存在的过度愈合"的结果(Haddow 1972),或者是"没有愈合的伤口"(Dvorak 1986),并有人指出肿瘤生长和伤口愈合过程(如成纤维细胞活化、白细胞吸引、细胞增殖和血管生成)之间存在明显的相似性。在过去的二十多年间,这个观点被分子生物学研究结果证实是成立的,再次印证了炎症产生过程对肿瘤发生和转移起根本的作用(Karin 2006;Guerra et al. 2007)。对于肿瘤的病因学而言,生殖细胞突变在肿瘤的生长方面起次要的作用,实际上,多达90%的肿瘤是与获得性体细胞突变相关的,后者主要通过环境和生活方式因素获得。全球30%的恶性肿瘤归因于吸烟,35%是由于包括过度肥胖在内的膳食原因造成的

N. Woller _ F. Kühnel (✉)
Clinic for Gastroenterology, Hepatology, and Endocrinology, Hannover Medical School,
Carl-Neuberg-Str. 1, 30625, Hannover, Germany
e-mail: Kuehnel.Florian@mh-hannover.de

（Aggarwal et al. 2009）。据估计，全球肿瘤发生数量中的 20%~25%与病原体造成的炎症有关，绝大部分是由于持续的、非可控性的病毒感染导致炎症发生（Hussain and Harris 2007；Parkin 2006）。而且，在肿瘤的微环境中也存在炎症因素，这与流行病学意义上的传统病原体感染没有关系，而是与其他环境危险因素有关，如吸烟或吸入石英纤维，因此阐明了致癌机制中炎症的总体作用。在本文中，我们将总结病毒导致感染以及炎症在肿瘤发生中的关键作用，同时要讨论可直接应用的措施来预防感染相关性肿瘤。据此，我们将集中讨论致癌作用中感染导致炎症的过程，或许可以在肿瘤预防和治疗方面提供有效的药理学分子靶点。在本章第 1 节中，我们将简单介绍临床上能导致慢性组织炎症和肿瘤的最常见的病毒类型。

1 引起肿瘤的慢性病毒感染

病毒感染是肿瘤最重要的病因之一（de Martel and Franceschi 2009）。就全球健康问题而言，与病毒感染相关的肿瘤中，在肝脏和宫颈发生的实体瘤是最典型的。前一种主要是由乙型肝炎病毒和丙型肝炎病毒（HBV 和 HCV）引起的，后一种主要与人乳头状瘤病毒（HPV）有关。HBV 是嗜肝 DNA 病毒科中的一种小型的 DNA 病毒，主要通过血液或性接触传播。HBV 的肝脏感染经常会导致严重的并发症，例如，包括肝功能衰竭在内的急性肝炎，以及在持续感染下更进一步导致肝硬化和肝细胞癌（HCC）。HBV 和 HCC 生长之间的因果关系已经得到清晰的了解（Chen et al. 2006），保守估计肝癌病例中 54%是由于 HBV 感染造成的。尽管二十多年前就发明了一种有效的疫苗，但 HBV 仍然是造成健康问题的一个主要因素，因为全世界大约有 3.6 亿慢性 HBV 携带者（Shepard et al. 2006；Custer et al. 2004）。作为肝脏感染晚期并发症的 HCC，其发生的风险与病毒介导的炎症持续时间密切相关，涉及的几种病理机制包括乙肝病毒蛋白（如 HBx）介导的致瘤效应、突变性整合于宿主细胞基因组中，以及 T 细胞依赖性自身免疫（Farazi and DePinho 2006）。

能导致肝癌的另一种比较重要的病毒是丙型肝炎病毒（HCV），它属于黄病毒科，是单链 RNA 病毒。HCV 感染是一种基于血液传播的疾病，全球人口中的 3%遭受慢性感染（Shepard et al. 2005）。HCV 阳性的个体发生 HCC 的风险很高（Donato et al. 1998），大约有 31%的肝癌病例是由于慢性 HCV 感染造成的。其发生的病理学机制目前还未完全了解。就像 HBV 那样，通过长时间并发的炎症、细胞死亡和组织更新，HCV 能导致持续性感染和恶性转化。分子研究结果显示，有几种 HCV 蛋白（如 NS3、NS4B、NS5A 和核心蛋白）具有潜在的致瘤作用（Farazi and DePinho 2006；Barth et al. 2008）。

人类乳头状瘤病毒（HPV）也是引起感染与炎症相关性实体瘤的病因（Parkin and Bray 2006）。HPV 是一种无包膜的 DNA 病毒，它可以引起皮肤和黏膜的良性或恶性损伤。感染的过程通常是无症状的，对于大多数个体，其局部免疫会导致病毒清除（Plummer et al. 2007）。HPV 会在大约 10%的被感染妇女中持续感染，从而提高了发生宫颈癌的风险。在 100 种不同的基因型中，有几种被认为是高风险毒株，这是由于它们与宫颈癌的发生具有因果相关性。其中，最具致瘤风险性的 HPV-16 和 HPV-18 基因型与大多数宫颈肿瘤的发生相关（Smith et al. 2007）。基于 HPV 介导的肿瘤发生的病理学机制得到了较好的研究。慢性 HPV 感染和病毒 DNA 序列整合入宿主细胞的 DNA 中是相伴发生的。整合后的早期病毒基因（如 E6/E7）的表达会干扰抑癌基因（如 p53 和 Rb）的活性，从而激活细胞周期和抑制细胞凋亡。其他免疫学或诱变影响因素也会进一步促成细胞转化和肿瘤生长。

EB 病毒（EBV）是临床上发现的致瘤病毒的典型例子，它与几种血液恶性肿瘤有关，如伯基特淋巴瘤、霍奇金淋巴瘤、非霍奇金淋巴瘤。其他与肿瘤相关的病毒还有人类疱疹病毒 8 型（HHV-8），它是卡波西肉瘤相关性病原；此外还有人类 T 淋巴细胞白血病病毒 1 型（HTLV-1）和梅克尔细胞多瘤病毒。

2 炎症与肿瘤

2.1 炎症与肿瘤生长的内在联系

在正常状态下，组织完整性和细胞更新的维护是由宿主严密控制的。一旦组织完整性受到病原体感染或组织损伤的破坏，就会引起急性炎症，这是一种局部、及时而有限的免疫机制在起作用，从而可以有效清除病原体并产生伤口愈合反应。尽管急性炎症以重建无病原体的完整组织为目标，但是，最终感染并不容易被急性炎症机制彻底清除。接下来会导致慢性炎症反应，即和病原体共处于平衡状态中。有两种事件本质上会导致病毒介导的慢性感染。第一，与肿瘤相关的病毒必须找到一些途径来击溃宿主抗病毒免疫的防御机制，或者撤退到免疫逃逸状态以便维持后期的感染状态。第二，抗病毒免疫反应的程度必须调整到一定的水平，控制病毒得以局限在感染器官，病毒血症得到遏制，并能预防严重的免疫病理发生。这些持续性感染会导致轻微的慢性炎症。持续性感染情况下，细胞不仅是病毒致癌转化的主体，而且在慢性炎症中，容易导致肿瘤的遗传变异的累积过程也会被强化的细胞更新提速。这两种情况，即慢性炎症和细胞的病毒性转化，是肿瘤发生过程中的重要事件（Rakoff-Nahoum and Medzhitov 2009）。而且，炎症被认为在致瘤过程中的每一个环节起重要作用（Karin 2006）。关于炎症在初始的细胞转化中的作用也是一个值得讨论的话题。有研究表明，即使在没有出现确定性外在诱因的情况下，炎症也可能增加组织中的突变频率（Sato et al. 2006；Bielas et al. 2006）。炎症机制在"免疫监视"过程中起一定作用，因为免疫监视在极早期阶段可以有效地限制肿瘤的生长。受到异常的致癌基因活化的诱发，通过 CD4 T 细胞和 M1 巨噬细胞的协调作用，还可诱导肝细胞衰老并最终导致衰老细胞的清除（Kang et al. 2011）。另外，衰老过程中发生的免疫抑制、免疫克服及免疫逃逸，通过炎症机制（如分泌与衰老相关的细胞因子），会进一步促进早期的肿瘤形成。

一旦早期的肿瘤结节形成，会吸引几种白细胞和间充质细胞，这将建立肿瘤的微环境，给癌细胞提供起辅助作用的生长刺激和细胞因子。这种郁积的、伴随炎症的肿瘤微环境在肿瘤生长中起到核心作用，通常被认为是肿瘤的另一个显著标志（Hanahan and Weinberg 2011）。这些发现还引起其他更进一步的研究，如非恶性细胞对肿瘤微环境的贡献作用、它们的相互影响、释放的信号分子和起中心作用的分子途径。

2.2 肿瘤相关性炎症过程中细胞因子信号机制和分子途径

肿瘤相关性炎症与肿瘤生长过程具有密切的相互作用，其因果机制是：炎症发生过程是造成恶性肿瘤的主要驱动因素。通过各种研究，已经确定了炎症中与肿瘤发生相关的主要内源性因素，如信号转导与转录激活因子 3（STAT-3）、转录因子 NF-κB。这些转录激活因子在信号转导和/或炎症性细胞因子表达中起实质性作用。产生的肿瘤相关性炎症因子如 TNF-α、IL-6、IL-1β、IL-11 和 IL-23（Grivennikov et al. 2009；Fukuda et al. 2011；Lesina et al. 2011；Voronov et al. 2003；Langowski et al. 2006）。NF-κB 被广泛认为是先天免疫和炎症反应过程中的核心调节者，在肿瘤细胞和与炎症相关的免疫细胞中被活化。NF-κB 将整套外部和内部的危险信号表达成特定的基因活化。NF-κB 处于 Toll 样受体（TLR）-MyD88 依赖途径的下游，处理来自于炎症细胞因子（如 TNF-α 和 IL-1β）受体的信号。另外，癌细胞中的内源性遗传学改变可以使 NF-κB 上调。在上游信号中，NF-κB 可激活促炎因子的表达，如细胞因子、黏附分子、NO 合成酶、血管生成刺激因子，以及 COX2（前列腺素合成中的一种核心酶）。NF-κB 和 STAT3 通过凋亡抑制因子（如 Bcl-2、Bcl-XL、Mcl-1、c-Flip、生存素和 IAP）的表达促进细胞存活，从而抵抗肿瘤监视中的抗肿瘤免疫反应。另外，针对 NF-κB 活化和低氧反应之间的关系也有研究（Rius et al. 2008）。NF-κB 和 STAT3 还会干扰 p53 在基因组监测、DNA 损伤反应和内源性凋亡等方面的功能（Colotta et al. 2009；Ryan et al. 2000）。

2.3 炎症过程中的肿瘤微环境

被免疫系统招募到肿瘤微环境中的大多数细胞是肿瘤相关性巨噬细胞（TAM）。这种细胞类型代表单核巨噬细胞系中的一个亚类，在肿瘤侵袭、转移和血管生成过程中可能是必要的（Condeelis and Pollard 2006）。由于这些细胞的可塑性和多样性，这里只区分两种基本的表型。经典的 M1 活化由 TLR 配体和 IFN-γ 介导，而 M2 活化由 IL-4/IL-13 刺激。M1-M2 的极化反映了 Th1-Th2 T 细胞的极化。M1 巨噬细胞促进 Th1 反应并释放高浓度的促炎细胞因子、活性氧类和活性氮中间体，而 M2 极化的巨噬细胞表现免疫调节功能，促进组织重塑，呈现"清道夫"受体的高表达（Gordon and Martinez 2010；Biswas and Mantovani 2010；Mantovani et al. 2002）。在晚期肿瘤生长过程中发现的 TAM 通常显现类似 M2 的表型，其特点是促肿瘤活动相关的组织重塑、血管生成及 IL-10 的高表达。上述巨噬细胞被不同来源的淋巴细胞所极化。对于在不同器官发生的肿瘤，其淋巴细胞有所不同（Biswas and Mantovani 2010）。在乳腺癌发生过程中，浆细胞促进 TAM 极化（DeNardo et al. 2009；Pedroza-Gonzalez et al. 2011），而在皮肤癌发生过程中，分泌 IL-4 的 Th2 细胞诱导类似 M2 的表型（Schioppa et al. 2011；Andreu et al. 2010）。另外，通过分泌不同的成分，肿瘤细胞能够直接影响巨噬细胞进入促肿瘤模式。这些成分包括细胞外间质、细胞因子 M-CSF 和 IL-10，以及如 CCL2、CCl17、CCL18 和 CXCL4 这样的趋化因子（Mantovani et al. 2008；Erler et al. 2009；Kim et al. 2009；Roca et al. 2009）。有研究表明，高度 TAM 浸润与不良预后相关（Murdoch et al. 2008）。

除了 TAM 扮演的中心角色之外，肿瘤微环境中还发现了其他几种先天和获得性免疫细胞，这些细胞几乎都呈现促癌作用。这些细胞包括 T 细胞、B 细胞、树突状细胞、肥大细胞、髓源性抑制细胞和中性粒细胞。目前只知道 NK 细胞缺乏支持肿瘤生长的功能。实体瘤中出现的成熟 T 细胞归类于细胞毒性 CD8 T 细胞（CTL）和 CD4 辅助细胞（Th）。后者进一步划分成 Th1、Th2、Th17 和调节性 T 细胞（Treg）。这些细胞的极化决定了 T 细胞亚类（包括 CD8 T 细胞）是否会促进肿瘤的生长和转移（Roberts et al. 2007）。另外，极化在一些肿瘤中与存活率相关，这归因于与肿瘤特异性的 CTL 和 Th1 细胞的入侵，如在黑色素瘤、胰腺癌、结肠癌和多发性骨髓瘤中显示的那样（Galon et al. 2006；Laghi et al. 2009；Swann and Smyth 2007）。而且，乳腺癌中出现肿瘤浸润淋巴细胞（TIL）、高浓度 CD8/CD4 和 Th1/Th2，表明预后得以改善（Kohrt et al. 2005）。Treg 细胞通过抑制抗肿瘤免疫反应，被认为主要作用是调节肿瘤耐受性（Gallimore and Simon 2008）。但是，Erdman 和他的同事们揭示了 Treg 也可以抑制肿瘤相关的炎症，从而在恶性肿瘤中起抗肿瘤生成的作用（Erdman et al. 2005）。髓源性抑制细胞

（MDSC）通常被炎症-肿瘤微环境通过多种因子（如 IL-6、IL-1β 和 VEGF）招募和激活（Gabrilovich and Nagaraj 2009）。活化的 MDSC 进而释放促炎因子，这样形成了一个正反馈回路，促进肿瘤相关性炎症的发生。MDSC 不仅能抑制获得性免疫反应，而且能影响巨噬细胞的细胞因子的生产（Sinha et al. 2007）。肿瘤相关性中性粒细胞（TAN）已经被认为在肿瘤相关的炎症中起一定的作用（Cassatella et al. 2009；Mantovani 2009）。根据 TGF-β 极化情况的不同，这些细胞以前未被注意到的可塑性能够发挥肿瘤促进或溶瘤作用（Fridlender et al. 2009）。

肿瘤相关成纤维细胞（CAF）是肿瘤基质的一个主要成分，也是肿瘤相关性炎症环境中的一个组成部分。它们激活 IL-1，与伤口愈合过程中的活化成纤维细胞有许多共同点。CAF 具有促炎特征，可以促进肿瘤生长和血管生成（Erez et al. 2010）。

在肿瘤形成过程中，恶性细胞经常通过与免疫细胞相互作用，导致后者被极化成支持肿瘤的表型。肿瘤微环境在很大程度上是由这些促肿瘤免疫细胞的反馈产生的，最终通过肿瘤微环境中的浸润淋巴细胞的适应性和操控作用，调节其耐受性。

在肿瘤生长过程中，大多数先天性和获得性免疫细胞的作用都或多或少地表现出显著的可塑性，在某些条件下甚至可以被逆转（Sharma et al. 2010；Fridlender et al. 2009）。因此，可以假定，肿瘤相关性炎症和抗肿瘤免疫可以并存，从而在肿瘤生长过程中相互影响。但是，逐步增长的肿瘤最终会击败抗肿瘤免疫作用，进而在后期的肿瘤发展阶段获得完全的免疫逃逸（Koebel et al. 2007）。

2.4 肿瘤生长过程中的炎症、缺氧和血管生成

缺氧状况通常出现在实体恶性肿瘤中，当生长的肿瘤对氧气和营养的需求超过血液能够供应的数量时就会出现这种情况。首先，细胞响应产生缺氧诱导因子（HIF1α），后者会改变葡萄糖代谢、血管生成，进一步导致细胞存活和侵袭（Staller et al. 2003）。缺氧状况还会引起肿瘤中心的坏死性细胞死亡。这些走向死亡的细胞能诱导促炎介质 IL-1 和 HMGB1 的产生，进而触发血管生成并给肿瘤内环境提供更多的生长因子（Vakkila and Lotze 2004）。但是，除了缺氧之外，肿瘤血管形成会受到肿瘤相关巨噬细胞（TAM）驱动，TAM 能识别缺氧条件，然后通过释放血管生成素 2 和 VEGF 发生反应。需要注意的是，TAM 和其他细胞类型中的促血管生成基因是通过 AP1、STAT3 和 NF-κB 途径调节的（Kujawski et al. 2008；Rius et al. 2008）。目前还不清楚缺氧是否诱导血管形成，或者受缺氧活化的炎症介质是否是导致血管生成的关键驱动因素。

2.5 慢性病毒感染和恶性肿瘤中的 T 细胞耗竭

CD8 T 细胞在抗肿瘤免疫反应方面起重要作用。成熟的细胞毒性 T 细胞能够侵入受感染组织或肿瘤组织，并以抗原特异性方式直接溶解靶细胞。特异性是由 αβ T 细胞受体介导的，该受体能识别变异、过度表达的自身抗原或病毒源性抗原，这些病毒源性抗原提呈在假想的靶细胞表面的主要组织相容性复合物（MHC）分子上。低级抗原特异性 CD8 T 细胞在急性病毒感染之后会大量繁殖。首先，它们被高级抗原提呈细胞（APC）活化，抗原提呈细胞诸如树突状细胞（DC），会交叉提呈俘获的病毒多肽并提供共刺激的必要信号。在初始抗原刺激之后，低级病毒特异性 T 细胞会伴随着效应子功能的获得、趋化因子的产生，以及能迁移到感染部位的能力。病原体特异性 CD8 T 细胞的大量扩增通常有助于清除病毒，当达到克隆扩增的顶峰之后，病毒特定的 T 细胞数量会快速缩减，这时大多数 T 细胞面临凋亡。这类细胞中有一小部分能存活下来，并建立长久记忆性 CD8 T 细胞库，根据表型标志物（CD62L 和 CCR7）的不同，后者进一步细分为效应记忆性（EM）T 细胞和中心记忆性（CM）T 细胞。在接受刺激试验时，记忆细胞会快速繁殖并实施效应子功能，从而提供保护性免疫。

与急性感染后保护性 CD8 T 细胞免疫功能形成对比的是，慢性感染和肿瘤中的 CD8 T 细胞的行为截然不同。在慢性疾病早期，低级病原体或疾病特异性 T 细胞处于致敏状态，并从开始即获得效应子功能。但是，它们通常不能分化成功能性记忆细胞，效应子功能会逐步丧失。这种功能丧失也叫做 T 细胞耗竭。这个过程遵循层次结构顺序，耗竭的 T 细胞阻碍 IL-2 生成和增殖，然后获得不适当的溶细胞功能，合成更少的 TNF。最后，完全耗竭的 T 细胞甚至会丧失分泌 IFN-γ 的能力（Zajac et al. 1998；Fuller and Zajac 2003；Wherry et al. 2003）。

在耗竭过程中，CD8 T 细胞会持续性上调抑制性受体，如 PD-1、Tim-3、LAG3、CD160 和 2B4（Barber et al. 2006；Blackburn et al. 2009；Fourcade et al. 2010）。通常情况下，T 细胞耗竭的必然性可以用如下方式解释，即针对病毒抗原的免疫系统的炎症反应的调整，这样一方面可以限制病毒复制，另一方面，如果宿主不能完全清除病毒的话，可以避免长期感染组织中因炎症引起的持久性组织损伤。

恶性肿瘤疾病中的 CD8 T 细胞反应直接靶向肿瘤表达的抗原，这在黑色素瘤患者中常见（Boon et al. 2006）。自发性产生的肿瘤特异性免疫反应及进一步发展中的疾病二者并存，这也表明 T 细胞中存在肿瘤诱导的功能障碍。在肿瘤患者中，肿瘤特异性 T 细胞的诱导不会遵循与急性病毒感染一致的机制。肿瘤耐受性机制主动干扰抗肿瘤免疫反应，在肿瘤细胞中，肿瘤抗原进一步失去病原相关性分子伴侣（PAMP）。这会导致细胞毒性 T 细胞的不完全活化和效应许可。此外，主要抗原攻击和炎症耐受性介导下的肿瘤环境进一步导致耗竭 T 细胞的功能丧失

（Fourcade et al. 2010；Baitsch et al. 2011）。

在患者中发现的肿瘤相关性抗原（TAA）通常是肿瘤胚系抗原（CGA），它是通过不同来源的肿瘤细胞表达的，而不是通过非肿瘤细胞所表达（睾丸组织细胞除外）。CGA NY-ESO-1 通常遭受自发的细胞和体液反应攻击，这在晚期 NY-ESO-1 表达的肿瘤患者中可以检测到（Stockert et al. 1998；Mandic et al. 2005；Fourcade et al. 2008）。近期关于自发肿瘤抗原特异性 CD8 T 细胞的研究揭示了老鼠和黑色素瘤患者中 PD-1 和 Tim-3 的上调现象（Fourcade et al. 2010；Sakuishi et al. 2010；Baitsch et al. 2011）。这两种负向调节或免疫监视分子在肿瘤疾病中是非常重要的 T 细胞耗竭标志物。PD-1 阻止 T 细胞受体信号传递，Tim-3 在促使 MDSC 产生和调节髓细胞来源的细胞因子反应方面起作用（Dardalhon et al. 2010；Zhang et al. 2012）。

除此之外，PD-1 还能控制 NY-ESO-1 特异性 CD8 T 细胞的扩增。与患者中的单阳性 CD8 T 细胞相比，PD-1/Tim-3 双阳性细胞能产生少量的 IFN-γ、IL-2 和 TNF，从而具有更易耗竭的表型（Fourcade et al. 2010）。在动物模型中，通过阻断 PD-1 和 Tim-3，可以部分恢复 T 细胞功能，而且组合的靶向 Tim-3 和 PD-1 途径比单一途径在抑制肿瘤生长方面更有效（Sakuishi et al. 2010）。

有趣的是，在使用 CpG 和 Melan-A/MART-1 接种后的黑色素瘤患者体内，发现 TAA 特异性 CD8 细胞及其效应子共存于循环系统中，耗竭的 T 细胞则出现在转移肿瘤环境中（Baitsch et al. 2011）。

3 炎症与转移

转移在临床肿瘤学中是非常重要的一个方面，因为超过 90%的肿瘤死亡病例归因于转移。转移的发生是很复杂的过程，包括肿瘤细胞的运动性产生、内渗到循环系统、通过血液或淋巴系统扩散和外渗，最终植入新的组织和器官中并增生肿瘤结节。进入循环系统中的肿瘤细胞大约只有 0.01%会成功发生微转移（Joyce and Pollard 2009）。早期转移的肿瘤细胞增加的运动性和侵袭力是由于上皮-间质转化（EMT）造成的。在 EMT 过程中，上皮细胞获得类似成纤维细胞的属性，从而增加其运动性，并有助于侵入上皮屏障和穿越基底膜进入循环系统（Kalluri and Weinberg 2009）。前期转移细胞的外渗是通过整合素介导的，接着与免疫和基质细胞之间产生对话（crosstalk），进而允许细胞的增殖（Polyak and Weinberg 2009）。有研究显示，白细胞能够为转移前龛的形成做准备（Erler et al. 2009；Hiratsuka et al. 2006；Kaplan et al. 2006；Kaplan et al. 2005；Padua et al. 2008），炎症刺激进一步受细胞外基质成分的多能蛋白聚糖介导，活化巨噬细胞并致其分泌促转移细胞因子 TNF-α（Kim et al. 2009）。另一种促转移和抗炎细胞因子是

TGF-β。它通过诱导血管生成素 4 来介导跨内皮细胞迁移和肿瘤转移,该细胞因子可由肿瘤细胞、髓系细胞和 T 淋巴细胞分泌。TGF-β 水平的增加通常指示预后不良(Yang and Weinberg 2008)。

4 炎症相关性肿瘤的预防

治疗与慢性病毒感染相关的肿瘤,可以在肿瘤生长过程的不同阶段进行干预处理(可行的方法总结在图 3-1 中)。首先,有效的疫苗是根本性的需求,这不仅可以预防急性感染相关的疾病,而且,由于肿瘤是病毒感染导致的后期并发症,因此也可以最终预防肿瘤的产生。如果患者在一生中曾经受到病毒感染,并且这种病毒会造成高致癌风险的话,他/她必须定期接受监测以防发生慢性变化。需要前沿的药物学治疗方法尽可能减少慢性感染患者体内的病毒量,或者最好能治愈感染。慢性感染患者还需要接受仔细检查,排除受影响组织部位是否有肿瘤发生

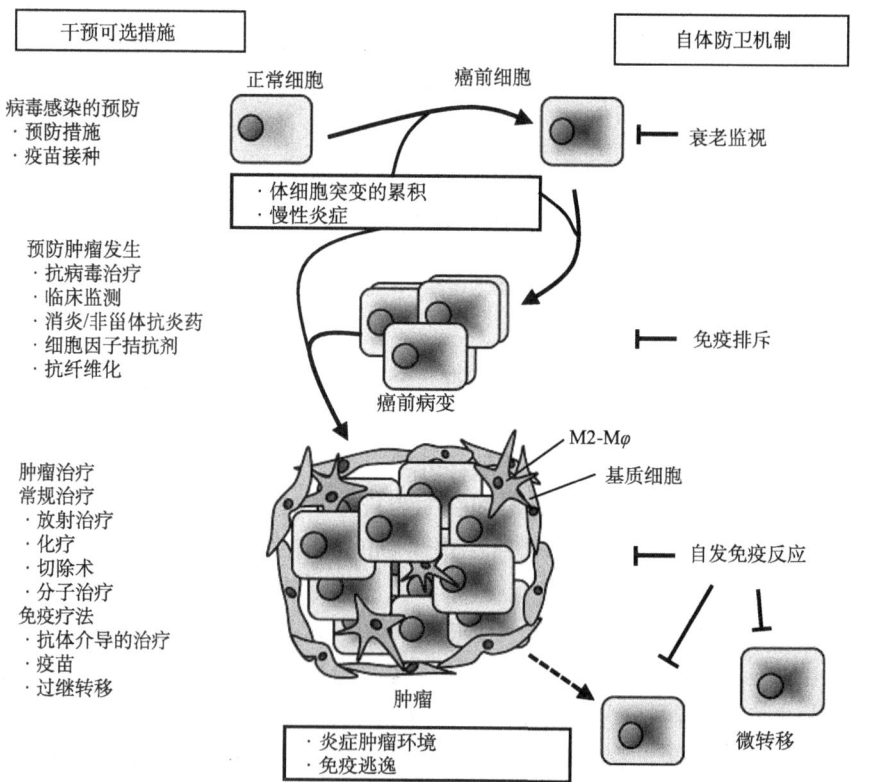

图 3-1 炎症相关性肿瘤的多阶段发生过程和对应的免疫防御机制及其适应的预防与干预措施。

前的损伤现象。在这种情况下，应该考虑使用治疗干预手段来抑制，甚至是逆转组织的结构，特别是对那些具有肿瘤遗传倾向的个体。由于慢性炎症会促使肿瘤生成和扩散，长期使用消炎剂的治疗方案对受感染患者是一个合理的预防肿瘤的选择。关于以上提到的预防病毒介导的肿瘤的选择方案，其具体处理方法将在下文讨论。

4.1 抗病毒疫苗和治疗

在与慢性病毒感染相关性炎症有关的实体瘤中，HBV、HCV 和 HPV 感染是其中大多数肿瘤的病因。

预防 HBV 相关性 HCC 的方案是阻止高风险人群中所发生的慢性 HBV 感染，这个人群包括如通过静脉注射的吸毒成瘾者或接受输血的个体。事实上，抵抗 HBV 的有效疫苗在二十多年前就已经存在了。给其母亲受到 HBV 感染的孩子实施"接触后预防"也是预防措施之一，儿童时期接受被动免疫等的免疫项目已经大大降低了 HBV 携带者数量，从而减少 HCC 发生（Chang et al. 1997）。HBV 疫苗作为国家婴儿免疫计划的一部分，在 162 个国家中开展实施，这是肿瘤预防疫苗的第一个例子。但是，针对 HBV 相关性 HCC 以阻止患者死亡的疫苗接种项目，其实际临床效果需要几十年后才能体现出来（Zanetti et al. 2008）。另外，定期对献血者做 HBsAg（乙型肝炎病毒表面抗原）筛查，有助于降低因输血传播 HBV 的可能性（Schreiber et al. 1996）。至于已经是慢性感染 HBV 的众多患者，HBV 疫苗并不能有效预防 HCC。这种情况下，控制 HBV 病毒血症是主要的治疗目标，目的是减少肝脏炎症及防止病症向肝硬化和 HCC 方向发展。如果对慢性 HBV 携带者的肝脏组织学诊断结果表明需要进行干预治疗，可以使用干扰素-α 和/或核苷类似物控制体内的病毒量，有利于避免 HCC 发生。但是，对核苷类似物的耐药性仍是一个问题（Colombo and Donato 2005）。

不幸的是，尚没有针对 HCV 的功能性疫苗用来预防 HCV 相关性 HCC。只有几种候选疫苗开始进入 I/II 期临床试验阶段，但是还不确定这些候选疫苗能否最终应用到临床中（Torresi et al. 2011）。尽管有效的疫苗接种策略还需要继续研究，但是在治疗急性和慢性 HCV 感染方面已经取得了显著的进展。目前的医学治疗方案是使用基于聚乙二醇化干扰素 IFN-α 和利巴韦林，大约 50%的患者可以治愈。近期研制的"病毒直接作用制剂"（DAA），如 NS3/4A 蛋白酶抑制剂或亲环素 B 抑制剂，有望通过取得持续性病毒学反应而进一步治疗 HCV 感染（Patel and Heathcote 2011；Kronenberger and Zeuzem 2012；McHutchison et al. 2009）。

就 HPV 而言，有效疫苗的出现，使得在全球预防宫颈癌方面取得了里程碑式的进展。从空病毒衣壳（病毒样颗粒）提取的二价和四价疫苗能有效预防高风险 HPV 基因型 16 和 18 的感染，而后者能导致发生 70%的宫颈癌病例（Garland et al.

2007；Paavonen et al. 2007）。也有报道表明，这种疫苗在一定程度上还可以预防其他与 16/18 相关的基因型（Joura et al. 2007）。

4.2 抗纤维化治疗

暂时的纤维化和晚期逆转性的纤维瘢痕化是伤口愈合的一个重要特征。在肝脏慢性组织损伤情况下产生的永久性纤维化及其导致的致命后果这方面，尽管人们还没完全弄清楚，但已经有广泛的研究成果。在肝组织纤维化重组的晚期阶段发生的肝硬化常常是慢性 HBV 或 HCV 感染产生的并发症。肝硬化与以下情况有关：门静脉血压过高、减弱的肝脏功能、发生 HCC 的风险高。来源于肝星状细胞（HSC）的非均质促肝纤维化肌成纤维细胞（MFB）群被认为能够调节肝脏的纤维化作用（Lee and Friedman 2011）。在肝脏受到损伤和发生炎症后，导致发生纤维化的一个主要事件是沉寂的 HSC 被活化，这个过程可由相邻肝细胞的旁分泌刺激、Kupffer 细胞和肝窦内皮细胞（LSEC）触发如下几个因素，包括活化氧类、TLR4 配体、凋亡小体的吸收。永久性的 MFB 纤维化基因型主要来源于特定的微环境，其中，促肝纤维化细胞因子和生长因子（如 TGF-β 和 PDGF）占主要成分。活化的胆管细胞被确定是这些促肝纤维化介质的重要来源。活化的 MFB 的表型标志物有：α 平滑肌肌动蛋白（SMA）的表达、胶原蛋白的高表达、增强的繁殖能力和可使组织硬化的脂质含量增加。就特异性基因调节而言，研究表明血管收缩素 2 可活化转录因子 NF-κB，从而使 MFB 在诱导凋亡和促使细胞成活方面降低敏感性（Oakley et al. 2009）。最近的数据表明，在老鼠肝细胞中活化 NF-κB 信号通路会诱导肝脏纤维化（Sunami et al. 2012）。细胞外基质（ECM）的累积是导致纤维化发生的另一个特征，ECM 累积可引起组织硬化。ECM 的主要调节者是基质金属蛋白酶类（MMP），后者是负责基质降解和伤疤组织清除的酶。ECM 的净产量是由于 MMP 表达失衡及其特异性抑制剂（金属蛋白酶类组织抑制剂或 TIMP）的分泌造成的。在生理性再生和肝损伤修复过程中，存在一定的机制，使得一旦启动原因得到控制，即可调节纤维瘢痕组织的消退。在这个过程中，由于表型逆转、衰老和被自然杀伤细胞清除，MFB 最终从肝脏受害部位消失。据此，纤维化组织通过增强的 MMP 活动和降低的 TIMP 浓度被清除掉。研究表明，肝巨噬细胞在这个调节和瘢痕组织重塑的过程中具有一定的作用。

抗纤维化治疗的理想方法包括清除潜在的疾病触发因素。在慢性 HBV 或 HCV 感染中，清除病毒会造成纤维化消退，甚至能增加肝硬化患者的肝脏功能。对于那些不能对抗病毒治疗产生有效反应的患者而言，特异性抗纤维化治疗需要尽快实施，以降低发生纤维化的速度，并且降低晚期并发症和 HCC 的发生。具有发生纤维化高风险的患者应该接受有针对性的筛查。例如，基因中具有特异性多态性的"七个基因标志物"与纤维化发生高风险有关；TGF-β、TNF-α 或 IL-10

在慢性 HCV 患者肝脏纤维化发生评估中具有显著的价值（肝硬化风险数值）（Huang et al. 2007）。随后对这些患者需要纤维化进展的监测。未来，像超声诊断仪（通过超声描记术评估肝脏的硬度）这样的无创方法会成为替代肝脏组织活检的疗法。与血清学标志物（如甲胎蛋白）结合的话，可以在可能治愈的早期阶段检测到 HCC（Mok et al. 2005）。至于抗纤维化治疗，凡是能引起纤维化发生或消退的所有分子因素或者机制都可以考虑成为合适的靶点（Fallowfield 2011）。由于炎症和氧化应激产生的肝脏损伤可以用所谓的保肝药来治疗，部分药物的肝脏保护功能可以归结为它们能够抑制 NF-κB 的炎症活化功能。有很多天然药物可以长期大量地服用，这些药物具有抗氧化和保肝效果，如白藜芦醇（来自红葡萄酒）、水飞蓟素（来自乳蓟）、咖啡和维生素 E。

肝细胞生长因子（HGF）被认为能够刺激肝细胞的生成，在动物模型实验中显示能有效抑制纤维化（Xia et al. 2006）。但是，由于 HGF 是肝细胞的强力分裂素，因此还应考虑其存在潜在的致瘤风险。一个进一步的潜在目标是在肝脏炎症发生过程中减少凋亡细胞的失误。肝细胞的凋亡会直接或通过 Kupffer 细胞活化 HSC。在动物模型中，泛硫胱胺酸蛋白酶抑制剂 VX-166 显示具有抗纤维化功能（Witek et al. 2009）。相比而言，如果可以在活化的 HSC 中选择性诱导细胞死亡的话，促使细胞凋亡的策略也是另一种选择。为达到此目的，使用促凋亡的 IkB 抑制剂胶霉素与抗突触小泡蛋白的单链抗体结合。突触小泡蛋白能在细胞上选择性表达。这个方法在 CCl₄ 老鼠中毒模型中能降低纤维化（Douglass et al. 2008）。作为对活化 HSC 诱导凋亡的另一个策略，干扰大麻素受体信号在动物纤维化模型中显示具有良好的效果（Teixeira-Clerc et al. 2006），但是在临床试验中显示出引起幻觉的副作用。其他防止 HSC 活化的策略在实验模型中已经显示出抗纤维化活性，但需要在临床试验中得到确认，这些策略包括过氧化物酶体增殖物-活化剂受体-γ 的配体（"格列酮类"）、法尼酯衍生物 X 受体激动剂、HMG-CoA 还原酶抑制剂（"他汀类药物"）。血管紧张素系统抑制剂即将在临床中得到应用。血管紧张素转换酶抑制剂和血管紧张素 1 受体拮抗剂（"沙坦类药物"）在动物中可以抑制纤维化。重要的是，AT1R 拮抗剂氯沙坦对于慢性 HCV 患者可以降低纤维化进程。将来的进一步策略是靶向 TGF-β 途径。对中和抗体、诱饵受体和 siRNA 都有过研究，但是还不能应用到临床。吡非尼酮作为一种抑制 TFG-β 生成的制剂，在非受控性预试验研究中显示出良好的前景（Armendariz-Borunda et al. 2006）。αvβ6 整合素在局部微环境中能活化无活性的、与基质相连的 TFG-β。这种策略的诱人之处在于，对整合素的特异性抑制作用可以避免因产生系统性 TGF-β 抑制带来的副作用。在胆源性和非胆源性纤维化模型中，抵抗 αvβ6 整合素的中和抗体会抑制胆管上皮细胞活化和胶原沉积（Popov et al. 2008）。刺激 MMP 的溶胶原活性的制剂，如口服生物碱卤夫酮，在动物模型中显示结果良好，但在临床患者仍需要进一步研究。值得注意的是，目前临床中取得的成功和动物实验模型中的抗纤维化效果并不具相关性，这表明现有的动物纤维化模型并不能完全反映对 ECM 成熟过程的影响（Rockey 2008）。ECM 成熟是通过纤维化过程中的交联和潜在的"无回头路"实现的。然而，功能性抗纤维化治疗仍是迫切需要的，并且其临床应用已显现初步成效。

4.3 抗炎治疗

由于慢性炎症导致肿瘤生成和扩散，因此一旦受感染患者被诊断发生病毒介导的组织损伤，消炎药应该是一种有效的预防措施。促进肿瘤相关的炎症过程的几个因素已经被确定，因此，这些因素也是预防高风险患者发生肿瘤的合理的分子靶点。有几种消炎药，如果用作预防用药，已经显示可以降低肿瘤的发生概率；如果作为治疗用药，可以减弱肿瘤生长速度并提高生存率，这在结直肠癌中有研究（Gupta and DuBois 2001）。首先，经典的非甾体类抗炎药（NSAID），如阿司匹林，就不愧为预防用药的一个较好的选择（Cuzick et al. 2009；Langley et al. 2011）。NSAID 价格低廉、无专利权、应用已久，并且长期的临床实践表明其可以低剂量预防血栓。研究显示，预防性阿司匹林治疗方法可以显著降低发生结直肠癌的风险（Flossmann and Rothwell 2007；Rothwell et al. 2010）。一项大规模的荟萃分析显示，在几种主要的胃肠道实体肿瘤中可以降低发生癌症的风险，如在胃癌、食道癌、结肠直肠癌和胰腺癌中；此外还有肺癌（Rothwell et al. 2011）。其带来的益处与服用阿司匹林的时间长久和个体的年龄增长有相关性。值得注意的是，阿司匹林对治疗血液恶性肿瘤并没有带来益处，这与以下的假设是一致的，即抗炎治疗主要针对实体瘤慢性炎症微环境起作用。出于风险和效益的平衡考虑，Rothwell 研究结果表明，一方面，阿司匹林具有引起胃肠道出血的风险（包括致命性的出血）；另一方面，在每日服用阿司匹林 5~10 年后，由于各种原因造成的死亡率要减少 10%，这二者中后者要胜过前者。需要指出的是，这些研究中的患者并没有被区分对待，即没有考虑他们是否真正罹患炎症疾病。有研究显示，阿司匹林可以降低前列腺癌的发生风险，但只是在携带淋巴毒素 α 基因的一个特殊的多态等位基因（该基因可以导致增强的淋巴毒素表达）的患者中有效（Liu et al. 2006）。该观察报告说明，肿瘤高风险患者需要尽早接受基因筛查和/或监测炎症参数，这样有可能从抗炎治疗中获得最佳效益。为了减少长期治疗中产生的胃肠道并发症，选择性 COX-2 抑制剂可以作为预防性肿瘤治疗的另一个方法（Kawamori et al. 1998；Reddy et al. 2000）。在研究由遗传导致或致癌物质诱发的结肠癌、肠道癌、皮肤癌和膀胱癌的几个临床前期模型中，已经发现塞来昔布（celecoxib）可显著降低肿瘤发生概率（Fischer et al. 2011）。针对人类患者的研究显示，塞来昔布在预防自发性结直肠腺瘤方面也具有一定的应用前景，它可以减少家族性腺瘤息肉病中的息肉数量（Bertagnolli et al. 2006；Arber et al. 2006；Steinbach et al. 2000）。但需要注意的是，塞来昔布与发生不良心血管事件有一定的关联（Mukherjee et al. 2001）。

针对炎症发生过程中细胞因子或趋化因子信号中的特异性分子靶点的药物也是具有前景的。其中大多数制剂已经用于治疗慢性炎症疾病，如类风湿性关节炎、牛皮癣或炎性肠道疾病（IBD），或者尚处于治疗肿瘤的临床开发阶段。目前还不清楚这些制剂是否适合于长期治疗。有一种沙利度胺的结构类似物叫来那度胺，可以用来抑制几种炎症相关的细胞因子的产生，与地塞米松联合使用还可以有效治疗黑色素瘤（Weber et al. 2007）。

如前所述，NF-κB 和 STAT3 信号途径在肿瘤生成及抵抗治疗方面起关键作用，这表明靶向抑制剂在预防或治疗方面会有一定的潜力。但是，长期药理学抑制 NF-κB 会引起 IL-1β 浓度的增加，从而导致严重的免疫缺陷、中性粒细胞增多症和严重的急性炎症（Greten et al. 2007）。另一种比较有潜力的做法是，可以处理 NF-κB 的确定性上游靶标，这是因为多条外在和内在途径汇合到一起会激活该中央转录因子。已经研制出针对 STAT3 和 JAK2（在 STAT3 上游）的抑制剂，并在老鼠异体移植模型中显现出其在实体瘤内具有抑瘤活性（Hedvat et al. 2009）。处理 IL-6、IL-6 受体、CCR2、CCR4 和 CXCR4 的受体拮抗剂和封闭性抗体也正在临床开发中，有望用于治疗几种肿瘤。TNFα-抗体，如英夫利昔，对治疗 IBD 的效果具有突破性，更重要的是长期使用安全性好（Fidder et al. 2009）。第一批针对晚期癌症患者的 TNF-α 拮抗剂的临床研究结果显示，它具有稳定病情或部分反应的效果（Brown et al. 2008；Harrison et al. 2007）。进一步研究显示，英夫利昔在老鼠中可以减少结肠炎相关性肿瘤的发生（Kim et al. 2010），这表明对患者有预防肿瘤的益处。另外，TNF-α 参与清除病毒感染的过程（Trevejo et al. 2001），研究显示，它在动物体内对于诱导抗肿瘤的 T 细胞反应起至关重要的作用（Calzascia et al. 2007）。鉴于 TNF-α 生物学机制比较复杂而且有时有自相矛盾的结果，目前还难以评估 TNF-α 拮抗剂对于病毒介导炎症造成的肿瘤是否有较好的预防作用。从临床角度看，与原位瘤相比，转移瘤是恶性化疾病更具挑战性的形式。由于炎症是扩散的主要驱动力，应用抗炎药对防止发生转移应该是一种有效的干预措施。最近发现，原本开发用于治疗骨质疏松症的抗 RANKL 抗体狄诺塞麦，在前列腺和乳腺癌的晚期临床研究中可以延缓骨转移的发生（Stopeck et al. 2010；Smith et al. 2012）。通过抑制 TNF-α 来预防肿瘤转移也有一定的前景，因为小鼠试验显示，封闭 TNF-α 可以使炎症造成的肿瘤转移转变为 TRAIL 介导的肿瘤消退（Luo et al. 2004）。总之，这些例子表明，涉及肿瘤和扩散相关炎症的分子机制及信号途径是预防和治疗干预措施中的有效靶标。

5 展望：肿瘤免疫治疗的前景

无论是在肿瘤的预防还是治疗方面，抗癌免疫应答都正在成为焦点。抗癌免疫应答甚至可以由常见的化学治疗触发，同时也可能大大促进治疗结果（Casares et al. 2005；Apetoh et al. 2008）。我们目前所知的关于免疫应答的肿瘤免疫治疗方案主要有两种。一种方案是促进或恢复先天的、已经存在的适应性免疫应答，另一种则是通过治疗剂的干预而激活适应性的免疫应答。由于肿瘤已经可通过各种方式来逃避免疫攻击，这两种方式几乎是具有同样的挑战性。尽管我们已经能够阐释其中的根本作用机制并且已掌握许多治疗方法，我们仍然不能保证在个别情况下某一疗法不会被肿瘤的免疫抑制机制攻破。因此，理想的免疫治疗方案应着眼于肿瘤的致命要害并且能同时适用于所有实体瘤。

最近，在慢性炎症的肿瘤微环境对肿瘤维持和发展方面的重要性的发现已经引导我们通过使用抗炎药物来治疗癌症，而这种方法的基本优点在于它能使免疫细胞不易于产生抗药性。然而，这种抗炎治疗很有可能不能在癌细胞上体现足够的细胞毒性的效果，从而必须要配合以额外的治疗来体现有效的疗效。正如之前已经提到的，一些阶段 I、II 期的临床实验调查了抗 IL6 和抗 TNF-α 药物对多种癌症的功效（Balkwill 2009）。

在各种适应性免疫应答中，能直接介导转化细胞溶解的细胞毒性 T 细胞被广泛认为是癌症免疫治疗的最佳细胞种类。然而，肿瘤特异性的 CD8 T 细胞的有效应答却很难在带瘤宿主身上被感应到。像腺苷、前列腺素 E2、VEGF-A 和 TGF-β 这些旁分泌介质直接或间接地调节着抑制免疫力的活动，并且能作用于不同水平的免疫系统。研究表明，免疫抑制性的活动会由于 T 细胞的衰竭而引起迟钝、无意识的适应性应答(Fourcade et al. 2010；Sakuishi et al. 2010；Baitsch et al. 2011）；或者作用于树突状细胞（DC 细胞），通过抑制共刺激信号来引起缺陷的形成，从而使其无法为肿瘤靶向的 CD8 T 细胞应答做准备。因此，要想谨慎地设计出一种能引起有效的肿瘤靶向 CD8 T 细胞应答的疫苗，就必须要想到一种能阻止肿瘤反抗行为的策略。在黑色素瘤小鼠模型中，通过使用 1-甲基色氨酸阻断 IDO（吲哚胺-2,3-双氧化酶）介导的免疫抑制作用，借以保护 TDLN 中的 DC 细胞功能，从而诱导对 CD8 T 细胞疫苗的强效细胞毒性作用（Sharma et al. 2010）。另一个避免肿瘤介质免疫应答的途径是通过肿瘤结节里的裂解病毒实现的感染来调节，这种感染能破坏肿瘤结构并造成一种伴随有白细胞渗透和大量肿瘤细胞死亡的炎症。当肿瘤靶向的 DC 疫苗使用在病毒介导的炎症的这一时间点时，将触发强烈的细胞毒性 CD8 T 细胞应答，而在其他时间点接种疫苗并结合病毒治疗并没有显著的疗效。有趣的是，与真正的病毒感染相比，通过 Toll 样受体配体介导的炎症将无法促进由接种 DC 疫苗引发的有效的 CD8 T 细胞的感应,而这可能主要与被肿瘤感染的树突状细胞缺少肿瘤特异性抗原交叉提呈有关(Woller et al. 2011)。

近年来有关免疫治疗策略的临床转化实验为建立一个癌症治疗的新领域提供了希望,而这个新领域也可能同样需要与传统的治疗方式相结合。一个关于表达粒性白细胞集落刺激因子(GM-CSF)和 TK(胸苷激酶)缺陷痘病毒的临床实验在肝细胞肿瘤上发现了明显的反应,这些结果给予了我们希望(Breitbach et al. 2011;Park et al. 2008)。在一次临床实验阶段 I、II 期中,不同来源的晚期实体瘤患者获得了抗 PD-1 的抗体来逆转耗竭的 T 细胞,有些可观察到的反应可以持续一年以上。然而,只有在肿瘤组织中有 PD-L1 阳性染色的患者身上才会有对于阻塞 PD-1 抗体治疗的客观反应(Topalian et al. 2012)。

这些实验以及许多其他的实验都阐明了癌症免疫治疗新奇的干预能力和治疗的可能性,而它们都是以所积累的关于免疫系统、癌症生物学及二者相互作用的知识为基础的。这些特殊的重新指向肿瘤的免疫反应感应现象,似乎为恶性疾病的治疗打开了一扇振奋人心的大门。此外,仍有许多奥秘等待我们去探索,而从目前的实验方法到明确的治疗方案也仍有漫漫长路等待着我们。

(卢建红,周诠 译)

参 考 文 献

Aggarwal BB, Vijayalekshmi RV, Sung B (2009) Targeting inflammatory pathways for prevention and therapy of cancer: short-term friend, long-term foe. Clin Cancer Res 15:425–430

Andreu P, Johansson M, Affara NI, Pucci F, Tan T, Junankar S, Korets L, Lam J, Tawfik D, DeNardo DG, Naldini L, de Visser KE, De PM, Coussens LM (2010) FcRgamma activation regulates inflammation-associated squamous carcinogenesis. Cancer Cell 17:121–134

Apetoh L, Tesniere A, Ghiringhelli F, Kroemer G, Zitvogel L (2008) Molecular interactions between dying tumor cells and the innate immune system determine the efficacy of conventional anticancer therapies. Cancer Res 68:4026–4030

Arber N, Eagle CJ, Spicak J, Racz I, Dite P, Hajer J, Zavoral M, Lechuga MJ, Gerletti P, Tang J, Rosenstein RB, Macdonald K, Bhadra P, Fowler R, Wittes J, Zauber AG, Solomon SD, Levin B (2006) Celecoxib for the prevention of colorectal adenomatous polyps. N Engl J Med 355:885–895

Armendariz-Borunda J, Islas-Carbajal MC, Meza-Garcia E, Rincon AR, Lucano S, Sandoval AS, Salazar A, Berumen J, Alvarez A, Covarrubias A, Arechiga G, Garcia L (2006) A pilot study in patients with established advanced liver fibrosis using pirfenidone. Gut 55:1663–1665

Baitsch L, Baumgaertner P, Devevre E, Raghav SK, Legat A, Barba L, Wieckowski S, Bouzourene

H, Deplancke B, Romero P, Rufer N, Speiser DE (2011) Exhaustion of tumor- specific CD8(+) T cells in metastases from melanoma patients. J Clin Invest 121:2350–2360

Balkwill F (2009) Tumour necrosis factor and cancer. Nat Rev Cancer 9:361–371

Balkwill F, Mantovani A (2001) Inflammation and cancer: back to Virchow? Lancet 357:539–545

Barber DL, Wherry EJ, Masopust D, Zhu B, Allison JP, Sharpe AH, Freeman GJ, Ahmed R (2006) Restoring function in exhausted CD8 T cells during chronic viral infection. Nature 439:682–687

Barth H, Robinet E, Liang TJ, Baumert TF (2008) Mouse models for the study of HCV infection and virus-host interactions. J Hepatol 49:134–142

Bertagnolli MM, Eagle CJ, Zauber AG, Redston M, Solomon SD, Kim K, Tang J, Rosenstein RB, Wittes J, Corle D, Hess TM, Woloj GM, Boisserie F, Anderson WF, Viner JL, Bagheri D, Burn J, Chung DC, Dewar T, Foley TR, Hoffman N, Macrae F, Pruitt RE, Saltzman JR, Salzberg B, Sylwestrowicz T, Gordon GB, Hawk ET (2006) Celecoxib for the prevention of sporadic colorectal adenomas. N Engl J Med 355:873–884

Bielas JH, Loeb KR, Rubin BP, True LD, Loeb LA (2006) Human cancers express a mutator phenotype. Proc Natl Acad Sci U S A 103:18238–18242

Biswas SK, Mantovani A (2010) Macrophage plasticity and interaction with lymphocyte subsets: cancer as a paradigm. Nat Immunol 11:889–896

Blackburn SD, Shin H, Haining WN, Zou T, Workman CJ, Polley A, Betts MR, Freeman GJ, Vignali DA, Wherry EJ (2009) Coregulation of CD8+T cell exhaustion by multiple inhibitory receptors during chronic viral infection. Nat Immunol 10:29–37

Boon T, Coulie PG, Van den Eynde BJ, van der Bruggen P (2006) Human T cell responses against melanoma. Annu Rev Immunol 24:175–208

Breitbach CJ, Burke J, Jonker D, Stephenson J, Haas AR, Chow LQ, Nieva J, Hwang TH, Moon A, Patt R, Pelusio A, Le Boeuf F, Burns J, Evgin L, De Silva N, Cvancic S, Robertson T, Je JE, Lee YS, Parato K, Diallo JS, Fenster A, Daneshmand M, Bell JC, Kirn DH (2011) Intravenous delivery of a multi-mechanistic cancer-targeted oncolytic poxvirus in humans. Nature 477:99–102

Brown ER, Charles KA, Hoare SA, Rye RL, Jodrell DI, Aird RE, Vora R, Prabhakar U, Nakada M, Corringham RE, DeWitte M, Sturgeon C, Propper D, Balkwill FR, Smyth JF (2008) A clinical study assessing the tolerability and biological effects of infliximab, a TNF-alpha inhibitor, in patients with advanced cancer. Ann Oncol 19:1340–1346

Calzascia T, Pellegrini M, Hall H, Sabbagh L, Ono N, Elford AR, Mak TW, Ohashi PS (2007) TNF-alpha is critical for antitumor but not antiviral T cell immunity in mice. J Clin Invest 117:3833–3845

Casares N, Pequignot MO, Tesniere A, Ghiringhelli F, Roux S, Chaput N, Schmitt E, Hamai A,

Hervas-Stubbs S, Obeid M, Coutant F, Metivier D, Pichard E, Aucouturier P, Pierron G, Garrido C, Zitvogel L, Kroemer G (2005) Caspase-dependent immunogenicity of doxorubicin-induced tumor cell death. J Exp Med 202:1691–1701

Cassatella MA, Locati M, Mantovani A (2009) Never underestimate the power of a neutrophil. Immunity 31:698–700

Chang MH, Chen CJ, Lai MS, Hsu HM, Wu TC, Kong MS, Liang DC, Shau WY, Chen DS (1997) Universal hepatitis B vaccination in Taiwan and the incidence of hepatocellular carcinoma in children. Taiwan Childhood Hepatoma Study Group [see comments]. N Engl J Med 336:1855–1859

Chen CJ, Yang HI, Su J, Jen CL, You SL, Lu SN, Huang GT, Iloeje UH (2006) Risk of hepatocellular carcinoma across a biological gradient of serum hepatitis B virus DNA level. JAMA 295:65–73

Colombo M, Donato MF (2005) Prevention of hepatocellular carcinoma. Semin Liver Dis 25:155–161

Colotta F, Allavena P, Sica A, Garlanda C, Mantovani A (2009) Cancer-related inflammation, the seventh hallmark of cancer: links to genetic instability. Carcinogenesis 30:1073–1081

Condeelis J, Pollard JW (2006) Macrophages: obligate partners for tumor cell migration, invasion, and metastasis. Cell 124:263–266

Custer B, Sullivan SD, Hazlet TK, Iloeje U, Veenstra DL, Kowdley KV (2004) Global epidemiology of hepatitis B virus. J Clin Gastroenterol 38:S158–S168

Cuzick J, Otto F, Baron JA, Brown PH, Burn J, Greenwald P, Jankowski J, La VC, Meyskens F, Senn HJ, Thun M (2009) Aspirin and non-steroidal anti-inflammatory drugs for cancer prevention: an international consensus statement. Lancet Oncol 10:501–507

Dardalhon V, Anderson AC, Karman J, Apetoh L, Chandwaskar R, Lee DH, Cornejo M, Nishi N, Yamauchi A, Quintana FJ, Sobel RA, Hirashima M, Kuchroo VK (2010) Tim-3/galectin-9 pathway: regulation of Th1 immunity through promotion of CD11b ? Ly-6G ? myeloid cells. J Immunol 185:1383–1392

de Martel C, Franceschi S (2009) Infections and cancer: established associations and new hypotheses. Crit Rev Oncol Hematol 70:183–194

DeNardo DG, Barreto JB, Andreu P, Vasquez L, Tawfik D, Kolhatkar N, Coussens LM (2009) CD4(+) T cells regulate pulmonary metastasis of mammary carcinomas by enhancing protumor properties of macrophages. Cancer Cell 16:91–102

Donato F, Boffetta P, Puoti M (1998) A meta-analysis of epidemiological studies on the combined effect of hepatitis B and C virus infections in causing hepatocellular carcinoma. Int J Cancer 75:347–354

Douglass A, Wallace K, Parr R, Park J, Durward E, Broadbent I, Barelle C, Porter AJ, Wright MC

(2008) Antibody-targeted myofibroblast apoptosis reduces fibrosis during sustained liver injury. J Hepatol 49:88–98

Dvorak HF (1986) Tumors: wounds that do not heal. Similarities between tumor stroma generation and wound healing. N Engl J Med 315:1650–1659

Erdman SE, Sohn JJ, Rao VP, Nambiar PR, Ge Z, Fox JG, Schauer DB (2005) CD4？CD25？regulatory lymphocytes induce regression of intestinal tumors in ApcMin/+ mice. Cancer Res 65:3998–4004

Erez N, Truitt M, Olson P, Arron ST, Hanahan D (2010) Cancer-Associated Fibroblasts Are Activated in Incipient Neoplasia to Orchestrate Tumor-Promoting Inflammation in an NF-kappaB-Dependent Manner. Cancer Cell 17:135–147

Erler JT, Bennewith KL, Cox TR, Lang G, Bird D, Koong A, Le QT, Giaccia AJ (2009) Hypoxia-induced lysyl oxidase is a critical mediator of bone marrow cell recruitment to form the premetastatic niche. Cancer Cell 15:35–44

Fallowfield JA (2011) Therapeutic targets in liver fibrosis. Am J Physiol Gastrointest Liver Physiol 300:G709–G715

Farazi PA, DePinho RA (2006) Hepatocellular carcinoma pathogenesis: from genes to environment. Nat Rev Cancer 6:674–687

Fidder H, Schnitzler F, Ferrante M, Noman M, Katsanos K, Segaert S, Henckaerts L, Van AG, Vermeire S, Rutgeerts P (2009) Long-term safety of infliximab for the treatment of inflammatory bowel disease: a single-centre cohort study. Gut 58:501–508

Fischer SM, Hawk ET, Lubet RA (2011) Coxibs and other nonsteroidal anti-inflammatory drugs in animal models of cancer chemoprevention. Cancer Prev Res (Phila) 4:1728–1735

Flossmann E, Rothwell PM (2007) Effect of aspirin on long-term risk of colorectal cancer: consistent evidence from randomised and observational studies. Lancet 369:1603–1613

Fourcade J, Kudela P, Andrade Filho PA, Janjic B, Land SR, Sander C, Krieg A, Donnenberg A, Shen H, Kirkwood JM, Zarour HM (2008) Immunization with analog peptide in combination with CpG and montanide expands tumor antigen-specific CD8？T cells in melanoma patients. J Immunother 31:781–791

Fourcade J, Sun Z, Benallaoua M, Guillaume P, Luescher IF, Sander C, Kirkwood JM, Kuchroo V, Zarour HM (2010) Upregulation of Tim-3 and PD-1 expression is associated with tumor antigen-specific CD8？T cell dysfunction in melanoma patients. J Exp Med 207:2175–2186

Fridlender ZG, Sun J, Kim S, Kapoor V, Cheng G, Ling L, Worthen GS, Albelda SM (2009) Polarization of tumor-associated neutrophil phenotype by TGF-beta: "N1" versus "N2" TAN. Cancer Cell 16:183–194

Fukuda A, Wang SC, Morris JP, Folias AE, Liou A, Kim GE, Akira S, Boucher KM, Firpo MA, Mulvihill SJ, Hebrok M (2011) Stat3 and MMP7 contribute to pancreatic ductal adenocarcinoma initiation and progression. Cancer Cell 19:441–455

Fuller MJ, Zajac AJ (2003) Ablation of CD8 and CD4 T cell responses by high viral loads. J Immunol 170:477–486

Gabrilovich DI, Nagaraj S (2009) Myeloid-derived suppressor cells as regulators of the immune system. Nat Rev Immunol 9:162–174

Gallimore AM, Simon AK (2008) Positive and negative influences of regulatory T cells on tumour immunity. Oncogene 27:5886–5893

Galon J, Costes A, Sanchez-Cabo F, Kirilovsky A, Mlecnik B, Lagorce-Pages C, Tosolini M, Camus M, Berger A, Wind P, Zinzindohoue F, Bruneval P, Cugnenc PH, Trajanoski Z, Fridman WH, Pages F (2006) Type, density, and location of immune cells within human colorectal tumors predict clinical outcome. Science 313:1960–1964

Garland SM, Hernandez-Avila M, Wheeler CM, Perez G, Harper DM, Leodolter S, Tang GW, Ferris DG, Steben M, Bryan J, Taddeo FJ, Railkar R, Esser MT, Sings HL, Nelson M, Boslego J, Sattler C, Barr E, Koutsky LA (2007) Quadrivalent vaccine against human papillomavirus to prevent anogenital diseases. N Engl J Med 356:1928–1943

Gordon S, Martinez FO (2010) Alternative activation of macrophages: mechanism and functions. Immunity 32:593–604

Greten FR, Arkan MC, Bollrath J, Hsu LC, Goode J, Miething C, Goktuna SI, Neuenhahn M, Fierer J, Paxian S, Van RN, Xu Y, O'Cain T, Jaffee BB, Busch DH, Duyster J, Schmid RM, Eckmann L, Karin M (2007) NF-kappaB is a negative regulator of IL-1beta secretion as revealed by genetic and pharmacological inhibition of IKKbeta. Cell 130:918–931

Grivennikov S, Karin E, Terzic J, Mucida D, Yu GY, Vallabhapurapu S, Scheller J, Rose-John S, Cheroutre H, Eckmann L, Karin M (2009) IL-6 and Stat3 are required for survival of intestinal epithelial cells and development of colitis-associated cancer. Cancer Cell 15:103–113

Guerra C, Schuhmacher AJ, Canamero M, Grippo PJ, Verdaguer L, Perez-Gallego L, Dubus P, Sandgren EP, Barbacid M (2007) Chronic pancreatitis is essential for induction of pancreatic ductal adenocarcinoma by K-Ras oncogenes in adult mice. Cancer Cell 11:291–302

Gupta RA, DuBois RN (2001) Colorectal cancer prevention and treatment by inhibition of cyclooxygenase-2. Nat Rev Cancer 1:11–21

Haddow A (1972) Molecular repair, wound healing, and carcinogenesis: tumor production a possible overhealing? Adv Cancer Res 16:181–234

Hanahan D, Weinberg RA (2011) Hallmarks of cancer: the next generation. Cell 144:646–674
Harrison ML, Obermueller E, Maisey NR, Hoare S, Edmonds K, Li NF, Chao D, Hall K, Lee C, Timotheadou E, Charles K, Ahern R, King DM, Eisen T, Corringham R, DeWitte M, Balkwill F, Gore M (2007) Tumor necrosis factor alpha as a new target for renal cell carcinoma: two sequential phase II trials of infliximab at standard and high dose. J Clin Oncol 25:4542–4549

Hedvat M, Huszar D, Herrmann A, Gozgit JM, Schroeder A, Sheehy A, Buettner R, Proia D, Kowolik CM, Xin H, Armstrong B, Bebernitz G, Weng S, Wang L, Ye M, McEachern K, Chen H, Morosini D, Bell K, Alimzhanov M, Ioannidis S, McCoon P, Cao ZA, Yu H, Jove R, Zinda M (2009) The JAK2 inhibitor AZD1480 potently blocks Stat3 signaling and oncogenesis in solid tumors. Cancer Cell 16:487–497

Hiratsuka S, Watanabe A, Aburatani H, Maru Y (2006) Tumour-mediated upregulation of chemoattractants and recruitment of myeloid cells predetermines lung metastasis. Nat Cell Biol 8:1369–1375

Huang H, Shiffman ML, Friedman S, Venkatesh R, Bzowej N, Abar OT, Rowland CM, Catanese JJ, Leong DU, Sninsky JJ, Layden TJ, Wright TL, White T, Cheung RC (2007) A 7 gene signature identifies the risk of developing cirrhosis in patients with chronic hepatitis C. Hepatology 46:297–306

Hussain SP, Harris CC (2007) Inflammation and cancer: an ancient link with novel potentials. Int J Cancer 121:2373–2380

Joura EA, Leodolter S, Hernandez-Avila M, Wheeler CM, Perez G, Koutsky LA, Garland SM, Harper DM, Tang GW, Ferris DG, Steben M, Jones RW, Bryan J, Taddeo FJ, Bautista OM, Esser MT, Sings HL, Nelson M, Boslego JW, Sattler C, Barr E, Paavonen J (2007) Efficacy of a quadrivalent prophylactic human papillomavirus (types 6, 11, 16, and 18) L1 virus-like-particle vaccine against high-grade vulval and vaginal lesions: a combined analysis of three randomised clinical trials. Lancet 369:1693–1702

Joyce JA, Pollard JW (2009) Microenvironmental regulation of metastasis. Nat Rev Cancer 9:239–252

Kalluri R, Weinberg RA (2009) The basics of epithelial-mesenchymal transition. J Clin Invest 119:1420–1428

Kang TW, Yevsa T, Woller N, Hoenicke L, Wuestefeld T, Dauch D, Hohmeyer A, Gereke M, Rudalska R, Potapova A, Iken M, Vucur M, Weiss S, Heikenwalder M, Khan S, Gil J, Bruder D, Manns M, Schirmacher P, Tacke F, Ott M, Luedde T, Longerich T, Kubicka S, Zender L (2011) Senescence surveillance of pre-malignant hepatocytes limits liver cancer development. Nature 479:547–551

Kaplan RN, Riba RD, Zacharoulis S, Bramley AH, Vincent L, Costa C, MacDonald DD, Jin DK, Shido K, Kerns SA, Zhu Z, Hicklin D, Wu Y, Port JL, Altorki N, Port ER, Ruggero D, Shmelkov SV, Jensen KK, Rafii S, Lyden D (2005) VEGFR1-positive haematopoietic bone marrow progenitors initiate the pre-metastatic niche. Nature 438:820–827

Kaplan RN, Rafii S, Lyden D (2006) Preparing the "soil": the premetastatic niche. Cancer Res 66:11089–11093

Karin M (2006) Nuclear factor-kappaB in cancer development and progression. Nature 441:431–

436

Kawamori T, Rao CV, Seibert K, Reddy BS (1998) Chemopreventive activity of celecoxib, a specific cyclooxygenase-2 inhibitor, against colon carcinogenesis. Cancer Res 58:409–412

Kim S, Takahashi H, Lin WW, Descargues P, Grivennikov S, Kim Y, Luo JL, Karin M (2009) Carcinoma-produced factors activate myeloid cells through TLR2 to stimulate metastasis. Nature 457:102–106

Kim YJ, Hong KS, Chung JW, Kim JH, Hahm KB (2010) Prevention of colitis-associated carcinogenesis with infliximab. Cancer Prev Res (Phila) 3:1314–1333

Koebel CM, Vermi W, Swann JB, Zerafa N, Rodig SJ, Old LJ, Smyth MJ, Schreiber RD (2007) Adaptive immunity maintains occult cancer in an equilibrium state. Nature 450:903–907

Kohrt HE, Nouri N, Nowels K, Johnson D, Holmes S, Lee PP (2005) Profile of immune cells in axillary lymph nodes predicts disease-free survival in breast cancer. PLoS Med 2:e284

Kronenberger B, Zeuzem S (2012) New developments in HCV therapy. J Viral Hepat 19(Suppl 1):48–51

Kujawski M, Kortylewski M, Lee H, Herrmann A, Kay H, Yu H (2008) Stat3 mediates myeloid cell-dependent tumor angiogenesis in mice. J Clin Invest 118:3367–3377

Laghi L, Bianchi P, Miranda E, Balladore E, Pacetti V, Grizzi F, Allavena P, Torri V, Repici A, Santoro A, Mantovani A, Roncalli M, Malesci A (2009) CD3+cells at the invasive margin of deeply invading (pT3-T4) colorectal cancer and risk of post-surgical metastasis: a longitudinal study. Lancet Oncol 10:877–884

Langley RE, Burdett S, Tierney JF, Cafferty F, Parmar MK, Venning G (2011) Aspirin and cancer: has aspirin been overlooked as an adjuvant therapy? Br J Cancer 105:1107–1113

Langowski JL, Zhang X, Wu L, Mattson JD, Chen T, Smith K, Basham B, McClanahan T, Kastelein RA, Oft M (2006) IL-23 promotes tumour incidence and growth. Nature 442:461–465

Lee UE, Friedman SL (2011) Mechanisms of hepatic fibrogenesis. Best Pract Res Clin Gastroenterol 25:195–206

Lesina M, Kurkowski MU, Ludes K, Rose-John S, Treiber M, Kloppel G, Yoshimura A, Reindl W, Sipos B, Akira S, Schmid RM, Algul H (2011) Stat3/Socs3 activation by IL-6 transsignaling promotes progression of pancreatic intraepithelial neoplasia and development of pancreatic cancer. Cancer Cell 19:456–469

Liu X, Plummer SJ, Nock NL, Casey G, Witte JS (2006) Nonsteroidal antiinflammatory drugs and decreased risk of advanced prostate cancer: modification by lymphotoxin alpha. Am J Epidemiol 164:984–989

Luo JL, Maeda S, Hsu LC, Yagita H, Karin M (2004) Inhibition of NF-kappaB in cancer cells converts inflammation-induced tumor growth mediated by TNFalpha to TRAIL-mediated tumor regression. Cancer Cell 6:297–305

Mandic M, Castelli F, Janjic B, Almunia C, Andrade P, Gillet D, Brusic V, Kirkwood JM, Maillere B, Zarour HM (2005) One NY-ESO-1-derived epitope that promiscuously binds to multiple HLA-DR and HLA-DP4 molecules and stimulates autologous CD4 ? T cells from patients with NY-ESO-1-expressing melanoma. J Immunol 174:1751–1759

Mantovani A (2009) The yin-yang of tumor-associated neutrophils. Cancer Cell 16:173–174 Mantovani A, Sozzani S, Locati M, Allavena P, Sica A (2002) Macrophage polarization: tumor-associated macrophages as a paradigm for polarized M2 mononuclear phagocytes. Trends Immunol 23:549–555

Mantovani A, Allavena P, Sica A, Balkwill F (2008) Cancer-related inflammation. Nature 454:436–444

McHutchison JG, Everson GT, Gordon SC, Jacobson IM, Sulkowski M, Kauffman R, McNair L, Alam J, Muir AJ (2009) Telaprevir with peginterferon and ribavirin for chronic HCV genotype 1 infection. N Engl J Med 360:1827–1838

Mok TS, Yeo W, Yu S, Lai P, Chan HL, Chan AT, Lau JW, Wong H, Leung N, Hui EP, Sung J, Koh J, Mo F, Zee B, Johnson PJ (2005) An intensive surveillance program detected a high incidence of hepatocellular carcinoma among hepatitis B virus carriers with abnormal alpha-fetoprotein levels or abdominal ultrasonography results. J Clin Oncol 23:8041–8047

Mukherjee D, Nissen SE, Topol EJ (2001) Risk of cardiovascular events associated with selective COX-2 inhibitors. JAMA 286:954–959

Murdoch C, Muthana M, Coffelt SB, Lewis CE (2008) The role of myeloid cells in the promotion of tumour angiogenesis. Nat Rev Cancer 8:618–631

Oakley F, Teoh V, Ching AS, Bataller R, Colmenero J, Jonsson JR, Eliopoulos AG, Watson MR, Manas D, Mann DA (2009) Angiotensin II activates I kappaB kinase phosphorylation of RelA at Ser 536 to promote myofibroblast survival and liver fibrosis. Gastroenterology 136:2334–2344

Paavonen J, Jenkins D, Bosch FX, Naud P, Salmeron J, Wheeler CM, Chow SN, Apter DL, Kitchener HC, Castellsague X, de Carvalho NS, Skinner SR, Harper DM, Hedrick JA, Jaisamrarn U, Limson GA, Dionne M, Quint W, Spiessens B, Peeters P, Struyf F, Wieting SL, Lehtinen MO, Dubin G (2007) Efficacy of a prophylactic adjuvanted bivalent L1 virus-like-particle vaccine against infection with human papillomavirus types 16 and 18 in young women: an interim analysis of a phase III double-blind, randomised controlled trial. Lancet 369:2161–2170

Padua D, Zhang XH, Wang Q, Nadal C, Gerald WL, Gomis RR, Massague J (2008) TGFbeta primes breast tumors for lung metastasis seeding through angiopoietin-like 4. Cell 133:66–77

Park BH, Hwang T, Liu TC, Sze DY, Kim JS, Kwon HC, Oh SY, Han SY, Yoon JH, Hong SH,

Moon A, Speth K, Park C, Ahn YJ, Daneshmand M, Rhee BG, Pinedo HM, Bell JC, Kirn DH (2008) Use of a targeted oncolytic poxvirus, JX-594, in patients with refractory primary or metastatic liver cancer: a phase I trial. Lancet Oncol 9:533–542

Parkin DM (2006) The global health burden of infection-associated cancers in the year 2002. Int J Cancer 118:3030–3044

Parkin DM, Bray F (2006) Chapter 2: The burden of HPV-related cancers. Vaccine 24 (Suppl 3):S3-11–S3/25

Patel H, Heathcote EJ (2011) Sustained virological response with 29 days of Debio 025 monotherapy in hepatitis C virus genotype 3. Gut 60:879

Pedroza-Gonzalez A, Xu K, Wu TC, Aspord C, Tindle S, Marches F, Gallegos M, Burton EC, Savino D, Hori T, Tanaka Y, Zurawski S, Zurawski G, Bover L, Liu YJ, Banchereau J, Palucka AK (2011) Thymic stromal lymphopoietin fosters human breast tumor growth by promoting type 2 inflammation. J Exp Med 208:479–490

Plummer M, Schiffman M, Castle PE, Maucort-Boulch D, Wheeler CM (2007) A 2-year prospective study of human papillomavirus persistence among women with a cytological diagnosis of atypical squamous cells of undetermined significance or low-grade squamous intraepithelial lesion. J Infect Dis 195:1582–1589

Polyak K, Weinberg RA (2009) Transitions between epithelial and mesenchymal states: acquisition of malignant and stem cell traits. Nat Rev Cancer 9:265–273

Popov Y, Patsenker E, Stickel F, Zaks J, Bhaskar KR, Niedobitek G, Kolb A, Friess H, Schuppan D (2008) Integrin alphavbeta6 is a marker of the progression of biliary and portal liver fibrosis and a novel target for antifibrotic therapies. J Hepatol 48:453–464

Rakoff-Nahoum S, Medzhitov R (2009) Toll-like receptors and cancer. Nat Rev Cancer 9:57–63

Reddy BS, Hirose Y, Lubet R, Steele V, Kelloff G, Paulson S, Seibert K, Rao CV (2000) Chemoprevention of colon cancer by specific cyclooxygenase-2 inhibitor, celecoxib, administered during different stages of carcinogenesis. Cancer Res 60:293–297

Rius J, Guma M, Schachtrup C, Akassoglou K, Zinkernagel AS, Nizet V, Johnson RS, Haddad GG, Karin M (2008) NF-kappaB links innate immunity to the hypoxic response through transcriptional regulation of HIF-1alpha. Nature 453:807–811

Roberts SJ, Ng BY, Filler RB, Lewis J, Glusac EJ, Hayday AC, Tigelaar RE, Girardi M (2007) Characterizing tumor-promoting T cells in chemically induced cutaneous carcinogenesis. Proc Natl Acad Sci U S A 104:6770–6775

Roca H, Varsos ZS, Sud S, Craig MJ, Ying C, Pienta KJ (2009) CCL2 and interleukin-6 promote survival of human CD11b+peripheral blood mononuclear cells and induce M2-type macrophage polarization. J Biol Chem 284:34342–34354

Rockey DC (2008) Current and future anti-fibrotic therapies for chronic liver disease. Clin Liver Dis

12:939–962, xi

Rodier F, Coppe JP, Patil CK, Hoeijmakers WA, Munoz DP, Raza SR, Freund A, Campeau E, Davalos AR, Campisi J (2009) Persistent DNA damage signalling triggers senescence-associated inflammatory cytokine secretion. Nat Cell Biol 11:973–979

Rothwell PM, Wilson M, Elwin CE, Norrving B, Algra A, Warlow CP, Meade TW (2010) Long- term effect of aspirin on colorectal cancer incidence and mortality: 20-year follow-up of five randomised trials. Lancet 376:1741–1750

Rothwell PM, Fowkes FG, Belch JF, Ogawa H, Warlow CP, Meade TW (2011) Effect of daily aspirin on long-term risk of death due to cancer: analysis of individual patient data from randomised trials. Lancet 377:31–41

Ryan KM, Ernst MK, Rice NR, Vousden KH (2000) Role of NF-kappaB in p53-mediated programmed cell death. Nature 404:892–897

Sakuishi K, Apetoh L, Sullivan JM, Blazar BR, Kuchroo VK, Anderson AC (2010) Targeting Tim-3 and PD-1 pathways to reverse T cell exhaustion and restore anti-tumor immunity. J Exp Med 207:2187–2194

Sato Y, Takahashi S, Kinouchi Y, Shiraki M, Endo K, Matsumura Y, Kakuta Y, Tosa M, Motida A, Abe H, Imai G, Yokoyama H, Nomura E, Negoro K, Takagi S, Aihara H, Masumura K, Nohmi T, Shimosegawa T (2006) IL-10 deficiency leads to somatic mutations in a model of IBD. Carcinogenesis 27:1068–1073

Schioppa T, Moore R, Thompson RG, Rosser EC, Kulbe H, Nedospasov S, Mauri C, Coussens LM, Balkwill FR (2011) B regulatory cells and the tumor-promoting actions of TNF-alpha during squamous carcinogenesis. Proc Natl Acad Sci U S A 108:10662–10667

Schreiber GB, Busch MP, Kleinman SH, Korelitz JJ (1996) The risk of transfusion-transmitted viral infections. The Retrovirus Epidemiology Donor Study. N Engl J Med 334:1685–1690

Sharma MD, Hou DY, Baban B, Koni PA, He Y, Chandler PR, Blazar BR, Mellor AL, Munn DH (2010) Reprogrammed foxp3(+) regulatory T cells provide essential help to support cross-presentation and CD8(+) T cell priming in naive mice. Immunity 33:942–954

Shepard CW, Finelli L, Alter MJ (2005) Global epidemiology of hepatitis C virus infection. Lancet Infect Dis 5:558–567

Shepard CW, Simard EP, Finelli L, Fiore AE, Bell BP (2006) Hepatitis B virus infection: epidemiology and vaccination. Epidemiol Rev 28:112–125

Sinha P, Clements VK, Bunt SK, Albelda SM, Ostrand-Rosenberg S (2007) Cross-talk between myeloid-derived suppressor cells and macrophages subverts tumor immunity toward a type 2 response. J Immunol 179:977–983

Smith JS, Lindsay L, Hoots B, Keys J, Franceschi S, Winer R, Clifford GM (2007) Human papillomavirus type distribution in invasive cervical cancer and high-grade cervical lesions: a meta-analysis update. Int J Cancer 121:621–632

Smith MR, Saad F, Coleman R, Shore N, Fizazi K, Tombal B, Miller K, Sieber P, Karsh L, Damiao R, Tammela TL, Egerdie B, Van PH, Chin J, Morote J, Gomez-Veiga F, Borkowski T, Ye Z, Kupic A, Dansey R, Goessl C (2012) Denosumab and bone-metastasis-free survival in men with castration-resistant prostate cancer: results of a phase 3, randomised, placebo-controlled trial. Lancet 379:39–46

Staller P, Sulitkova J, Lisztwan J, Moch H, Oakeley EJ, Krek W (2003) Chemokine receptor CXCR4 downregulated by von Hippel-Lindau tumour suppressor pVHL. Nature 425:307–311

Steinbach G, Lynch PM, Phillips RK, Wallace MH, Hawk E, Gordon GB, Wakabayashi N, Saunders B, Shen Y, Fujimura T, Su LK, Levin B (2000) The effect of celecoxib, a cyclooxygenase-2 inhibitor, in familial adenomatous polyposis. N Engl J Med 342:1946–1952

Stockert E, Jager E, Chen YT, Scanlan MJ, Gout I, Karbach J, Arand M, Knuth A, Old LJ (1998) A survey of the humoral immune response of cancer patients to a panel of human tumor antigens. J Exp Med 187:1349–1354

Stopeck AT, Lipton A, Body JJ, Steger GG, Tonkin K, de Boer RH, Lichinitser M, Fujiwara Y, Yardley DA, Viniegra M, Fan M, Jiang Q, Dansey R, Jun S, Braun A (2010) Denosumab compared with zoledronic acid for the treatment of bone metastases in patients with advanced breast cancer: a randomized, double-blind study. J Clin Oncol 28:5132–5139

Sunami Y, Leithauser F, Gul S, Fiedler K, Guldiken N, Espenlaub S, Holzmann KH, Hipp N, Sindrilaru A, Luedde T, Baumann B, Wissel S, Kreppel F, Schneider M, Scharffetter-Kochanek K, Kochanek S, Strnad P, Wirth T (2012) Hepatic activation of IKK/NF-kappaB signaling induces liver fibrosis via macrophage-mediated chronic inflammation. Hepatology 56:1117–1128

Swann JB, Smyth MJ (2007) Immune surveillance of tumors. J Clin Invest 117:1137–1146

Teixeira-Clerc F, Julien B, Grenard P, Van Tran NJ, Deveaux V, Li L, Serriere-Lanneau V, Ledent C, Mallat A, Lotersztajn S (2006) CB1 cannabinoid receptor antagonism: a new strategy for the treatment of liver fibrosis. Nat Med 12:671–676

Topalian SL, Hodi FS, Brahmer JR, Gettinger SN, Smith DC, McDermott DF, Powderly JD, Carvajal RD, Sosman JA, Atkins MB, Leming PD, Spigel DR, Antonia SJ, Horn L, Drake CG, Pardoll DM, Chen L, Sharfman WH, Anders RA, Taube JM, McMiller TL, Xu H, Korman AJ, Jure-Kunkel M, Agrawal S, McDonald D, Kollia GD, Gupta A, Wigginton JM, Sznol M (2012) Safety, Activity, and Immune Correlates of Anti-PD-1 Antibody in Cancer. N Engl J Med 366:2443–2454

Torresi J, Johnson D, Wedemeyer H (2011) Progress in the development of preventive and therapeutic vaccines for hepatitis C virus. J Hepatol 54:1273–1285

Trevejo JM, Marino MW, Philpott N, Josien R, Richards EC, Elkon KB, Falck-Pedersen E (2001)

TNF-alpha -dependent maturation of local dendritic cells is critical for activating the adaptive immune response to virus infection. Proc Natl Acad Sci U S A 98:12162–12167

Vakkila J, Lotze MT (2004) Inflammation and necrosis promote tumour growth. Nat Rev Immunol 4:641–648

Voronov E, Shouval DS, Krelin Y, Cagnano E, Benharroch D, Iwakura Y, Dinarello CA, Apte RN (2003) IL-1 is required for tumor invasiveness and angiogenesis. Proc Natl Acad Sci U S A 100:2645–2650

Weber DM, Chen C, Niesvizky R, Wang M, Belch A, Stadtmauer EA, Siegel D, Borrello I, Rajkumar SV, Chanan-Khan AA, Lonial S, Yu Z, Patin J, Olesnyckyj M, Zeldis JB, Knight RD (2007) Lenalidomide plus dexamethasone for relapsed multiple myeloma in North America. N Engl J Med 357:2133–2142

Wherry EJ, Teichgraber V, Becker TC, Masopust D, Kaech SM, Antia R, von Andrian UH, Ahmed R (2003) Lineage relationship and protective immunity of memory CD8 T cell subsets. Nat Immunol 4:225–234

Witek RP, Stone WC, Karaca FG, Syn WK, Pereira TA, Agboola KM, Omenetti A, Jung Y, Teaberry V, Choi SS, Guy CD, Pollard J, Charlton P, Diehl AM (2009) Pan-caspase inhibitor VX-166 reduces fibrosis in an animal model of nonalcoholic steatohepatitis. Hepatology 50:1421–1430

Woller N, Knocke S, Mundt B, Gurlevik E, Struver N, Kloos A, Boozari B, Schache P, Manns MP, Malek NP, Sparwasser T, Zender L, Wirth TC, Kubicka S, Kuhnel F (2011) Virus- induced tumor inflammation facilitates effective DC cancer immunotherapy in a Treg- dependent manner in mice. J Clin Invest 121:2570–2582

Xia JL, Dai C, Michalopoulos GK, Liu Y (2006) Hepatocyte growth factor attenuates liver fibrosis induced by bile duct ligation. Am J Pathol 168:1500–1512

Yang J, Weinberg RA (2008) Epithelial-mesenchymal transition: at the crossroads of development and tumor metastasis. Dev Cell 14:818–829

Zajac AJ, Blattman JN, Murali-Krishna K, Sourdive DJ, Suresh M, Altman JD, Ahmed R (1998) Viral immune evasion due to persistence of activated T cells without effector function. J Exp Med 188:2205–2213

Zanetti AR, Van DP, Shouval D (2008) The global impact of vaccination against hepatitis B: a historical overview. Vaccine 26:6266–6273

Zhang Y, Ma CJ, Wang JM, Ji XJ, Wu XY, Moorman JP, Yao ZQ (2012) Tim-3 regulates pro- and anti-inflammatory cytokine expression in human CD14+monocytes. J Leukoc Biol 91:189–196

第4章 病毒感染与肿瘤微环境

摘 要 肿瘤细胞生存的周围环境称为肿瘤微环境。大量的研究表明,肿瘤微环境中的细胞和分子不仅促进肿瘤的生成,而且可积极促进肿瘤的起始、发展和转移过程。部分病毒与肿瘤相关,是肿瘤发生的病原学因素。病毒感染可引起宿主的炎症反应,通过与肿瘤细胞及免疫细胞的相互作用参与肿瘤微环境的形成。肿瘤微环境可能成为今后临床治疗肿瘤的新方向。了解病毒感染与肿瘤微环境之间的关系将为肿瘤的发生、治疗及预后等提供新的思路。上一章关于病毒感染、炎症与肿瘤的关系中也涉及肿瘤微环境的内容,本章将重点讨论病毒感染与肿瘤微环境的相互作用,以及几种病毒的感染与肿瘤微环境的形成。

关键词 病毒感染,肿瘤微环境,炎症,免疫

1 引言

有关肿瘤生长的"种子-土壤"假说(Paget 1889)最早提出是在1889年,但是,在过去的几十年间,由于肿瘤细胞中的瘤基因及抑瘤基因的进展,致使忽视了肿瘤生成过程中肿瘤微环境的作用。然而,肿瘤不仅仅是由一群转化的细胞构成。肿瘤细胞仅仅能在异常的肿瘤微环境中增殖。肿瘤微环境由细胞外基质及基质细胞组成。基质细胞包括免疫细胞、纤维细胞、上皮细胞、髓系抑制性细胞、干细胞和前体细胞等。已经发现几种病毒与肿瘤的发生密切相关,例如,乙型肝炎病毒(hepatitis B virus,HBV)能引起肝细胞癌(hepatocellular carcinoma,HCC);丙型肝炎病毒(hepatitis C virus,HCV)不仅能引起HCC,而且可能与某些淋巴瘤发生相关;人类乳头状瘤病毒(human papillomavirus,HPV)能引起宫颈癌(cervical cancer);EB病毒(Epstein-Barr virus,EBV)能引起鼻咽癌、淋巴瘤(lymphomas)等肿瘤。本章将讨论病毒感染后肿瘤微环境中的细胞和分子变化,以及它们与肿瘤的发生、发展和转移之间的关系,综述几种病毒引起的炎症、随病情进展,最终发展成肿瘤过程中微环境的形成。

2 病毒感染与肿瘤微环境的形成及其相互影响

病毒感染可引起局部的炎症、免疫细胞、microRNA、代谢等方面的反应和变

化（图4-1），以下将从这几个方面了解病毒感染与肿瘤微环境可能存在的联系。

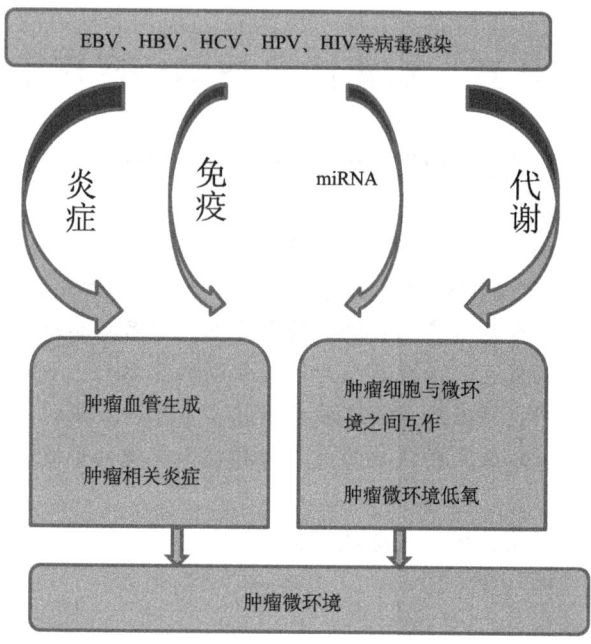

图4-1 病毒感染与肿瘤微环境的形成

2.1 炎症、癌变与肿瘤微环境

炎症发生于感染、自身免疫、微环境及肿瘤（Raposo et al. 2015）。当组织受到病原体感染或者损伤时，引起局部的、及时的急性反应，以有效清除病原体并产生伤口愈合反应。感染或损伤引起的急性反应如不能彻底被治愈，将逐渐转化成慢性炎症，即与病原体处于相平衡状态。这种状态也可称为非可控性炎症。持续的病毒感染，可致细胞发生形态改变及肿瘤的遗传变异累积，从而参与肿瘤的发生。故非可控性炎症和细胞的病毒性转化，是肿瘤发生过程中的重要事件（Rakoff-Nahoum and Medzhitov 2009）。除此之外，炎症细胞产生活性氧及活性氮中间产物，这些产物能提高细胞突变率，诱导 DNA 损伤及增加基因组的不稳定性（Waris and Ahsan 2006）。这些分子也能使基因的错配修复功能失去作用，从而进入肿瘤的起始阶段。在正反馈循环中，DNA 损伤能导致炎症，促进肿瘤的发生和发展（Ohnishi et al. 2013）。

大量研究显示，非可控性炎症在介导肿瘤发生中起关键作用。慢性炎症不可避免地促进肿瘤的起始、发展及进程。炎症分子的上调和过表达通常是作为肿瘤患者预后的标志物（Chai et al. 2015）。例如，趋化因子 CXC 水平增加，不仅仅与药物抗性有关，而且可能预示患者预后较差。

基质细胞与肿瘤细胞组成的肿瘤微环境，是多种炎性生长因子、细胞因子、趋化因子和蛋白质互相联系，通过复杂的对话方式进行的。趋化因子是具有趋化性的细胞因子，而趋化因子受体表达在肿瘤细胞和基质细胞上。趋化因子和它们同源的受体通过一种旁分泌或者自分泌的方式调控肿瘤的生长和转移。它们在炎症细胞的招募、微血管的形成，以及肿瘤细胞的生存、增殖、黏附、浸润和远处转移中起主要的作用。另外，新的钙结合蛋白家族 S100 由于在肿瘤进展和转移时对肿瘤微环境的调控发挥非同寻常的作用，受到越来越多的关注，可能成为癌症治疗和预防的一种潜在性的策略（Nasser et al. 2015）。

在细胞学或细胞因子网络分子的驱动下，肿瘤微环境在不同种类肿瘤中呈现各异。关于炎症和肿瘤之间的联系，最近有了一系列基因和分子的证据。从这个角度显示，大量报道的感染和慢性炎症能促进肿瘤的发展、浸润和转移。肿瘤来源的囊泡，尤其是外泌体，在招募和重组合肿瘤微环境成分上发挥极为重要的作用（Chiantore et al. 2015）。外泌体是一类分泌到细胞外的小囊泡体（30~100nm），已逐渐成为肿瘤细胞和肿瘤微环境之间如基质成纤维细胞、内皮细胞及浸润的免疫细胞等其他主要类型的一种重要的调节者和信息传播者（Tang and Wong 2015）。

2.2 免疫细胞与肿瘤微环境

近年来，关于病毒感染与癌症之间的关系已经引起了广泛的关注和研究，这有助于更好地理解感染、免疫在病毒介导的肿瘤发生、发展和转移进展中发挥的重要作用。研究已经显示，病毒介导的免疫学改变可能在肿瘤形成过程中为形成免疫耐受的微环境创造条件（Chiantore et al. 2015）。

肿瘤微环境中含有大量浸润的免疫细胞，包括 T 淋巴细胞、巨噬细胞、树突状细胞及肥大细胞等。这些细胞被招募到肿瘤的间质中，并且相互合作，促进肿瘤的起始、浸润、迁移及肿瘤的远端转移，或者引起抗肿瘤免疫（Song et al. 2014）。

T 淋巴细胞在细胞免疫中发挥主要作用。与肿瘤相关的巨噬细胞在肿瘤的发生中被招募至肿瘤部位，通过改变其自身功能表型，来应对产生于肿瘤和基质细胞的多种多样的微环境信号，并与临床不良预后相关（Chanmee et al. 2014）；树突状细胞是一群抗原提呈细胞，可识别、处理和加工肿瘤抗原，提呈给初始 T 淋巴细胞（Steinman and Banchereau 2007；Mildner and Jung 2014）；肥大细胞来源于造血干细胞或从骨髓中的粒细胞祖先中分化出来（Galli et al. 1999）。肥大细胞可诱导血管生成前因子的释放，可作为抗原提呈细胞（Shelburne et al. 2009），聚集嗜酸性粒细胞和中性粒细胞，激活抗肿瘤的 T 细胞及 B 细胞反应。肿瘤微环境中浸润的肥大细胞已经成为一种新的预后标记物（Shurin et al. 2009）。

细胞因子 IL-27 是一种重要的多功能免疫调节分子，在免疫反应上具有双重效果。已有研究结果阐明,在一定条件下,中性 IL-27 或其亚型 IL-27 p28 可能是控制炎症的一种有用的策略,而且 IL-27 在其他一些免疫环境下,包括病毒感染和肿瘤免疫中,也具有很强的抑制功能(Duan et al. 2015)。IL-27 作为临床靶标的潜在趋势将引起更多的研究和探讨。

2.3 microRNA 与肿瘤微环境

microRNA(miRNA)是一群小分子、非编码的 RNA,参与调控肿瘤的进程,尤其是侵袭和转移过程。尽管早期对转移的研究集中于 miRNA 对肿瘤细胞内在性质的影响,然而最近的研究报道,miRNA 也可以参与肿瘤细胞与其相关的间质之间的联系(Zhang et al. 2014)。从肿瘤患者血清中检测到的 miRNA 能作为多种癌症如乳腺癌(Roth et al. 2010)、胰腺癌(Kawaguchi et al. 2013)、结肠癌(Cheng et al. 2011)及肺癌(Zheng et al. 2011)等的生物标记物。

关于 miRNA 作用的这种复杂性的原因,Zhang 等(2014)学者认为:首先,几种 miRNA 作为肿瘤转移的主要调控者,同时也调控侵袭转移级联反应的多个过程;其次,尽管单个的 miRNA 通常能调控数百个不同的 mRNA 基因,选择不同的靶基因的能力可能是基于一种特定的细胞环境,甚至存在于同样的转移过程中;最后,在不同转移阶段,由特定的细胞环境决定的 miRNA 可能作用于同样的靶基因,但是导致不同的表型结果。

2.4 肿瘤细胞代谢与肿瘤微环境

肿瘤细胞通常优先利用糖酵解,而不是氧化磷酸化来代谢,甚至在有氧存在的情况下也是如此。这种有氧糖酵解的方式,被称为"瓦登堡效应",普遍存在于许多肿瘤中。最近的研究(Justus et al. 2015)显示,癌基因和抑癌基因,以及肿瘤微环境因素,如组织缺氧、酸中毒能够调节肿瘤细胞的糖代谢。与此相反,改变了的肿瘤细胞代谢能调控在肿瘤演变、转移及治疗中发挥重要作用的肿瘤微环境。

肿瘤细胞必须适应低氧环境,以维持肿瘤的生长。低氧环境能促进代谢的分子学改变,如产生缺氧诱导因子(HIF)等(Labiano et al. 2015)。这些改变能上调糖酵解酶的表达,抑制氧化磷酸化、线粒体选择性自我吞噬及葡萄糖依赖的柠檬酸盐的合成,从而改变葡萄糖代谢、血管生成,进一步导致细胞存活及获得侵袭能力(Staller et al. 2003)。

人体正常的 pH 约为 7.4,而肿瘤微环境中的 pH 为 5.5~7.4,呈偏酸性环境。减少的血液灌注增加无氧代谢,导致乳酸产生增加。即使在有氧存在时,癌细胞优先利用糖酵解产生大量的乳酸导致酸中毒。这是由于以下几个方面的原因:酸中毒能激活 p53,通过抑制糖酵解而刺激柠檬酸循环(Schwartzenberg-Bar-Yoseph et al. 2004);酸中毒增加葡萄糖-6-磷酸脱氢酶和谷氨酰胺酶的表达(Lamonte et al. 2013);激活的 p53 可能诱导与帕金森病相关的基因的表达,减少糖代谢的活动 (Zhang et al. 2011)。激活的 p53 通过减弱糖酵解、增强氧化磷酸化作用,从而调控肿瘤细胞的代谢,这个作用,结合 p53 刺激性减少活性氧等的作用,对于理解酸中毒引起肿瘤细胞代谢的改变具有十分重要的意义。因此,代谢研究有可能成为肿瘤微环境研究的全新的方向。

3 几种病毒的感染与肿瘤微环境

3.1 EBV 与肿瘤微环境

近年来,人们已认识到肿瘤微环境在淋巴瘤的发展中发挥的积极作用,而我们仅仅才开始了解淋巴细胞和基质细胞或淋巴瘤生成不同阶段的细胞成分之间的复杂联系。这些联系可能对于调控淋巴细胞的归巢、生长、生存、对宿主免疫的反应和治疗都是极为重要的(Scott and Gascoyne 2014;Shain et al. 2015)。

EB 病毒感染和多种人类肿瘤相关,尤其是一些与病毒潜伏感染的 B 淋巴系统有关,包括免疫功能低下的淋巴增生性疾病如霍奇金淋巴瘤、Burkitt 淋巴瘤及特殊类型的弥漫大 B 细胞淋巴瘤;其他 EBV 相关性肿瘤则发生在其他的靶组织,如鼻腔 T/NK 细胞淋巴瘤、未分化的鼻咽部肿瘤以及少部分的胃癌(Rickinson 2014)。Riccardo Dolcetti 认为 EBV 可上调几种能促进肿瘤生长及淋巴细胞生存的因子(如 EBV 编码的潜伏性蛋白,包括 6 种 EBV 核抗原 EBNA 和 3 种潜伏性膜蛋白 LMP-1、LMP-2A 及 LMP-2B),并调控支持肿瘤免疫逃逸的复杂机制,且 EBV 感染的 B 淋巴细胞可分泌外泌体(Dolcetti 2015)。外泌体是一团来自于内吞体膜的细胞外囊泡,可运输各类蛋白质、生长因子、受体、受体配体及核酸,近年来常被作为肿瘤细胞和肿瘤微环境中的基质细胞之间内部联系的关键介质(Webber et al. 2015)。

另外,EBV 还可促进血管生成。淋巴瘤生长的起始和进程阶段,依赖功能性血管网络的建立来支持淋巴瘤的增生,而淋巴瘤细胞产生的血管生长因子与淋巴瘤的恶性行为密切相关。血管内皮生长因子是生理性与病理性血管生成中最重要的血管生成前的因子。事实上,EBV 编码的蛋白质能上调一些促进血管生成的因子的表达,如 LMP-1 能诱导 VEGF、IL-8 和成纤维生长因子-2 的表达及细胞外释放,从而促进肿瘤的血管生成、肿瘤的浸润和扩散(Vacca et al. 1998;Ceccarelli et al. 2007;Wang et al. 2010)。LMP-1 在 EBV 感染的肿瘤中发挥重要作用。LMP-1 在细胞表型上的影响包含通过直接的细胞联系或者通过可溶性因子增加与肿瘤微环境的互动(Dolcetti et al. 2013)。因此,最佳的治疗策略不仅针对 EBV,而且也需要强调肿瘤微环境的因子。

Ahmed 等（2014）研究发现，EBV 编码的 RNA（EBER）可在 EBV 转染的细胞释放的外泌体碎片中存在，而且纯的外泌体碎片同样也包含 EBER 结合的蛋白质（La），表明 EBER 很可能在 EBV 感染细胞的外泌体中以 EBER-La 复合体的形式被释放出来。然而，至今还未完全确定是由于 EBER 或者其他分泌的细胞因子，还是病毒成分导致这样的结果，具体原因尚有待进一步研究发现。

在淋巴瘤发病机理的研究中，对肿瘤微环境中角色的阐释可为临床进行针对淋巴瘤细胞和肿瘤微环境成分有效而新奇的治疗提供策略。

3.2 HBV 与肿瘤微环境

肝脏具有复杂的功能，包括吸收营养及处理血液中的代谢产物和病原微生物。肝细胞癌是全球最常见的肿瘤之一，每年有将近 70 万新发病例，并且预后很差，易发生肝内转移和复发（Portolani et al. 2006；Yang and Roberts 2010）。在中国，HBV 感染是引发肝细胞癌最主要的病因（Chen et al. 2006；Chen et al. 2007）。与 HBV 相关的免疫反应在介导肿瘤发生方面有重要作用。肝脏的微环境通常被认为对抑制炎症具有重要作用。IL-10 在 Toll 样受体（TLR）配体（如 LPS）刺激下大量产生，LPS 可通过 TLR4 信号影响肝细胞癌中的肿瘤细胞和 Kupffer 细胞，从而调控 IL-10 的产生（Knolle et al. 1995）。Shi 等研究发现，与高 IL-10 组相比较，低 IL-10 对 TLR 配体的刺激更不敏感，研究显示在 HBV 诱导的肝细胞癌（HCC）中，IL-10 的产生能力和肿瘤浸润的淋巴结（tumor-infiltrating lymphocytes，TIL）增殖能力有关（Shi et al. 2015）。

与 HBV 感染相关的 HCC 一般经历了长时间"慢性肝炎—肝硬化—肝癌"三步的缓慢变化，HBV 在招募炎症细胞及激活肿瘤微环境中的细胞（如免疫细胞、纤维母细胞等）与非细胞成分（如细胞因子、生长因子等）方面发挥至关重要的作用。Yang 等（2014）认为肿瘤微环境是一个复杂的系统，能促进致癌因素的诱导作用。肝细胞癌主要是由于慢性炎症的长期刺激及周围组织纤维化，肝脏的肿瘤微环境成分比其他许多种类的肿瘤更加复杂，包括肿瘤细胞、间质细胞及细胞外基质中分泌的蛋白质。因此，HBV 感染引起炎症和纤维化，以及大量伴随的产物、刺激产生的细胞因子、趋化因子和生长因子，同时还有白细胞的活化、自身免疫的激活及成纤维细胞的数目，因此，它提供了一个动态的肿瘤微环境，促进不同阶段的肝细胞癌的发展。Li 等（Yang et al. 2012）研究发现，HBV 感染和肝细胞癌的患者存在门静脉癌栓的因果联系。他们认为，肝组织中 HBV 持续存在，能提高 TGF-β 的活性，抑制 microRNA-34a 的表达，从而导致趋化因子 CCL22 的产生增加，而 CCL22 可招募调节性 T 细胞，致使肿瘤发生免疫逃逸。这些发现强烈地支持了 HBV 感染和 TGF-β-miR-34a-CCL22 通路作为潜在的致病因素，能使肝细胞癌患者出现门静脉癌栓,可能是通过对免疫有害的肿瘤微环境,使扩散的肝癌细胞侵犯至门静脉系统。在这种情况下,CCL22 作为一种分泌的小分子,能够同时作用于肿瘤和免疫细胞,可能将成为肝细胞癌一种潜在性的、有效的治疗靶点。

3.3　HCV 与肿瘤微环境

慢性 HCV 感染是进程性的肝脏疾病,包括肝纤维化、肝硬化及肝细胞癌的一个主要的危险因素(Buhler and Bartenschlager 2012)。然而,由慢性 HCV 感染怎样发展到这些肝疾病的机制还不清楚。TGF-β 是一种多功能的细胞因子,调控免疫反应、细胞周期、细胞分化及凋亡等生理功能。Benzoubir 等(2013)发现由 HCV 核心蛋白调控 *TGF-β1* 基因。在肝细胞中过表达核心蛋白可诱导 *TGF-β1* 靶基因的表达,并且诱导细胞信号转导分子的磷酸化,从而使 TGF-β 信号通路激活。同时,表达 HCV 核心蛋白的肝细胞也能激活细胞培养系中的肝星状细胞,且这种激活是依赖于 TGF-β 的。这表明 HCV 核心蛋白可诱导 TGF-β 依赖的上皮-间质转化,这个过程可通过影响 TGF-β 信号通路促进肿瘤细胞的浸润和转移实现。

HCV 在肝细胞长期的隐性感染可能意味着该病毒对 HCC 间接的作用。肝细胞中由病毒核心蛋白引起持续的细胞应激反应,可通过调控微环境发挥作用。大量的报道也强调了感染细胞和细胞外基质在纤维化、上皮-间质转化、肿瘤浸润及转移过程中的关键效应,因而在肝疾病中对宿主蛋白的研究成为了热点(Irshad and Dhar 2006)。

HCV 引起约 25%的肝细胞癌,且在全世界范围内是肿瘤致死的常见原因之一(Perz et al. 2006;Altekruse et al. 2009;Jemal et al. 2011)。有研究(Allison et al. 2015)发现,慢性 HCV 感染人群,相较于一般人群,更易发展并死于非肝脏肿瘤疾病,如胰腺肿瘤(2.5%)、直肠癌(2.1%)、肾细胞癌(1.7%)、非霍奇金淋巴瘤(1.6%)和肺癌(1.6%),并且发病年龄呈现年轻化趋势。例如,Carbone 和 Gloghini(2013)通过对与 HBV 感染相关的淋巴瘤的研究,认为与 HCV 相关的边缘区淋巴瘤,以及与黏膜相关的淋巴组织淋巴瘤,都与它们的肿瘤微环境存在相互作用、相互依赖的关系。在这些淋巴瘤里,肿瘤细胞与微环境因子通常共同存在。起初,肿瘤的发生和肿瘤细胞的生长主要依赖于来自微环境的外部刺激,如病毒抗原、细胞因子及细胞与细胞之间的联系。边缘区淋巴瘤和弥漫大 B 型淋巴瘤是与 HBV 感染关系最密切的组织学类型。HCV 可诱导淋巴瘤产生,其原因可能是 HCV 抗原的刺激为混合性的冷球蛋白血症和 B 细胞淋巴瘤中 B 淋巴细胞的增殖奠定了基础。而且,抗病毒的治疗及敲除 HCV-RNA 的临床效果也为 HCV 和淋巴组织增生的因果联系提供了强有力的证据(Hermine et al. 2002;Peveling-Oberhag et al. 2013)。然而,目前关于 HBV 感染与 B 细胞淋巴瘤的因果关系的机制还有待进一步探究。

3.4 HPV 与肿瘤微环境

HPV 是宫颈癌的主要致病因素。与 HPV 感染相关的肿瘤众多，包括宫颈癌、肛门与生殖器肿瘤及口咽部肿瘤，在发展中国家已经造成了主要的公共健康问题（Stone et al. 2014）。肿瘤微环境中炎症是一个重要的组成部分，在肿瘤进程中发挥主要作用。Stone 等（2014）的研究显示，HPV 阳性细胞系在肿瘤微环境中招募白细胞，以及增加骨髓和脾脏中的粒细胞的能力强于 HPV 阴性的细胞系，同时，他们还注意到 HPV 阳性细胞系显著高表达 IL-6 和 IL-8，而 HPV 阴性细胞系显著高表达 IL-16 和 IL-17。尽管肿瘤细胞分泌不同的细胞因子，白细胞浸润 HPV 阳性细胞系后，呈现极微量的 STAT3，且没有 NF-κB 的磷酸化作用。只有 HPV 阴性细胞系诱导的肿瘤炎性浸润具有 NF-κB 和 STAT3 的表达。不同的细胞系呈现了肿瘤炎症的不同表达，这对于宫颈癌的免疫治疗具有十分重要的临床价值，也可能为 HPV 相关的其他肿瘤提供可能的方向。

结肠癌是全球继肺癌和乳腺癌之后的第三大最常见的肿瘤，其发病率、死亡率及五年生存率分别是 9.7%、8.5% 及 10.9%（Ferlay et al. 2013）。如今普遍流行的观点是，大部分的实体瘤，包括结肠直肠癌，直接或间接地与慢性炎症有联系（Gagliani et al. 2014）。由于肿瘤微环境中存在多种多样的炎性细胞和细胞因子，肿瘤通常被称为"不会愈合的伤口"（Grivennikov et al. 2010）。信号转导子和转录激活子 3（signal transducer and activator of transcription 3，Stat3）是一条关键的信号通路，可通过调控下游的促炎细胞因子及能促进肿瘤生长及浸润的因素，参与到肿瘤微环境的形成中（Yu et al. 2009）。IL-17 是一种由 Stat3 诱导、辅助性 T 淋巴细胞——Th17 细胞产生的一种必要的炎性细胞因子。Li 等（2015）的研究结果显示，HPV 感染在结肠癌中的发生率高达 48.4%，且 HPV 感染与在结肠直肠癌组织中强的 Stat3 的活动能力及高水平的 IL-17 存在极强的联系，而在癌旁组织中没有，故认为结肠直肠癌 Stat3 与 IL-17 共同作用，调控了炎性的肿瘤微环境，从而可能促进了肿瘤的生成，促进了结肠直肠癌的浸润。预防性地给青少年注射 HPV 疫苗可有效地减少 HPV 的感染，从而可能减少结肠直肠癌及相关肿瘤的发病率。

3.5 HIV 与肿瘤微环境

人类获得性免疫缺陷病毒（HIV）没有被列为严格意义上的致瘤病毒，但是 HIV 感染造成免疫缺陷，易发生艾滋相关性淋巴瘤（见第 5 章）。淋巴瘤的肿瘤微环境一直是研究的热点。尽管有高效的抗逆转录病毒疗法，与 HIV 感染相关的非霍奇金淋巴瘤仍然很常见（Achenbach et al. 2014），并且与 HIV 相关的经典霍奇金淋巴瘤发病率逐年升高（Taylor et al. 2015）。如前所述，B 细胞淋巴瘤的肿瘤微环境包括各种各样的免疫细胞、基质细胞、血管及细胞外基质。肿瘤微环境的范围、构成及空间排列包含了由恶性肿瘤细胞支持的基因的变异，这些成分仍然依赖于外部的刺激存活、增生、免疫侵犯，以及引起宿主的炎症反应。这些成分之间的内部联系产生了肿瘤微环境的广泛范围（De Paoli and Carbone 2015）。与病毒感染相关的淋巴瘤的研究不仅致力于 B 淋巴细胞，也注重对组成肿瘤微环境的免疫细胞（如反应的 T 淋巴细胞、B 淋巴细胞及巨噬细胞）与非免疫细胞（如内皮细胞）的研究。De Paoli 和 Carbone（2015）发现，HIV 阳性的弥漫大 B 细胞淋巴瘤组织包含更少的 $CD3^+T$ 细胞，$CD4^+T$ 细胞也明显减少，但 $CD8^+T$ 细胞是主要的作用细胞；在合并有人类获得性免疫缺陷的非霍奇金淋巴瘤研究中，对非免疫细胞成分的肿瘤微环境研究主要在于血管生成方面。

4　针对肿瘤微环境的靶向治疗及展望

肿瘤细胞与肿瘤微环境的联系机制较为复杂，主要有两类（Fang and DeClerck 2013）：依赖联系的机制（包括细胞-细胞、细胞-细胞外基质黏附分子）和不依赖于联系的机制。在不依赖于联系的机制里，可溶性的分子，如生长因子、细胞因子、趋化因子及可溶性的亚细胞器，包括小囊泡和外泌体。最终，通过近分泌和旁分泌的方式，肿瘤细胞和非肿瘤的基质细胞中的信号通路被激活。Fang 主要针对肿瘤微环境，讨论了 4 种不同的治疗策略：针对肿瘤血管；针对肿瘤相关炎症；针对肿瘤细胞和肿瘤微环境联系互动；针对肿瘤微环境中的低氧（Fang and DeClerck 2013）。

自 10 年前 FDA 批准 Avastin 作为第一个针对肿瘤微环境治疗的药剂以来，针对肿瘤微环境的临床前研究及临床试验不断在增长。一些药品已成为特殊肿瘤的治疗标准，然而一些还处于临床试验的早期阶段。目前，针对肿瘤血管的策略研究最为成功。针对病毒感染及其引起的微环境的变化，其治疗策略也应该是一样的原则，不过，这方面的研究仍然有很大的空间，并且有很长的路要走。

尽管更多针对肿瘤微环境的临床试验逐渐开展起来，仍然存在许多问题。例如，这些治疗单独应用于临床是否最有效，抑或是仍需要结合化疗、放疗以及其他分子靶向治疗的方法综合运用。最近的数据显示，肿瘤微环境是临床治疗的重要贡献者（Meads et al. 2009）。因此，针对肿瘤微环境治疗，对于预防存在药物抵抗的肿瘤细胞的微小残留至为重要。另外，这些治疗策略在肿瘤进展哪个阶段（如早期或者更晚期）更有效，也是需要探讨的。尽管如此，针对肿瘤微环境治疗策略的药物仍然是一个重要的方向。

（卢建红，刘灵芝　编）

参 考 文 献

Achenbach CJ, Buchanan AL, Cole SR et al (2014) HIV viremia and incidence of non-Hodgkin lymphoma in patients successfully treated with antiretroviral therapy. Clinical Infectious Diseases 58:1599-1608

Ahmed W, Philip PS, Tariq S, Khan G (2014) Epstein-Barr virus-encoded small RNAs (EBERs) are present in fractions related to exosomes released by EBV-transformed cells.Plos one 9:e99163

Allison RD, Tong X, Moorman AC et al (2015) Increased Incidence of Cancer and Cancer-related Mortality Among Persons with Chronic Hepatitis C Infection, 2006-2010. Journal of hepatology 63: 822–828

Altekruse SF, McGlynn KA, Reichman ME (2009) Hepatocellular carcinoma incidence, mortality, and survival trends in the United States from 1975 to 2005. Journal of clinical oncology 27: 1485–1491

Benzoubir N, Lejamtel C, Battaglia S et al (2013) HCV core-mediated activation of latent TGF-β via thrombospondin drives the crosstalk between hepatocytes and stromal environment. Journal of hepatolog 59: 1160-1168

Bühler S, Bartenschlager R (2012) Promotion of hepatocellular carcinoma by hepatitis C virus. Digestive diseases 30: 445-452

Carbone A, Gloghini A (2013) Relationships between lymphomas linked to hepatitis C virus infection and their microenvironment. World journal of gastroenterology 19: 7874-7879

Ceccarelli S, Visco V, Raffa S, Wakisaka N, Pagano JS, Torrisi MR (2007) Epstein‐Barr virus latent membrane protein 1 promotes concentration in multivesicular bodies of fibroblast growth factor 2 and its release through exosomes. International journal of cancer 121: 1494-1506

Chai EZ, Siveen KS, Shanmugam MK, Arfuso F, Sethi G (2015) Analysis of the intricate relationship between chronic inflammation and cancer." Biochem Journal 468: 1–15

Chanmee T, Ontong P, Konno K, Itano N (2014) Tumor-associated macrophages as major players in the tumor microenvironment. Cancers 6: 1670-1690

Chen C-J, Yang H-I, Su J et al (2006) Risk of hepatocellular carcinoma across a biological gradient of serum hepatitis B virus DNA level. Jama 295: 65-73

Chen C-J, Iloeje UH, Yang H-I (2007) Long-term outcomes in hepatitis B: the REVEAL-HBV study. Clinics in liver disease 11: 797-816

Cheng H, Zhang L, Cogdell DE et al (2011) Circulating plasma MiR-141 is a novel biomarker for metastatic colon cancer and predicts poor prognosis. PloS one 6: e17745

De Paoli P, Carbone A (2015) Microenvironmental abnormalities induced by viral cooperation: Impact on lymphomagenesis. Seminars in cancer biology [doi:10.1016/j.semcancer.2015.03.009]

Dolcetti R (2015) In Cross-talk between Epstein-Barr virus and microenvironment in the pathogenesis of lymphomas. Seminars in cancer biology [doi: 10.1016/j.semcancer. 2015.04. 006]

Dolcetti R, Dal Col J, Martorelli D, Carbone A, Klein E (2013) Interplay among viral antigens, cellular pathways and tumor microenvironment in the pathogenesis of EBV-driven lymphomas. Seminars in cancer biology 23: pp 441-456

Duan Y, Jia Y, Wang T, Wang Y, Han X, Liu L (2015) Potent therapeutic target of inflammation, virus and tumor: focus on interleukin-27. International immunopharmacology 26: 139-146

Fang H, DeClerck YA (2013) Targeting the tumor microenvironment: from understanding pathways to effective clinical trials. Cancer research 73: 4965-4977

Ferlay J, Soerjomataram I, Ervik M, Dikshit R, Eser S, Mathers C (2013) Globocan 2012 v1. 0, Cancer Incidence and Mortality Worldwide: IARC CancerBase No. 11 [documento en internet]. Lyon, France: International Agency for Research on Cancer

Gagliani N, Hu B, Huber S, Elinav E, Flavell RA (2014) The fire within: microbes inflame tumors. Cell 157: 776-783

Galli SJ, Maurer M, Lantz CS (1999) Mast cells as sentinels of innate immunity. Current opinion in immunology 11: 53-59

Grivennikov SI, Greten FR, Karin M (2010) Immunity, inflammation, and cancer. Cell 140: 883-899

Hermine O, Lefrère F, Bronowicki J-P et al (2002) Regression of splenic lymphoma with villous lymphocytes after treatment of hepatitis C virus infection. New England Journal of Medicine 347: 89-94

Irshad M, Dhar I (2006) Hepatitis C virus core protein: an update on its molecular biology, cellular functions and clinical implications. Medical Principles and Practice 15: 405-416

Jemal A, Bray F, Center MM, Ferlay J, Ward E, Forman D (2011) Global cancer statistics. CA: a cancer journal for clinicians 61: 69-90

Justus CR, Sanderlin EJ, Yang LV (2015) Molecular Connections between Cancer Cell Metabolism and the Tumor Microenvironment. International journal of molecular sciences 16: 11055-11086

Kawaguchi T, Komatsu S, Ichikawa D et al (2013) Clinical impact of circulating miR-221 in plasma of patients with pancreatic cancer. British journal of cancer 108: 361-369

Knoll P, Schlaak J, Uhrig A, Kempf P, zum Büschenfelde K-HM, Gerken G (1995) Human Kupffer cells secrete IL-10 in response to lipopolysaccharide (LPS) challenge. Journal of hepatology 22: 226-229

Labiano S Palazon A and Melero I (2015) In Immune Response Regulation in the Tumor Microenvironment by Hypoxia. Seminars in oncology 42:378-386

LaMonte G, Tang X, Chen J et al (2013) Acidosis induces reprogramming of cellular metabolism to mitigate oxidative stress. Cancer Metab 1: 23

Li YX, Zhang L, Simayi D et al (2015) Human Papillomavirus Infection Correlates with Inflammatory Stat3 Signaling Activity and IL-17 Level in Patients with Colorectal Cancer. PloS one 10: e0118391

Meads MB, Gatenby RA, Dalton WS (2009) Environment-mediated drug resistance: a major contributor to minimal residual disease. Nature Reviews Cancer 9: 665-674

Mildner A, Jung S (2014) Development and function of dendritic cell subsets. Immunity 40: 642-656

Nasser MW, Elbaz M, Ahirwar DK, Ganju RK (2015) Conditioning solid tumor microenvironment through inflammatory chemokines and S100 family proteins. Cancer letters 365:11-22

Ohnishi S, Ma N, Thanan R et al (2013) DNA damage in inflammation-related carcinogenesis and cancer stem cells. Oxidative medicine and cellular longevity 2013: 387014

Paget S (1889) The distribution of secondary growths in cancer of the breast. Cancer metastasis reviews 8: 98

Perz JF, Armstrong GL, Farrington LA, Hutin YJ, Bell BP (2006) The contributions of hepatitis B virus and hepatitis C virus infections to cirrhosis and primary liver cancer worldwide. Journal of hepatology 45: 529-538

Peveling-Oberhag J, Arcaini L, Hansmann M-L, Zeuzem S (2013) Hepatitis C-associated B-cell non-Hodgkin lymphomas. Epidemiology, molecular signature and clinical management. Journal of hepatology 59: 169-177

Portolani N, Coniglio A, Ghidoni S et al (2006) Early and late recurrence after liver resection for hepatocellular carcinoma: prognostic and therapeutic implications. Annals of surgery 243: 229-235

Rakoff-Nahoum S, Medzhitov R (2009) Toll-like receptors and cancer. Nature Reviews Cancer 9: 57-63

Raposo T, Beirão B, Pang L, Queiroga F, Argyle D (2015) Inflammation and cancer: Till death tears them apart. The Veterinary Journal 9:161-174

Rickinson A (2014) Co-infections, inflammation and oncogenesis: future directions for EBV research. Seminars in cancer biology 26:99-115

Roth C, Rack B, Müller V, Janni W, Pantel K, Schwarzenbach H (2010) Circulating microRNAs as blood-based markers for patients with primary and metastatic breast cancer. Breast Cancer Research 12: R90

Schwartzenberg-Bar-Yoseph F, Armoni M, Karnieli E (2004) The tumor suppressor p53 down-regulates glucose transporters GLUT1 and GLUT4 gene expression. Cancer research 64: 2627-2633

Scott DW, Gascoyne RD (2014) The tumour microenvironment in B cell lymphomas. Nature Reviews Cancer 14:517-534

Shain K, Dalton W, Tao J (2015) The tumor microenvironment shapes hallmarks of mature B-cell malignancies. Oncogene 34:4673-4682

Shelburne CP, Nakano H, John ALS et al (2009) Mast cells augment adaptive immunity by orchestrating dendritic cell trafficking through infected tissues. Cell host & microbe 6: 331-342

Shi Y, Song Q, Hu D, Zhuang X, Yu S (2015) Tumor-infiltrating lymphocyte activity is enhanced in tumors with low IL-10 production in HBV-induced hepatocellular carcinoma. Biochemical and biophysical research communications 461: 109-114

Shurin MR, Potapovich AI, Tyurina YY, Tourkova IL, Shurin GV, Kagan VE (2009) Recognition of live phosphatidylserine-labeled tumor cells by dendritic cells: a novel approach to immunotherapy of skin cancer. Cancer research 69: 2487-2496

Song N, Li T, Zhang XM (2014) Immune Cells in Tumor Microenvironment. Progress in Biochemistry and Biophysics 41: 1075-1084

Staller P, Sulitkova J, Lisztwan J, Moch H, Oakeley EJ, Krek W (2003) Chemokine receptor CXCR4 downregulated by von Hippel–Lindau tumour suppressor pVHL. Nature 425: 307-311

Steinman RM, Banchereau J (2007) Taking dendritic cells into medicine. Nature 449: 419-426

Stone SC, Rossetti RAM, Lima AM, Lepique AP (2014) HPV associated tumor cells control tumor microenvironment and leukocytosis in experimental models. Immunity, Inflammation and Disease 2: 63-75

Tang MK, Wong AS (2015) Exosomes: Emerging biomarkers and targets for ovarian cancer. Cancer letters 367: 26-33

Taylor JG, Liapis K, Gribben JG (2015) The role of the tumor microenvironment in HIV-associated lymphomas 9:473-482

Vacca A, Ribatti D, Iurlaro M et al (1998) Human lymphoblastoid cells produce extracellular matrix-degrading enzymes and induce endothelial cell proliferation, migration, morphogenesis, and angiogenesis. International Journal of Clinical and Laboratory Research 28: 55-68

Vincenza CM, Mangino G, Simona ZM et al (2015) Role of the Microenvironment in Tumourigenesis: Focus on Virus-Induced Tumors. Current medicinal chemistry 22: 958-974

Wang Z, Luo F, Li L et al (2010) STAT3 activation induced by Epstein-Barr virus latent membrane protein1 causes vascular endothelial growth factor expression and cellular invasiveness via JAK3 And ERK signaling. European journal of cancer 46: 2996-3006

Waris G, Ahsan H (2006) Reactive oxygen species: role in the development of cancer and various chronic conditions. Journal of carcinogenesis 5: 14

Webber J, Yeung V, Clayton A (2015) In Extracellular vesicles as modulators of the cancer microenvironment. Seminars in cell & developmental biology 40:27-34

Yang JD, Roberts LR (2010) Hepatocellular carcinoma: a global view. Nature Reviews Gastroenterology and Hepatology 7: 448-458

Yang P, Li Q J, Feng Y et al (2012) TGF-β-miR-34a-CCL22 signaling-induced Treg cell recruitment promotes venous metastases of HBV-positive hepatocellular carcinoma. Cancer cell 22: 291-303

Yang P, Markowitz GJ, Wang X F (2014) The hepatitis B virus-associated tumor microenvironment in hepatocellular carcinoma. National science review 1: 396-412

Yu H, Pardoll D, Jove R (2009) STATs in cancer inflammation and immunity: a leading role for STAT3. Nature Reviews Cancer 9: 798-809

Zhang C, Lin M, Wu R et al (2011) Parkin, a p53 target gene, mediates the role of p53 in glucose metabolism and the Warburg effect. Proceedings of the National Academy of Sciences 108: 16259-16264

Zhang Y, Yang P, Wang X F (2014) Microenvironmental regulation of cancer metastasis by miRNAs. Trends in cell biology 24: 153-160

Zheng D, Haddadin S, Wang Y et al (2011) Plasma microRNAs as novel biomarkers for early detection of lung cancer. International journal of clinical and experimental pathology 4: 575-588

第 5 章 EB 病毒的致瘤作用

摘　要　EB 病毒（Epstein-Barr virus，EBV）与多种人类淋巴细胞、上皮细胞起源的恶性肿瘤和疾病相关，包括鼻咽癌、胃癌、霍奇金淋巴瘤、伯基特淋巴瘤、AIDS 相关性淋巴瘤及移植后淋巴组织增生性疾病（PTLD）等。在免疫功能齐全的患者中，EB 病毒具有潜在的高致瘤性，是引发侵袭性肿瘤的病因，每年新增病例约 20 万。目前，EB 病毒的致瘤机制尚不十分清楚，但是已经明确 EBV 潜伏感染基因组的存在和病毒量在相关肿瘤的发生发展中起重要作用。潜伏膜蛋白 1（LMP1）是 EBV 的癌蛋白，在 EBV 的致病作用中扮演重要角色。EBV 通过编码或诱导细胞 microRNA 的异常表达是 EBV 发挥致瘤作用的一个重要表现。

关键词　EB 病毒，鼻咽癌，B 细胞淋巴瘤，癌症，潜伏膜蛋白 1

1　引言

EB 病毒（EBV）属于 γ 疱疹病毒家族成员，是第一个被发现对人类致癌的病毒（Schiller and Lowy 2010）。1964 年，EBV 由 Michael Epstein 和 Yvonne Barr 从伯基特（Burkitt's）淋巴瘤来源的细胞中通过电镜首次发现（Epstein and Barr 1964）。全球每年有超过二十多万新发肿瘤病例与 EBV 感染有关。EBV 相关性肿瘤也可以由于免疫缺陷造成，如移植后淋巴组织增生性疾病（PTLD）和艾滋病（AIDS）相关性淋巴瘤。在非免疫缺陷的患者中，EBV 的高致瘤性潜能可以引起严重的肿瘤，如胃癌、鼻咽癌、伯基特淋巴瘤和霍奇金（Hodgkin's）恶性淋巴瘤。

EBV 普遍存在，它会感染超过 90%的未成年人群（Steven 1997；Cohen 1999）。原发感染经常发生在儿童早期，表现为无症状的或者表现轻微的非特异性症状。在青少年和年轻成人中，EBV 感染与传染性单核细胞增多症（IM）有关，IM 的症状通常被描述为对病毒免疫反应的结果。EBV 的自然感染过程中的第一步是裂解期，主要感染口咽部的上皮细胞，由于病毒复制而导致新病毒的产生和受感染细胞的死亡。原发感染之后，EBV 的裂解复制在健康的携带者中通常是不活跃的，但是在某些条件下（如免疫抑制）可能会重新活化。伴随着病毒裂解复制期，B 淋巴细胞中的潜伏感染则会促进终身感染，导致 EBV 感染的 B 淋巴母细胞的形成。在 B 淋巴母细胞中，EBV 基因组以附加体形式整合至宿主基因组，并随宿主细胞的复制而增殖。早期受感染母细胞的扩增对于病毒存活可能是很重要的。潜伏的EBV具有很复杂的生存策略，这包括：①合成可以转化人类细胞或抑制抗原加工的病毒蛋白；②分泌细胞因子和可溶性受体，从而抵制细胞毒性细胞免疫；③下调自身的基因表达水平（Liebowitz 1998；Rickinson 1998；Cohen 1999）。在这种潜伏途径中，EBV是一种具有潜在转化能力的病毒，它的致癌作用与它逃避免疫监视的能力密切相关（Schiller and Lowy 2010；Okano and Gross 2012）。然而，只有少数具有免疫功能的EBV感染个体会发生肿瘤，这个事实说明单独的感染不足以致瘤，还有其他的因素起作用（遗传的、表观遗传的、环境因素及病毒载量等）。最后，一些受EBV感染的B淋巴母细胞会分化为记忆B细胞，后者不再呈现更多的病毒特异性抗原，从而无细胞免疫发生，这时就建立了EBV的最终保存库（Steven 1997）。

关于EBV感染与相关性肿瘤的流行病学、与炎症和微环境的关系等方面，在前面章节有涉及，其中的一些内容本章不再赘述。

2　EB病毒的感染与复制

EBV与多种人类恶性肿瘤相关，主要有上皮肿瘤和淋巴瘤，而EBV相关的上皮肿瘤占据了EBV相关恶性肿瘤的80%（Cohen et al. 2011）。在EBV相关上皮肿瘤中，几乎每个细胞都可以检测到EBV基因组及一部分潜伏基因的表达产物，因此，可以推测EBV在这些肿瘤的发生发展中扮演了重要角色。EBV主要通过人类宿主的唾液传播，它穿过口腔黏膜上皮细胞而感染B淋巴细胞，再通过一系列病毒潜伏转录程序使B淋巴细胞转变为静息的记忆B细胞，从而建立终生潜伏感染。当记忆B细胞分化为浆细胞时，可引起EBV裂解性感染并释放病毒颗粒，释放的病毒颗粒可进一步感染口咽上皮细胞，从而促进病毒的复制及传播（Thorley-Lawson et al. 2013）。我们现在对EBV所了解的知识大部分都是通过研究类淋巴母细胞（LCL）而来的，它是在体外用EBV感染初始B淋巴细胞而获得的。EBV的原发感染通常发生在幼年时期，这种感染是无症状的，感染个体成为EBV的终生携带者。与此不同，若原发感染发生在青年期，则会引起30%~50%的感染个体发生传染性单核细胞增多症（IM），这是一种急性自限制性疾病（Young and Rickinson 2004），主要症状为发热或者持续数周的咽炎、淋巴结病、全身性不适等。

2.1　EB病毒的感染与进入细胞

EBV感染有潜伏感染和裂解感染两种形式。裂解感染可发生于舌咽部的B淋巴细胞和上皮细胞内，而潜伏感染主要存在于B淋巴细胞中。EBV在体内可感染完整的上皮细胞，原发感染在口咽部，之后通过上皮组织中的血管运输到达B淋巴细胞，并处于潜伏感染状态。裂解感染时，EBV 表达其全部基因组、扩增其DNA 并产生高滴度的子代病毒颗粒以进行新一轮的感染，最终杀死宿主细胞。而潜伏感染时，EBV 基因组以游离体 DNA 形式存在且只有部分基因表达，没有病毒颗粒的产生。在 EBV 相关的癌症中，大部分 EBV 都是以潜伏感染形式存在的。根据 EBV 潜伏基因表达的不同，主要将其分为 4 种潜伏感染模式（Kang and Kieff 2015）：0 型潜伏感染表达产物为 EBER，主要发生在静息记忆 B 细胞中，即健康的携带者当中；Ⅰ型潜伏感染表达产物有 EBNA1、EBER 和 BART，主要出现在伯基特淋巴瘤（BL）中；Ⅱ型潜伏感染表达产物有 EBNA1、EBER、LMP 和 BART，主要出现在霍奇金病（HD）、自然杀伤 T 细胞淋巴瘤、鼻咽癌和胃癌当中；Ⅲ型潜伏感染表达 6 种核抗原（EBNA1、EBNA2、EBNA3A、EBNA3B、EBNA3C 和 LP）、3 种潜伏膜蛋白（LMP1、LMP 2A 和 LMP2B）和 2 种 EBER（EBER1 和 EBER2），主要出现在 PTLD、潜伏感染的类淋巴母细胞（LCL）和艾滋病相关性淋巴瘤。

免疫力低下人群的 EBV 感染通常会导致较严重疾病的发生。PTLD 是实体器官和造血干细胞移植后发生的最严重的并发症（Petrara et al. 2015），是移植后因免疫功能障碍导致从多克隆增生到非霍奇金淋巴瘤的一种疾病（Hao et al. 2013）。目前已经明确，引起移植后淋巴瘤的主要原因是免疫抑制和 EBV 的感染。一般情况下，EBV 感染的 B 细胞受控于细胞毒 T 细胞（Nowakowska et al. 2015），此时 B 细胞的生长和死亡处于平衡状态。PTLD 大多是移植后患者在长期的免疫抑制状态下，EBV 诱导 B 细胞增殖而发生的。在这个过程中，EBV 编码的 LMP1 蛋白通过激活宿主细胞的肿瘤坏死因子家族成员而导致 B 细胞的生长和转化。系统性红斑狼疮（SLE）是一种多发于青年女性、累及多脏器的自身免疫性炎症性结缔组织病。许多研究都将 SLE 的发生发展与 EBV 关联起来。SLE 患者外周血单核细胞中的病毒量是正常人的 10~40 倍之多（Yu et al. 2005），而且有 42%的 SLE 患者血清中发现 EBV DNA 的升高，而在健康对照中只有 3%的升高（Lu et al. 2007）。在 SLE 患者中还发现部分病毒 mRNA 的异常高表达，这些 mRNA 主要表达 BZLF1、gp350、病毒 IL10、LMP1、LMP2 和 EBNA1 蛋白，而这些蛋白质的表达意味着 EBV 的激活、被感染 B 细胞的扩增、免疫逃逸能力的增强、感染细胞生存能力的增强等（Poole et al. 2009）。此外，SLE 患者中的 IgG、IgA 等抗体水平的升高及细胞介导的免疫力下降，都说明 SLE 患者对 EBV 持续激活的控制能力下降（Draborg et al. 2013）。艾滋病是由于人体感染人类免疫缺陷病毒（HIV）后造成机体免疫功能严重受损而引起的。与 HIV/AIDS 相关的淋巴瘤称为 AIDS 相关性淋巴瘤（AIDS-related lymphoma，ARL）。有研究表明，ARL 与 EBV 的感染相关，ARL 样本的全转录组测序也检测到了 EBV 的存在（Arvey et al. 2015），可见 EBV 在 ARL 中扮演重要角色，其具体的机制仍有待进一步的阐明。

EBV 优先感染 B 淋巴细胞。人们对于 EBV 在 B 淋巴细胞内的生活周期已经有了很好的了解，但对于其在上皮细胞内的生活周期却知之甚少，这是因为在体外 EBV 能有效地感染 B 淋巴细胞，但是却很难感染上皮细胞。上皮细胞是一种复层结构，在体外很难模拟出相似的生长环境，但也有研究者在体外成功培养了角质细胞的复层上皮，继而用 EBV 感染，结果发现 EBV 仅能感染复层上皮的基底上层，并且能够进行有效的复制（Temple et al. 2014）。EB 病毒有效地进入 B 淋巴细胞至少需要 5 种病毒包膜糖蛋白和 3 种细胞蛋白。首先，EBV 包膜糖蛋白 gp350 与 B 细胞表面受体 CR2 或称 CD21（the complement receptor type 2）相互作用，从而使 EBV 附着于 B 细胞表面。再通过 EBV 糖蛋白 gB、gH 和 gL 的作用，使包膜与细胞膜融合，随后，通过胞吞作用使 EBV 进入一个较低 pH 的环境。gB 和 gH 都是膜锚定蛋白，而 gL 仅有一个断裂的信号肽。EBV 进入 B 细胞还需要病毒糖蛋白 gp42 的作用，gp42 能直接结合 gH，使二聚体 gHgL 转变为 gHgLgp42 三聚体复合物。gp42 还能与人类白细胞抗原 II（HLA II）相互作用，并且这种相互作用可以活化膜融合过程。上皮细胞表面由于缺乏 CR2 受体和 HLA II，在体外也很难建立 EBV 感染的上皮细胞系，因此，对于 EBV 进入上皮细胞的机制并不十分清楚。研究表明，EB 病毒的 gHgL 复合物可与上皮细胞的整合素复合物（αvβ6 和 αvβ8）相互作用，从而引起 EBV 包膜蛋白与细胞膜的融合，促进病毒的穿入（Hutt-Fletcher 2007）。中山大学的研究发现，在鼻咽癌组织和细胞系中癌蛋白 Bim-1 表达异常，而且 Bim-1 的高表达与鼻咽癌患者不良预后相关。通过过表达 Bim-1 永生化原代人鼻咽上皮细胞，建立由机体本身基因表达异常而永生化的细胞系，为研究鼻咽癌发病机制提供了较好的研究模型（Song et al. 2006）。最近发现，宿主非肌性肌球蛋白重链 IIA 能够在体外和体内环境下，与 EBV 病毒的 gHgL 结合，发生相互作用，介导 EBV 感染鼻咽上皮细胞（Xiong et al. 2015）。EBV 糖蛋白 gB 在 EBV 感染 B 细胞和上皮细胞过程中，是一个非常关键的融合蛋白，决定 EBV 对非 B 细胞的易感性。神经纤维蛋白 1（neuropilin 1，NRP1）能够与 EBVgB 结合，并介导 EBV 活化的 EGFR / RAS / ERK 信号通路，以及 NRP1 依赖受体酪氨酸激酶（RTK）信号通路，促进 EBV 的感染。但是，NRP2 和 NRP1 同源物不能促进 EBV 感染鼻咽上皮细胞（Wang et al. 2015）。Gp42 通过干扰与 gHgL 复合物的结合而阻止 EBV 进入上皮细胞。有趣的是，上皮细胞释放的 EB 病毒颗粒富含 gp42，可以促进 B 细胞的感染却不能促进上皮细胞的感染。相反，B 细胞释放的 EB 病毒颗粒缺乏 gp42，能够促进它们感染上皮细胞。这种双重细胞趋性暗示在 EBV 感染周期中，EB 病毒不断地在 B 细胞与上皮细胞之间穿梭，这对于 EBV 在人类中持续感染的建立可能是非常重要的（Tsao et al. 2015）。

EB 病毒侵入上皮细胞要比侵入 B 淋巴细胞复杂得多，这是由于绝大多数上皮细胞缺少 B 淋巴细胞表面受体 CR2，病毒不能与上皮细胞直接结合。EB 病毒可能主要通过三种模式进入上皮细胞：①EBV 经感染的 B 淋巴细胞或朗格汉斯细胞直接接触上皮细胞介导、通过 cell-to-cell 方式"转移感染"进入上皮细胞；②EBV 利用自身的相关蛋白与宿主相应的受体蛋白相结合后，通过膜的融合或内吞作用，感染上皮细胞；③感染 EBV 的上皮细胞经基底膜将病毒颗粒传递给邻近的细胞。在体外，EBV 也可通过 B 淋巴细胞等的介导作用而"转移感染"上皮细胞。有研究表明，将上皮细胞与 EBV 阳性的 Akata 细胞共培养可使上皮细胞成功地感染 EBV，并且感染效率要比单纯用 EBV 上清高得多（Imai et al. 1998）。最近有报道，淋巴细胞还可以通过 cell-in-cell 的方式感染上皮细胞（Ni et al. 2015）。本文作者在实验中尝试过这些感染方式，似乎并不是高效的，也许体外还受到各种条件的限制。作者也成功构建了含 EBV 全基因组的 293 细胞系，再通过共转 BZLF1、BALF4 两种质粒诱导 293 稳转的细胞系发生裂解性复制，从而产生感染性 EB 病毒颗粒；通过 B 淋巴细胞的介导作用使 EBV 病毒颗粒"转移感染"至鼻咽癌上皮细胞（Lu et al. 2010；Yu et al. 2012）。有研究表明，EBV 还可通过郎格汉斯细胞而感染上皮细胞（Walling et al. 2007）。郎格汉斯细胞是一种树突状抗原提呈细胞，分布在皮肤和黏膜上皮的基底层。骨髓来源的郎格汉斯细胞前体在血液循环的过程中能够迁移至上皮，并分化为郎格汉斯细胞。部分郎格汉斯细胞前体能够表达 CR2，在血液循环过程中，若受到 EBV 潜伏感染，则作为 EBV 的一种运输工具，使 EBV 随其迁移至上皮，分化为 EBV 感染的成熟郎格汉斯细胞。而这种细胞的触角存在于上皮组织中，当 EBV 裂解复制时，病毒颗粒能够与 CR2 阳性的上皮细胞结合，或者利用这些触角与周围上皮细胞接触，类似于 B 淋巴细胞，再通过内吞作用而侵入上皮细胞（Zuo et al. 2014）。

2.2 EB 病毒的主要编码产物

EBV 基因组很大，约 172kb，包含近 100 个基因，编码 200 多种蛋白质，但大多数基因的功能还不清楚。以下介绍几种 EBV 编码的、对其功能了解较多的潜伏期产物。

EBV 编码的核抗原 1（EBNA1）是唯一在所有 EBV 相关肿瘤中都表达的 EB 病毒潜伏蛋白。EBNA1 对于 EBV 病毒基因组 DNA 以附加体形式存在于细胞内及其复制至关重要，它通过其 DNA 结合活性与潜伏期 EB 病毒的复制原点 oriP 结合而发挥功能。在鼻咽癌和胃癌中，EBNA1 可诱导早幼粒白血病蛋白核体（PML nuclear body）的丢失、p53 活化降低，以及 DNA 损伤过程中减少凋亡（Sivachandran et al. 2012）。EBNA1 还可以诱导 let-7 microRNA 家族的表达，反过来可以降低 Dicer 酶的表达水平、抑制潜伏 EBV 的活化，可能增强转移的能力（Mansouri et al. 2014）。EBNA1 与宿主细胞染色体也有关联，以确保在细胞有丝分裂时 EB 病毒基因组得到复制和维持（Marechal et al. 1999）。EBNA1 既能作为转录激活因子激活其他的 EBV 潜伏基因的表达，又能作为一个负性调控因子抑制其自身的转录。用 EBNA1 的 DNA 反义寡核苷酸可以抑制 EBV 永生化细胞的增殖，而 EBNA1 的转基因鼠可诱发产生淋巴瘤，这些都说明 EBNA1 参与了 EBV 相关肿瘤的肿瘤发生过程（Wilson et al. 1996）。然而，另一个研究组报道他们的 EBNA1 转基因鼠并没有罹患淋巴瘤（Kang et al. 2005）。因此，是否能以转基因鼠为模式生物研究 EBNA1 的致瘤潜能仍具有争议。

EBV 感染 B 细胞后，EBNA2 和 EBNA-LP 很快共表达于细胞中（Alfieri et al. 1991），这两种蛋白质对于 EBV 高效地转化原代 B 淋巴细胞至类淋巴母细胞（LCL）是必需的。在 BL 和 P3HR1 细胞系中，EBV 基因组有一段包含 EBNA2 编码序列的区域缺失，这种突变使 EBV 失去了将原代 B 淋巴细胞转化成 LCL 的功能，但重新引入缺失的 DNA 片段可使转化功能得到恢复（Cohen et al. 1989）。EBNA-LP 和 EBNA2 共激活 EBNA2 调控的病毒基因启动子，如 Cp 和 LMP1 启动子。EBNA2 既可作为病毒基因的转录激活因子，又可作为宿主细胞基因的转录激活因子，它是通过反式激活其靶基因而不是直接结合相应的 DNA 元件而发挥作用的。LP 和 EBNA2 都可以与 cMyc 及 cMyc 调控基因的上游 DNA 元件结合，最终可导致细胞进入细胞周期而增殖（Portal et al. 2013）。

EBNA3A、EBNA3B 和 EBNA3C 属于同一基因家族，它们有相同的基因结构和部分同源的氨基酸序列。在三种 EBNA3 蛋白中，EBNA3A 和 EBNA3C 对于体外初始 B 淋巴细胞的转化是必需的，EBNA3A 和 EBNA3B 能够抑制促凋亡的肿瘤抑制基因（Bim）的表达（Anderton et al. 2008）。EBNA3 通过它的相互作用蛋白 RBP-JK/CBF1 而扮演转录抑制因子的角色。EBNA3 和 EBNA2 在 RBP-JK/CBF1 上有相同的结合位点，并且 EBNA3 可以抑制由 EBNA2 介导的潜伏启动子 Cp 的活化。在 LCL 中，所有 EBNA 的转录起始都是以 Cp 作为启动子的，因此，EBNA3 可能以负性调控的方式发挥作用。与这一观点相符的是，EBNA3A、EBNA3C 可与组蛋白去乙酰化酶和转录共抑制因子 CtBP（在转录水平上可使活性染色质逆转为沉默状态）相互作用。要阐明 EBNA3 和 CtBP 转录复合物的靶基因，还需要进一步的研究。

在过去的二三十年中，许多研究都表明潜伏膜蛋白 1（latent membrane protein 1，LMP1）是 EB 病毒的一个重要癌蛋白。LMP1 可诱导啮齿动物细胞发生锚定非依赖性生长（anchorage-independent growth），它对于 B 淋巴细胞的转化是必需的。无论是在体外还是动物模型中，它的表达与细胞增殖、抗凋亡和转化有关。LMP1 在 EBV 潜伏 II 和 III 期能被检测到，而且它与人类恶性肿瘤有非常密切的联系，包括 NPC、HD、PTLD 和 NHL（非霍奇金淋巴瘤）。在鼻咽癌（NPC）活检组织中，LMP1 的表达水平与肿瘤进程是相关的，如增强的侵袭与转移、DNA 甲基转移酶活性增强、黏附分子的下调等。总之，LMP1 的存在增加了细胞的转化能力，同时也提高了肿瘤的生存能力。LMP1 定位在脂筏或细胞膜上，它模拟肿瘤坏死因子受体（TNFR）家族成员的功能，包括 TNFR1 和 CD40，虽然它们几乎没有氨基酸同源序列。TNFR1 和 CD40 的激活需要配体的结合，而 LMP1 扮演的是不依赖于配体结合或调节的持续激活的受体样分子的角色。LMP1 可通过介导 NF-κB、p38/MAPK、JNK、JAK3、PI3K 等信号通路的活化而促进细胞的转化和肿瘤的发生。LMP1 还可以在转录和翻译水平上通过激活细胞 DNA 甲基转移酶而诱导上皮钙黏蛋白基因启动子的甲基化。近年来，LMP1 与肿瘤侵袭转移的关系也受到关注（Zhao et al. 2012）。LMP1 可通过诱导鼻咽癌细胞中 miR-10b 的过表达促进 NPC 的侵袭转移（Li et al. 2010；Allaya et al. 2015）。

LMP2 基因利用两种不同的启动子而编码两种 mRNA，结果是产生两种蛋白质——LMP2A 和 LMP2B。LMP2A 对于 EBV 潜伏状态的建立和维持，以及 EBV 相关疾病的发展是必需的，它在病毒相关肿瘤中是最广泛表达的 EBV 蛋白。过表达 LMP2A 能促进上皮细胞的转化、侵袭、迁移，能促进裸鼠的肿瘤形成能力，这些都表明 LMP2A 在 EBV 相关肿瘤形成中起着关键作用。LMP2B 被证实与 LMP2A 共存于细胞膜上，它们的羧基端可以相互作用并能调节彼此之间的活性。LMP2B 能够阻止 LMP2A 的聚集（Rovedo and Longnecker 2007），提示其与 LMP2A 所发挥的功能可能是相反的。LMP2B 所发挥的功能可能是诱导细胞进入 EBV 裂解性感染。

在 EBV 潜伏感染的细胞当中，EBV 编码的、小的、非多聚腺苷酸化的非编码 RNA（EBER）是表达最丰富的病毒转录本（Rymo 1979），每个细胞约有 10^7 个拷贝数。因此，可以通过原位杂交检测组织细胞中是否存在 EBER 而判断是否存在 EBV 感染。前期研究表明，EBER 在 EBV 的致瘤过程中发挥作用，表现为 B 淋巴细胞中 EBER 的表达可诱导在软琼脂上的克隆形成、促进裸鼠的肿瘤形成（Ruf et al. 2000）、对凋亡诱导物产生抗性，以及诱导 *bcl-2* 基因的表达。EBER 还可以诱导多种细胞因子的转录，例如，在伯基特淋巴瘤细胞中诱导白细胞介素 10（IL-10）的转录表达，上皮细胞中的胰岛素样生长因子 1（IGF1），T 细胞中的白细胞介素 9（IL-9）等，这些细胞因子随后在 EBV 感染的癌细胞中扮演自分泌生长因子而发挥作用（Iwakiri et al. 2005）。

此外，EBV 还编码 microRNA，将在下文中讨论。

2.3 EB 病毒的复制

EB 病毒感染进入细胞后，其复制可根据感染形式不同而分为潜伏期与裂解期。OriP 是潜伏期 EB 病毒的复制原点，大小为 1.7kb。在潜伏期核蛋白 EBNA1 作用下，oriP 对病毒 DNA 以附加体形式存在于细胞内及其复制至关重要。OriP 由两个功能不同的部分组成，一个是 120 bp 的、被称为双联体对称（dyad symmetry，

DS）的区域，它是功能性的复制子，含有 4 个 EBNA1 结合位点；另一个是 20 个 30 bp 重复序列家族（family of repeats，FR），且每个重复序列都含有一个 EBNA1 的结合位点。FR 的基本功能是防止潜伏期病毒附加体在细胞有丝分裂过程中丢失。潜伏感染时，EB 病毒附加体 DNA 在一个细胞周期中只复制一次，说明 oriP 的复制起始是受真核染色体复制许可（replication licensing）机制控制的。裂解期 EB 病毒 DNA 的复制受到病毒编码的转录因子 BZLF1 控制（Hammerschmidt and Sugden 2013）。BZLF1 可引起细胞基因的链式反应，并且可激活病毒的裂解性复制原点 oriLyt。OriLyt 位于 BHLF1 启动子及其基因之间，其中有两个核心元件为 oriLyt 最小的功能序列，分别称为上游 ZRE 元件和下游 TD 元件。由于 BHLF1 启动子分散分布，因此 ZRE 几乎完全位于 BHLF1 启动子区域内。BZLF1 蛋白可特异性识别 ZRE 位点并与之结合，而 TD 是一些细胞转录因子如 Sp1 和 ZBP-89 的结合位置。在裂解性感染时，共有 6 种病毒蛋白通过形成聚合酶复合物参与其基因组 DNA 的复制：DNA 聚合酶活性的 BALF5、聚合酶加工因子 BMRF1、单链 DNA 结合蛋白 BALF2、触发酶 BSLF1、触发酶相关蛋白 BBLF2/3，以及解旋酶 BBLF4。在 oriLyt 原点内，经过一系列蛋白质与蛋白质、蛋白质与 DNA 的相互作用，可促进 EB 病毒裂解期 DNA 复制的进行。其中，Sp1 和 ZBP-89 结合到下游元件后，与 DNA 聚合酶复合物的催化亚基 BALF5 及 BMRF1 接触，而 4 个 BZLF1 通过结合上游元件与 DNA 聚合酶辅助因子（BMRF1）、解旋酶及触发酶相互作用，在复制原点处形成环形结构，使 DNA 的 θ 复制得以进行。

3 EBV 相关性肿瘤和疾病

3.1　EBV 与上皮性肿瘤

EBV 与上皮细胞来源的鼻咽癌（NPC）高度相关，近年来也发现少部分的胃癌和乳腺癌与 EBV 存在相关性。

3.1.1　EBV 与鼻咽癌

人们普遍认可的与 EB 病毒感染最相关的恶性肿瘤是未分化的鼻咽癌，在东南亚和北非地区，EB 病毒与几乎 100% 的鼻咽癌相关，在中国南方的某些地区，鼻咽癌的发生率为每 10 万人中有 15~50 例，每年有 7.2 万新发鼻咽癌病例（Chan et al. 2002；Raab-Traub 2002；de Martel et al. 2012）。在 EB 病毒感染的鼻咽癌细胞中，基因表达模式为 II 型潜伏感染模式，主要表达 EB 病毒核抗原 EBNA1、潜伏膜蛋白（LMP1、LMP2A、LMP2B），以及几种 EB 病毒非编码 RNA（主要是 EBER1 和 EBER2）（Young et al. 1988；Brooks et al. 1992；Sam et al. 1993）。然而，EB 病毒在鼻咽癌中的作用机制尚不十分清楚，已明确的是这些病毒蛋白均具有独特的致瘤性，并可能有助于恶性 NPC 细胞的生存。

鼻咽癌的发病病因学是多方面的，包括遗传易感性、EB 病毒感染、环境致癌物（腌鱼、蔬菜摄入量少、烟草）。在亚洲有超过 80%的人患鼻咽癌，男性高发，且 40~50 岁是高发年龄段（Cao et al. 2011；Lee et al. 2012；Lee et al. 2012）。这是一种高度恶性疾病，早期通过淋巴传播，并能向远处转移。现代化的生活方式使鼻咽癌发生率明显降低 50%，死亡率下降 60%。然而，一级预防依然很难，这是由于在发病之前的很长一段时间里患者一直没有明显症状，所以一级预防的主要目标是尽早诊断。患者在患病的早期阶段（I 期和 II 期）的五年生存率高达 94%，在 III 期和 IV 期的五年生存率却是 80%。EB 病毒血清学检测是鼻咽癌筛选的基础，病毒衣壳蛋白（VCA）-IgA 的检测敏感性和特异性高。血清学和组织病理学的检查表明，在肿瘤的整个发生过程，尤其是在低分化和未分化的 NPC 上皮肿瘤组织中，均能检测到 EBV 基因组的存在（Pegtel et al. 2007；Zeng et al. 2007）。进行其他的血清学检测亦能提高预测的准确性，如进行 EB 病毒核蛋白 1、早期抗原（EA）-IgA 的检测。

3.1.2 EBV 与胃癌

在世界范围内与 EB 病毒感染有关的最普遍的恶性肿瘤可能是胃癌。胃癌的总体发生率为每年 100 万，已经证实的这些胃癌患者中与 EB 病毒感染有关的约 10%（Murphy et al. 2009；Fukayama 2010）。已经证实，EB 病毒与发生在胃部的淋巴上皮样肿瘤相关（Lee et al. 2009）。这些恶性肿瘤所表现出来的形态学现象与鼻咽癌相似，在亚洲地区和美国部分地区高发。EB 病毒潜伏感染的胃癌细胞有两种类型：淋巴上皮样瘤和普通的胃癌，临床特征包括男性高发、胃底部位高发、在早期有较少的患者患有淋巴瘤、与 EB 病毒阴性的胃癌相比预后较好（Chang and Kim 2005；Murphy et al. 2009；Truong et al. 2009；Chen et al. 2012）。与 EB 病毒相关的胃癌在胃切除手术后剩余胃部的发作率达到 25%（33%是进行胃空肠吻合术，12%是胃与十二指肠吻合术），这将会成为预防的一部分（Fukayama and Ushiku 2011）。发病机理是多种致瘤基因启动子区域的甲基化，包括 EB 病毒 LMP2A。研究表观遗传修饰将会为更好地进行特异性预防与治疗做出贡献，正如近期的一个例证，用甲基化转移酶抑制剂对 WNT5A 的表达进行遗传修饰（Liu et al. 2013）。

目前胃癌的治疗主要依赖化疗和手术，对于 EB 病毒感染诱发的胃癌一般使用药物进行局部的化学治疗（5-氟二氧嘧啶和多西他赛），这在体外实验中得到证实（Shin et al. 2011；Liu et al. 2013）。化学疗法的一个作用就是导致 EB 病毒从潜伏感染到病毒裂解性复制的转变，服用抗病毒药物如更昔洛韦将会增强疗效（Zhao et al. 2012）。

3.1.3 EB 病毒与乳腺癌

乳腺癌在世界范围内均为高发、常见肿瘤,根据乳腺癌组织的基因表达情况,可对乳腺癌进行分子分型。乳腺癌的异质性与多种因素有关,如遗传因素、环境因素、激素分泌和病原体感染等,尽管不同的研究所得出的结论并不完全一致,病毒参与肿瘤发生的病因之一。EB 病毒与乳腺癌的关系在 20 世纪 90 年代中期就有报道(Labrecque et al. 1995),EB 病毒阳性乳腺癌的发生率与检测技术及靶向的病毒基因组区域的不同有关(Joshi and Buehring 2012)。病毒相关的乳腺癌患者预后较差(Tsai et al. 2007),尤其是同时感染多种病毒的临床患者样本。研究发现,EB 病毒阳性的乳腺癌的侵袭性更强(Fina et al. 2001;Mazouni et al. 2011),但是 EB 病毒的存在对乳腺癌预后方面的作用机制仍不清楚。也有研究显示,EB 病毒的存在对乳腺癌的预后并没有不利的影响。目前还不能清楚地定义 EB 病毒在乳腺癌中是否为促癌因子,EB 病毒的存在和其在 DNA 水平上的作用之间的联系还有待深入研究。

3.2 EBV 与淋巴瘤

3.2.1 EBV 与 B 细胞淋巴瘤

EB 病毒与 B 细胞恶性肿瘤相关,包括霍奇金(Hodgkin's)淋巴瘤、伯基特(Burkitt's)淋巴瘤、大 B 细胞淋巴瘤(Mesri et al. 2014)和地方性 NK/T 细胞淋巴瘤(Harabuchi et al. 2009)。约有 30%~50%的霍奇金淋巴瘤与 EB 病毒感染有关,在典型的霍奇金淋巴瘤中更流行。早期感染单核细胞增多症与霍奇金淋巴瘤发生的风险增加有关(Hjalgrim et al. 2003;Gandhi et al. 2004)。霍奇金淋巴瘤在这些 B 细胞淋巴瘤中是独特的,因为霍奇金淋巴瘤中恶性的霍奇金-里德-斯泰伯格细胞由不足 1%的炎症细胞组成,而其他细胞主要由淋巴细胞浸润组成。最近,在 EBV 阳性和 EBV 阴性的霍奇金淋巴瘤中的分子研究已经逐渐表明,EB 病毒在促进霍奇金淋巴瘤的发展中起作用,证明 EB 病毒可以促进霍奇金淋巴瘤中恶性的霍奇金-里德-斯泰伯格细胞的致瘤性,而霍奇金-里德-斯泰伯格细胞又可以使 EB 病毒阴性的霍奇金淋巴瘤发生遗传改变(Green et al. 2012)。

EBV 阳性的伯基特淋巴瘤是一种地方病,在大多数国家很少见,主要发生在非洲和巴布亚新几内亚,在这些地区 100%的伯基特淋巴瘤与 EB 病毒有关。伯基特淋巴瘤主要发生在儿童早期,偶发于疟疾感染流行期。伯基特淋巴瘤与疟疾共流行的特性有助于慢性疟疾感染影响 EB 病毒特异的 T 细胞功能,促进感染 EB 病毒的 B 细胞的生长(Njie et al. 2009;Chattopadhyay et al. 2013)。伯基特淋巴瘤的基因表达谱主要为潜伏 I 型,即只有 EBNA1 的表达(Kelly et al. 2002)。对伯基特淋巴瘤和霍奇金淋巴瘤来说，预防主要依赖于早期诊断。根据疾病分期和危险因素，应该采取化学疗法和放射疗法进行治疗（Parker et al. 2010；Ansell 2012）。

EB 病毒阳性的大 B 细胞淋巴瘤是一种罕见的恶性肿瘤，发生在 50 岁以上的人群中。EB 病毒潜伏感染为 I 型或 II 型，通过检测某些大 B 细胞淋巴瘤患者的恶性细胞发现 EBNA2 和 EBNA3 的表达（Nguyen-Van et al. 2011；Liu et al. 2012；Ok et al. 2013）。与霍奇金淋巴瘤一样（Jarrett et al. 2005），EB 病毒阳性的大 B 细胞淋巴瘤的整体生存率比 EB 病毒阴性的大 B 细胞淋巴瘤的低（Park et al. 2007）。

3.2.2　EBV 与 AIDS 相关性淋巴瘤

AIDS 相关性淋巴瘤包括：①高度恶性淋巴瘤，主要为 Burkitt 淋巴瘤（BL）、弥漫性大 B 细胞淋巴瘤（DLBCL）；②罕见的淋巴瘤，如原发性渗出性淋巴瘤（PEL）、浆母细胞淋巴瘤（Carbone and Gloghini 2005）。尽管 HIV 感染的是 CD4 T 细胞，但至少 95%的 AIDS 相关淋巴瘤为 B 细胞来源，几乎所有的 B 细胞肿瘤均可见于 AIDS 患者。

AIDS 相关性淋巴瘤的发生是因为在 HIV 感染造成免疫抑制的情况下再感染了 EB 病毒（EBV），EBV 的致病作用在原发性中枢神经系统淋巴瘤中更为明确，它也可能与原发性渗出性淋巴瘤的发病有关。HHV-8 也被认为是原发性渗出性淋巴瘤重要的致病因子（Rohner et al. 2015）。许多 AIDS 相关的系统性淋巴瘤与 EBV 有关，并且两者的关联程度部分地与淋巴瘤组织的病理类型相关（Choi et al. 2015）。

在 AIDS 患者中，EBV 感染 B 淋巴细胞的发生率高可能与抗 EBV 的 T 细胞免疫功能缺乏有关。AIDS 患者发生淋巴瘤的危险性与 EBV 特异细胞毒 T 淋巴细胞的减少及感染 EBV 量增高呈正相关。免疫抑制和 EBV 感染容易使正在发生癌基因或抑癌基因改变的 B 细胞克隆增殖。在免疫母细胞性淋巴瘤中，这些基因包括 c-MYC 和 TCL1 癌基因。与没有发生淋巴瘤的 AIDS 患者比较，在 AIDS 相关的淋巴瘤患者中，血清可溶性 CD23（一种 B 细胞刺激因子）的水平明显升高，提示慢性 B 细胞刺激是诱导这类淋巴瘤的重要因素（Tsachouridou et al. 2015）。此外，HIV 能感染内皮细胞，从而增加了肿瘤性淋巴细胞与内皮细胞间的黏附性，使肿瘤细胞与内皮细胞产生的生长因子密切接触并加速肿瘤细胞的扩散。这是 AIDS 相关性淋巴瘤发生、发展和转移的另一重要因素（Lin et al. 2015）。

AIDS 患者发生非霍奇金淋巴瘤和霍奇金淋巴瘤的风险增加（Corti et al. 2014），尽管这些淋巴瘤的发病机理还不完全清楚，但是免疫力下降、遗传学改变、细胞因子产生在 HIV 相关性淋巴瘤的形成中发挥重要作用。淋巴瘤微环境对异质性淋巴瘤的形成、生长和发展起关键的作用。HIV 相关性淋巴瘤微环境的主要组分包括 EBV 和（或）HHV-8 同时感染、刺激炎症细胞的反应、肿瘤微血管生成和可溶性因子的产生。

3.3 EBV 与移植后淋巴组织增生性疾病

移植后淋巴组织增生性疾病（PTLD）发生在器官移植、骨髓干细胞移植后（Smets et al. 2000；Smets and Sokal 2002；Landgren et al. 2009；Gulley and Tang 2010；Reddy et al. 2011）。根据 2008 年世界卫生组织发布的数据（de Martel et al. 2012），PTLD 分为 4 类：早期病灶（浆细胞增生，IM）、多态性 PTLD、单态性 PTLD（B 细胞或 T 细胞淋巴瘤）和典型的霍奇金淋巴瘤样 PTLD（Campo et al. 2011）。早期病灶和多态性 PTLD 是很普遍的，经常发生在移植后的一年里，且大部分与 EBV 感染有关，然而单态性 PTLD 发生的较晚，且 EBV 阴性的患者达到 70%。发病率在不同发病类型和不同年龄有所不同，这暗示着潜在的致病机制和预后风险因素。在早期，免疫监督能力不足导致受 EBV 感染细胞的移植后淋巴组织增生。由于免疫抑制的影响，EBV 感染者在器官移植后不能发挥特异性免疫功能。进行骨髓干细胞移植后，在 T 细胞恢复免疫能力之前，PTLD 就发生了，随后，尽管免疫力足够强，但是由于病毒的免疫逃逸机制（抗原低表达基因突变和多态性）的存在，PTLD 依然能够发生。我们应该依据详细的肿瘤组织学进行诊断（包括淋巴细胞的类型、寻找单克隆性和 EBV 染色），根据临床表现进行体能状况的评价和疾病分期，临床表现包括放射学、骨髓和脑脊液检查等。

4 EBV 通过 microRNA 发挥致瘤作用

EBV 通过干扰细胞信号通路调控细胞的生长和存活，这在 EBV 与淋巴瘤等的发生中已有描述。近年来，microRNA（miRNA）的研究揭示了病毒致病作用的一些新机制。

miRNA 是一类 18~25nt 的非编码小 RNA 分子，能够抑制具有与其互补的序列的 mRNA 的表达，调控机体细胞增殖、分化、侵袭转移及病毒免疫逃逸等多种复杂的生命活动进程。包括肿瘤在内的多种疾病与 miRNA 的表达失调有关。EBV 不仅自身编码多种 miRNA 分子，如 miR-BART 和 miR-BHRF1（Klinke et al. 2014），还能诱导细胞内源性多种 miRNA 的异常表达。这些 miRNA 分子通过与下游各种不同的靶基因结合，以及 miRNA 之间间接或直接的相互作用，行使不同的生物学功能，影响肿瘤的发生发展（图 5-1）。

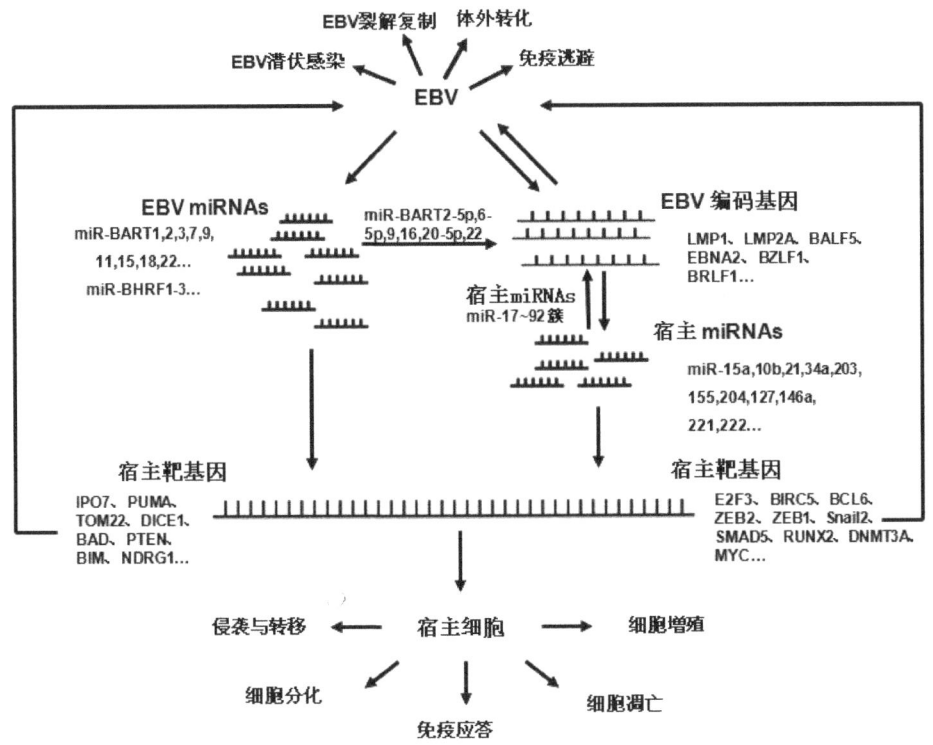

图 5-1　EBV 编码的 miRNA 与病毒诱导的 miRNA。EBV 编码的 miRNA 一方面可以直接作用于宿主细胞的靶基因；另一方面可以间接通过靶向 EBV 编码的病毒基因，诱导宿主 miRNAs 的表达，靶向宿主靶基因。通过这两种途径，miRNA 影响 EBV 本身潜伏感染、裂解复制、免疫逃逸和体外转化，以及影响宿主细胞增殖、分化、凋亡、侵袭转移等各个方面。此外，宿主 miRNA 分子也可以作用于 EBV 编码病毒基因。

4.1　EBV 编码的 miRNA

4.1.1　EBV miRNA 的分类

EBV 是鼻咽癌等恶性肿瘤的致病因子，其本身能够编码约 25 个前体 miRNA 分子。这些前体 miRNA 分子通过进一步剪切、加工，生成约 44 个成熟的 miRNA 分子行使不同的功能。EBV 编码的 miRNA 分子的基因主要定位于 BHRF1 的开放阅读框（miR-BHRF1）及 BART 区域（miR-BART），miR-BART 又分为 BART 簇 1 miRNA、BART 簇 2 miRNA 和 BART 2（图 5-2）。MiR-BHRF1 在 EBV 阳性的鼻咽癌、胃癌和伯基特淋巴瘤中，没有检测到 BHRF1 编码的 miRNA 分子，但能在 LCL 潜伏感染 III 型中检测到，如 miR-BHRF1-1 和 miR-BART1-5p 表达水平较高（Li et al. 2012）。但是 miR-BART 在几乎所有 EBV 相关肿瘤中都能检测到，且不同的 EBV 相关肿瘤，其 BART 区域表达的 miRNA 种类和表达水平是不一样的。在鼻咽癌中，EBV 编码的大多数 BART miRNA 分子，在鼻咽癌不同分期，表达水平不一样。在 LCL 中，缺乏 BART 簇 1 中 EBA-miR-BART15-3p，以及 BART 簇 2 中 EBA-BART18-3p、EBA-BART7-5p、EBA-BART9-5p、EBA-BART10-5p、EBA-BART10-3p、EBA-BART11-3p、EBA-BART20-5p、EBA-BART20-3p、EBA-BART13-5p 和 EBA-BART14-3p 的表达，miR-BART15-5p 和 miR-BART4-3p 处于低表达水平，而 miR-BART2-3p 处于低表达或不表达状态。

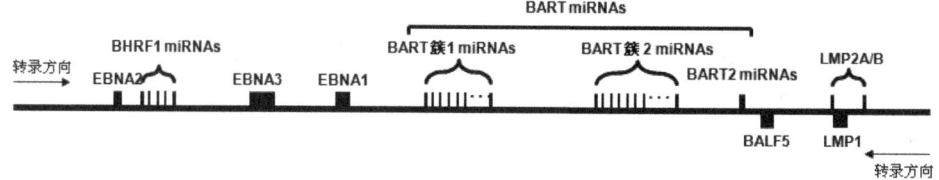

图 5-2 EBV miRNA 在病毒基因组的定位。EBV 编码的 miRNA 主要由两部分组成，一是 BHRF1 编码 3 个前体 miR-BHRF1-1、miR-BHRF1-2 和 miR-BHRF1-3，形成 4 个成熟 miRNA；二是 BART miRNA 分为 BART 簇 1 miRNA（编码 8 个 miRNA 前体）、BART 簇 2 miRNA（编码 13 个 miRNA 前体）和 BART 2。

4.1.2 EBV miRNA 作用的靶基因

4.1.2.1 EBV miRNA 靶向 EBV 编码基因

LMP1 癌蛋白是 EBV 编码的潜伏膜蛋白之一，能够活化多种信号通路，调控细胞增殖，抑制细胞凋亡，促进血管生成（Horikawa et al. 2001；Lo et al. 2004；Dawson et al. 2012）。LMP1 是 miR-BART1-5p、miR-BART9、miR-BART16、miR-BART17-5p 的靶基因，病毒编码的 miRNA 分子可以通过调节 LMP1 的表达，影响肿瘤的发生发展（Lo et al. 2007）。LMP2A 是病毒编码的另一种潜伏膜蛋白，通过调节 PI3K–AKT、RhoA 和 MAPK–ERK 信号通路，抑制细胞分化，促进细胞的存活（Scholle et al. 2000）。EBV-miR-BART22 的一个靶基因就是 LMP2A。miR-BART22 能够抑制 LMP2A 表达，保护 EBV 感染细胞不受免疫系统的攻击（Lung et al. 2009）。同时，miR-BART 分子可以抑制多种 EBV 裂解复制阶段基因，如 BZLF1、BRLF1、BALF5 的表达，促进 EBV 的潜伏感染，如 MiR-BART2-5p 能够抑制 BALF5 的表达（Barth et al. 2008）。

4.1.2.2　EBV miRNA 靶向宿主基因

miR-BART5 和 BART16 通过靶向促凋亡蛋白 PUMA、TOM22 和 BIM，抑制细胞凋亡（Choy et al. 2008）。miR-BART 分子可以保护 EBV 感染相关的癌变前或癌变后的上皮细胞免于机体免疫系统的识别与清除。MICB 能够通过活化 NK 细胞 CD8αβT 细胞、γT 细胞内的 NKG2D Ⅱ 型受体，启动免疫应答，清除感染细胞。miR-BART2-5p 抑制 MICB 的表达，使 EBV 感染的细胞不被识别或清除（Nachmani et al. 2009）。另外，EBV-miR-BART3 能够靶向入核受体 IPO7 的表达，削弱 IPO7 功能，有利于 EBV 的免疫逃避（Dolken et al. 2010）。在 293 细胞中，EBV-miR-BART3 通过靶向肿瘤抑制基因 DICE1，促进肿瘤细胞增殖，该结果在鼻咽癌中得到证实（Lei et al. 2013）；EBV-miR-BART9 能够靶向上皮细胞标志分子 E-Cadherin 来加强鼻咽癌细胞的侵袭与转移能力（Hsu et al. 2014）。Iizasa 等发现，在 EBV 感染的细胞中，miR-BART6-5p 能够沉默 Dicer、EBNA2、BZLF1 和 BRLF1 的表达；在 HeLa 细胞中，过表达 miR-BART6-5p，降低细胞内源 Dicer 的表达（Iizasa et al. 2010）。在胃癌中，miR-BART20-5p 靶向 BAD，抑制凋亡，促进细胞生长，影响 EBV 相关胃癌的发生发展（Kim et al. 2015）。miR-BART7-3p、miR-BART1 靶向肿瘤抑制因子 PTEN，调控 PI3K/Akt/GSK-3β 信号通路，使 Snail 和 β-catenin 高表达，促进 EMT（Cai et al. 2015）。

4.2　EBV 诱导宿主 miRNA 的异常表达

4.2.1　已确定的病毒蛋白诱导的宿主 miRNA

EBV 除了本身能够编码多个 miRNA 分子外，还能通过编码的多种病毒蛋白调控细胞内源 miRNA 分子的表达，影响肿瘤的发生与发展。LMP1 能够调控机体自身编码的多个 miRNA 分子的表达，影响下游靶基因的功能，进而影响肿瘤的发展进程。有研究表明，通过对 EBV 感染的细胞系的 miRNA 谱进行分析，发现能在上皮细胞中特异表达 miR-203 下调。在 EBV 感染的细胞中，LMP1 能够抑制 miR-203 的表达，促进细胞周期 G_1/S 转换及肿瘤细胞的增殖（Yu et al. 2012）。另一方面，LMP1 上调 miR-155 的表达，促进鼻咽癌细胞增殖、克隆形成、细胞迁移与侵袭能力（Zhu et al. 2014）。miR-10b 也能被 LMP1 所诱导。过表达 miR-10b，有利于鼻咽癌的转移，提高荷瘤裸鼠的死亡率（Li et al. 2010；Allaya et al. 2015）。此外，还有 miR-146a、miR-21（Yang et al. 2013）、miR-29b（Anastasiadou et al. 2010）、miR-34a（Forte et al. 2012）等 microRNA 分子被 LMP1 所诱导。EBV 编码的核抗原 1（EBNA1），在病毒复制及潜伏感染过程中有重要作用。在伯基特淋巴瘤中，EBNA1 能够诱导 miR-127 的表达，影响 B 细胞的分化（Onnis et al. 2012）。

Let-7a 抑制潜伏感染期的 EBV 活化进入裂解复制阶段，其能被 EBNA1 所诱导（Mansouri et al. 2014）。病毒编码的 EBNA2 诱导 miR-21 和 miR-146a 表达，有利于 EBV 对 B 淋巴细胞的转化，以及对机体固有免疫的抗病毒反应（Rosato et al. 2012）。EBNA3A 与 EBNA3C 共同诱导 miR-221/miR-222 表达（Bazot et al, 2015）；miR-155 除了能够被 LMP1 诱导以外，还能被 EBV 编码的另一种潜伏膜蛋白 2A（LMP2A）所诱导（Du et al. 2011）。

4.2.2 EBV 诱导的宿主 miRNA 靶基因功能

LMP1 诱导的 miR-203 下游存在多个靶基因，如 E2F3、CCNG1、Snail2、ZEB2。E2F3 属于 E2F 家族中的一员，在增生细胞的细胞周期进程中具有重要作用，能有效促进 G_1/S 期特异性基因的表达。另外，CCNG1 编码细胞中周期蛋白 G1，它也是细胞周期的调控分子之一。Snail2、ZEB2 是与 EMT 相关的转录因子，miR-203 通过抑制两者的表达，抑制细胞 EMT 的发生（Zhang et al. 2011; Yu et al. 2012）。MiR-21 的靶基因 *PTEN*、*RECK*、*TIMP3*，能够调控 ECM 重塑；而 TPM1、PDCD4 能够影响细胞增殖、凋亡及侵袭转移（Zhang et al. 2014）。*MMP2*、*MMP9* 是 miR-29b 靶基因，主要参与 ECM 重塑，抑制上皮细胞 EMT（Chou et al. 2013; Wang et al. 2013）。MiR-34a 的靶基因 *Snail1* 也与 EMT 相关，靶基因 *CCL22* 则与免疫逃逸、基质细胞的招募有关。EBNA1 诱导的 Let-7a 抑制 Dicer、A2、HMGA2 及 RAS 的表达，改变肿瘤细胞的增殖与生长，抑制病毒裂解、复制活化（Trang et al. 2010; Smits et al. 2011）。

4.3 EBV 相关的 miRNA 调控共同的靶基因

miRNA 能与多个基因 mRNA 3′-UTR 区结合，同时，一个基因也能被多个 miRNA 抑制，因此，不同的 miRNA 可能调控相同的靶基因。EBV 编码的 miR-BART2-5p 能够抑制 *BALF5*、*C1orf109*、*MICB* 等基因的表达；miR-BART20-5p 则能够与 *BZLF1*、*BRLF1* 和 *BAD* 等基因结合；miR-BART1-5p、miR-BART 9、miR-BART 16-5p、miR-BART 17-5p 能够与 EBV 编码基因 *LMP1* 3′-UTR 结合，通过抑制 LMP1 表达，参与调控细胞多项生命活动过程（Lo et al. 2007）；在多肿瘤中，如胶质母细胞瘤、乳腺癌、肺癌、头颈部鳞状细胞癌、淋巴瘤，基因 *PTEN* 异常存在，是与肿瘤发生关系密切的抑癌基因。该基因能够同时与 miR-29b、miR-21、miR-221、miR-222、miR-BART1、miR-BART7-3p 结合，即在 EBV 相关肿瘤中，能够被 miR-29b、miR-21、miR-221、miR-222、miR-BART1、miR-BART7-3p 所抑制（Cai et al. 2015; Cai et al. 2015）。Let-7a 与 EBV 编码的 miR-BART6-5p 共同靶向 Dicer，影响病毒的裂解复制；miR-BART22 除了能够与 LMP2A 结合，还能抑制 NDRG1 的表达，进而调控 EBV 的潜伏感染、裂解复制、

免疫逃逸及细胞侵袭转移等方面。MiRNA 能够调控一大群基因的转录表达，通过这些靶基因，参与机体各个方面的生命活动过程，如细胞增殖、凋亡、免疫反应、转录与侵袭等。

由此可见，在机体中，miRNA 发挥功能的作用机制是复杂的，一个 miRNA 分子就能够影响机体大量基因的转录表达，而其中某些基因同时受到其他的多个 miRNA 分子的调控。在机体细胞某一生命活动过程中，miRNA 分子之间在功能上是存在着相互作用的。这就意味着，在将 miRNA 作为其肿瘤相关的分子治疗靶标时，需要考虑相关联的 miRNA，以及这些 miRNA 的靶基因群，使得肿瘤治疗更稳定、安全、有效。

4.4 EBV 相关的 miRNA 与免疫逃逸

EBV 能够感染绝大多数人类，并能长时间潜伏在宿主细胞中，而不被机体免疫系统识别清除，即 EBV 能够逃避机体的免疫监控，或干扰、抑制细胞免疫应答。在鼻咽癌肿瘤中，存在着大量的 $CD8^+$ 和 $CD4^+$ T 细胞、B 细胞、NK 细胞及巨噬细胞，但是从鼻咽癌组织中分离的 EBV 特异性 CTL 缺乏细胞毒活性，不能诱导产生能够增加细胞免疫功能的 IFN-γ。在 EBV 相关肿瘤中，miRNA 参与病毒免疫逃逸过程。MICB 是 NKG2D 的配体，而 NKG2D 是 NK 细胞上的潜在活化受体，以及 γ/δT 细胞和 $CD8^+$ T 细胞上的一个协同刺激受体。在病毒感染和肿瘤性增殖情况下，MICB 表达增加，通过对 MICB 的识别，NK 细胞和 T 细胞活化后启动免疫反应（Diefenbach et al. 2000；Lisnic et al. 2010）。EBV-miR-BART2-5p 抑制 MICB 的表达，使得 NK 细胞不能识别 EBV 感染的细胞，减弱宿主细胞介导的免疫反应（Nachmani et al. 2009）。IPO7（importin 7）是 EBV-miR-BART3-3p 的靶基因，与活化 T 细胞的早期基因表达相关，且能与一个参与调控免疫耐受的转录因子 Aire 相互作用。EBV-miR-BART3-3p 与 IPO7 相互作用，抑制 IPO7 表达，削弱细胞毒性作用（Abramson et al. 2010；Dolken et al. 2010）。miR-BART22 抑制 EBV 编码的 LMP2A 的表达（Lung et al. 2009）。在 NPC 中，LMP2A 具有较高的免疫原性，miR-BART22 调控 LMP2A 的表达，使 NPC 细胞免受免疫系统的攻击（Straathof 2005；Hislop et al. 2007）。miR-BART9 能够靶向 LMP1，影响淋巴瘤中 NK T 细胞的增长（Ramakrishnan et al. 2011）。研究发现，EBV 阳性的 LCL、C666-1 细胞，以及 NPC 细胞来源的外泌体都含有 EBV miRNA，推测肿瘤细胞通过这些外泌体输送 EBVmiRNA 到邻近或免疫细胞，进而抑制宿主免疫反应（Gourzones 2010；Meckes 2010；Pegtel 2010）。miR-155 通过靶向黄酮体，抑制 TLR 触发的免疫反应；在 TLR3 配体存在情况下，miR-21 在 C666-1 及 NPC 组织中表达上调，进而增加 B 淋巴细胞中 IL-10 的表达，抑制 $CD8^+$ T 细胞的活化（Sun et al. 2012；Miao et al. 2014）。STAT3 可以促进大量的免疫抑制因子（IL-10，VEGR）的表达，而这些免疫抑制因子又可以激活 STAT3。STAT3 能够与 miR-146a 启动子结合，诱导 miR-146a 的表达。MiR-146a 通过靶向免疫相关的靶基因 IRAK1、TRAF6，发挥其在免疫反应过程中的功能。IRAK1S 是 IRAK 激酶家族中一种关键的固有免疫信号调节分子，具有激酶活性，参与调控 TLR/IL-1R 两个受体家族的信号级联反应，调节 TNF-α、Ⅰ型 IFN 及 AP-1 等炎症因子的表达。TRAF6 则通过 TLR 受体和 IFN-γ 信号转导途径参与细胞免疫反应（Sun et al. 2015）。miR-222、miR-223、miR-17-92、miR-155 与 T 细胞的分化有关（Riley et al. 2012；Saki et al. 2015）。

4.5 EBV 相关的 miRNA 与炎症和肿瘤微环境

在机体肿瘤周围有多种基质细胞，如纤维细胞、免疫细胞、血管内皮细胞，这些细胞与肿瘤细胞相互作用，以及分泌多种细胞因子、炎症因子等形成肿瘤微环境（the tumor microenvironment，TME）。而炎症性的肿瘤微环境在肿瘤的发生发展及转移过程中扮演重要的角色，例如，形成含氧低的环境，利于血管生成、细胞侵袭，改变 miRNA 的表达，增加肿瘤细胞的干细胞表型。EBV 感染的 B 淋巴细胞能够分泌含有 EBV-miR-BART15 的外泌体，靶向 NLRP3，抑制 NLRP3 炎症小体的形成，进而影响 IL-1β 与 IL-18 的表达。NLRP3 炎症小体是一种由 NLRP3、ASC 和 Caspase-1 相互结合形成的蛋白复合物，在天然免疫系统中有重要作用（Haneklaus et al. 2012）。IL-6（interleukin-6）是免疫细胞分泌的促炎因子，在 IL-6 存在的情况下，肿瘤细胞能够分泌循环的 miR-21 和 miR-29b，进一步诱导免疫细胞 IL-6 的产生（Patel 2015）。内源性 miR-155 和 miR-146a 是两个调控炎症反应非常重要的 miRNA 分子，前者能够加强炎症相关基因的表达，后者则降低炎症相关基因的表达（Alexander et al. 2015）。在炎症肿瘤微环境下，小胶质细胞中的 miR-let-7a 减少小硝酸盐的形成，以及降低 iNOS（inducible nitric oxide synthase）和 IL-6 的表达，增强 IL-4 和 IL-10 的表达（Cho and Song 2015）。在炎症反应中，miR-21 可以作为一个免疫反应回路开关，控制初始促炎反应与之后的免疫调节、抗炎反应之间的平衡，利于研究炎症性疾病（肿瘤与感染）的发病机理（Sheedy 2015）。在炎症肿瘤微环境中，EMT 也受到 miRNA 分子的调控作用。miR-203、miR-21、miR-155、miR-146a、miR-17-92 等多个 miRNA 能够靶向 EMT 相关分子，如 Snail2、ZEB2、Slug、Smad7、Smad 4、ZEB1 等（Eileen and Heinrich 2012；Wang et al. 2014）。EMT 非常重要的上皮细胞标志分子 E-Cadherin 能被 miR-BART9 所抑制，进而加强 NPC 细胞的侵袭与转移能力（Hsu et al. 2014）。

4.6 EBV 相关的 miRNA 与临床应用

在多种 EBV 相关肿瘤中，miRNA 存在特异性的表达，而这些特异性表达的 miRNA 能够作为肿瘤诊断、治疗和预后的潜在生物标志物。在 EBV 阳性鼻咽癌组织中 miR-203 特异性表达降低，且 miR-203 表达水平与鼻咽癌预后也存在相关性。miR-29 在乳腺癌中表达异常，其能通过靶向甲基化转移酶 3a 和 3b，改变下游基因的甲基化状态，影响基因的表达（Fabbri and Garzon 2007）。通过对 89 例 NPC 患者、28 例健康人、18 例非 NPC 患者 EBV miRNA 检测发现，循环过程中的 EBV-miR-BART7 和 EBV-miR-BART13 可以作为 NPC 治疗的分子靶标（Zhang et al. 2015）。

5 小结

自 1964 年 EB 病毒被发现以来，对它的研究已有 50 年。EBV 与多种肿瘤相关，但是人类对 EBV 的致瘤机制仍然不是十分了解。EBV 在大部分肿瘤中都是以潜伏状态存在的，了解 EBV 潜伏基因的表达及其与宿主细胞之间的相互作用将有助于对 EBV 致病机制的了解。EBV 编码或诱导细胞 miRNA 的异常表达是其发挥致瘤作用的一个重要途径。miRNA 能够调节细胞增殖、分化、凋亡、侵袭与转移及免疫应答，影响 EBV 潜伏感染、裂解复制和免疫逃逸。在将 EBV 编码的 miRNA，以及 EBV 相关肿瘤中特异表达的宿主细胞 miRNA 作为肿瘤潜在的或已经应用于诊断治疗的分子靶标时，也应注意其他相关 miRNA 分子的功能。深入地对 miRNA 功能进行研究，有利于进一步发现 EBV 致病的分子机制，为 EBV 相关性肿瘤的诊断和治疗提供新的依据。

（卢建红，左埒莲 编）

参 考 文 献

Abramson J, Giraud M, Benoist C et al (2010) Aire's partners in the molecular control of immunological tolerance. Cell 140: 123-135

Alexander M, Hu R, Runtsch MC et al (2015) Exosome-delivered microRNAs modulate the inflammatory response to endotoxin. Nat Commun 6: 7321-7336

Alfieri C, Birkenbach M, Kieff E (1991) Early events in Epstein-Barr virus infection of human B lymphocytes. Virology 181: 595-608

Allaya N, Khabir A, Sallemi-Boudawara T et al (2015) Over-expression of miR-10b in NPC patients: correlation with LMP1 and Twist1. Tumour Biol 36: 3807-3814

Anastasiadou E, Boccellato F, Vincenti S et al (2010) Epstein-Barr virus encoded LMP1 downregulates TCL1 oncogene through miR-29b. Oncogene 29: 1316−1328

Anderton E, Yee J, Smith P et al (2008) Two Epstein-Barr virus (EBV) oncoproteins cooperate to repress expression of the proapoptotic tumour-suppressor Bim: clues to the pathogenesis of Burkitt's lymphoma. Oncogene 27: 421−433

Ansell SM (2012) Hodgkin lymphoma: 2012 update on diagnosis, risk-stratification, and management. Am J Hematol 87:1096−1103

Arvey A, Ojesina AI, Pedamallu CS et al (2015) The tumor virus landscape of AIDS-related lymphomas. Blood 125: e14−22

Barth S, Pfuhl T, Mamiani A et al (2008) Epstein-Barr virus-encoded microRNA miR-BART2 down-regulates the viral DNA polymerase BALF5. Nucleic Acids Res 36: 666−675

Bazot Q, Paschos K, Skalska L et al (2015) Epstein-Barr Virus Proteins EBNA3A and EBNA3C Together Induce Expression of the Oncogenic MicroRNA Cluster miR-221/miR-222 and Ablate Expression of Its Target p57KIP2. PLoS Pathog 11: e1005031

Brooks L, Yao QY, Rickinson AB et al (1992) Epstein-Barr virus latent gene transcription in nasopharyngeal carcinoma cells: coexpression of EBNA1, LMP1, and LMP2 transcripts. J Virol 66:2689−2697

Cai L, Ye Y, Jiang Q et al (2015) Epstein-Barr virus-encoded microRNA BART1 induces tumour metastasis by regulating PTEN-dependent pathways in nasopharyngeal carcinoma.Nat Commun 6: 7353 doi: 10.1038/ncomms8353

Cai LM, Lyu XM, Luo WR et al (2015) EBV-miR-BART7-3p promotes the EMT and metastasis of nasopharyngeal carcinoma cells by suppressing the tumor suppressor PTEN. Oncogene 34: 2156−2166

Campo E, Swerdlow SH, Harris NL et al (2011) The 2008 WHO classification of lymphoid neoplasms and beyond: evolving concepts and practical applications. Blood 117:5019−5032

Cao SM, Simons MJ, Qian CN (2011) The prevalence and prevention of nasopharyngeal carcinoma in China. Chin J Cancer 30:114−119

Carbone A, Gloghini A (2005) AIDS-related lymphomas: from pathogenesis to pathology. Br J Haematol 130:662−670

Chan AT, Teo PM, Johnson PJ (2002) Nasopharyngeal carcinoma. Ann Oncol 13:1007−1015

Chang MS, Kim WH (2005) Epstein-Barr virus in human malignancy: a special reference to Epstein-Barr virus associated gastric carcinoma. Cancer Res Treat 37:257−267

Chattopadhyay PK, Chelimo K, Embury PB et al (2013) Holoendemic malaria exposure is associated with altered Epstein-Barr virus-specific CD8 (+) T-cell differentiation. J Virol 87:1779−1788

Chen JN, He D, Tang F et al (2012) Epstein-Barr virus-associated gastric carcinoma: a newly defined entity. J Clin Gastroenterol 46:262−271

Cho KJ, Song J, Oh Y et al (2015) MicroRNA-Let-7a regulates the function of microglia in inflammation. Mol Cell Neurosci 68: 167-176

Choi JW, Kim Y, Lee JH et al (2015) Human Herpesvirus 8-Negative and Epstein-Barr Virus-Positive Effusion-Based Lymphoma in a Patient with Human Immunodeficiency Virus. J Pathol Transl Med doi: 10.4132/jptm

Chou J, Lin JH, Brenot A et al (2013) GATA3 suppresses metastasis and modulates the tumour microenvironment by regulating microRNA-29b expression. Nat Cell Biol 15: 201-213

Choy EY, Siu KL, Kok KH et al (2008) An Epstein-Barr virus-encoded microRNA targets PUMA to promote host cell survival. J Exp Med 205: 2551-2560

Cohen JI (1999) The biology of Epstein-Barr virus: lessons learned from the virus and the host. Curr Opin Immunol 11:365-370

Cohen JI, Fauci AS, Varmus H et al (2011) Epstein-Barr virus: an important vaccine target for cancer prevention. Sci Transl Med 3: 107fs7 doi: 10.1126/scitranslmed.3002878

Cohen JI, Wang F, Mannick J et al (1989) Epstein-Barr virus nuclear protein 2 is a key determinant of lymphocyte transformation. Proc Natl Acad Sci 86: 9558-9562

Corti M, Villafane M, Bistmans A et al (2014) Primary extranodal non-hodgkin lymphoma of the head and neck in patients with acquired immunodeficiency syndrome: a clinicopathologic study of 24 patients in a single hospital of infectious diseases in Argentina. Int Arch Otorhinolaryngol 18:260-265

Dawson CW, Port RJ, Young LS (2012) The role of the EBV-encoded latent membrane proteins LMP1 and LMP2 in the pathogenesis of nasopharyngeal carcinoma (NPC). Semin Cancer Biol 22: 144-153

de Martel C, Ferlay J, Franceschi S et al (2012) Global burden of cancers attributable to infections in 2008: a review and synthetic analysis. Lancet Oncol 13:607-615

Diefenbach A, Jamieson AM, Liu SD et al (2000) Ligands for the murine NKG2D receptor: expression by tumor cells and activation of NK cells and macrophages. Nat Immunol 1: 119-126

Dolken L, Malterer G, Erhard F et al (2010) Systematic analysis of viral and cellular microRNA targets in cells latently infected with human gamma-herpesviruses by RISC immunoprecipitation assay. Cell Host Microbe 7: 324-334

Draborg AH, Duus K, Houen G (2013) Epstein-Barr virus in systemic autoimmune diseases. Clin Dev Immunol 2013: 535738 doi: 10.1155/2013/535738

Du ZM, Hu LF, Wang HY et al (2011) Upregulation of MiR-155 in nasopharyngeal carcinoma is partly driven by LMP1 and LMP2A and downregulates a negative prognostic marker JMJD1A. PLoS One 6: e19137

Epstein MA, Achong BG, Barr YM (1964) virus particles in cultured lymphoblasts from Burkitt's lymphoma. Lancet 1: 702-703

Fabbri M, Garzon R, Cimmino A et al (2007) MicroRNA-29 family reverts aberrant methylation in lung cancer by targeting DNA methyltransferases 3A and 3B. Proc Natl Acad Sci 104: 15805-15810

Fina F, Romain S, Ouafik L et al (2001) Frequency and genome load of Epstein-Barr virus in 509 breast cancers from different geographical areas. Br J Cancer 84:783-790

Forte E, Salinas RE, Chang C et al (2012) The Epstein-Barr virus (EBV) -induced tumor suppressor microRNA MiR-34a is growth promoting in EBV-infected B cells. J Virol 86: 6889-6898

Fukayama M (2010) Epstein-Barr virus and gastric carcinoma. Pathol Int 60:337-350

Fukayama M, Ushiku T (2011) Epstein-Barr virus-associated gastric carcinoma. Pathol Res Pract 207:529-537

Gandhi MK, Tellam JT, Khanna R (2004) Epstein-Barr virus-associated Hodgkin's lymphoma. Br J Haematol 125:267-281

Gourzones C, Gelin A, Bombik I et al (2010) Extra-cellular release and blood diffusion of BART viral micro-RNAs produced by EBV-infected nasopharyngeal carcinoma cells. Virol J 15: 271 doi: 10.1186/1743-422X-7-271

Green MR, Rodig S, Juszczynski P et al (2012) Constitutive AP-1 activity and EBV infection induce PD-L1 in Hodgkin lymphomas and posttransplant lymphoproliferative disorders: implications for targeted therapy. Clin Cancer Res 18:1611-1618

Gulley ML, Tang W (2010) Using Epstein-Barr viral load assays to diagnose, monitor, and prevent posttransplant lymphoproliferative disorder. Clin Microbiol Rev 23:350-366

Hammerschmidt W, Sugden B (2013) Replication of Epstein-Barr viral DNA. Cold Spring Harb Perspect Biol 5: a013029

Haneklaus M, Gerlic M, Kurowska-Stolarska M et al (2012) Cutting edge: miR-223 and EBV miR-BART15 regulate the NLRP3 inflammasome and IL-1beta production. J Immunol 189: 3795-3799

Hao QF, Sheng GY, Luan Z (2013) Latest update on immunotherapy of Epstein-Barr virus-associated post-transplantation lymphoproliferative disease. Zhongguo Dang Dai Er Ke Za Zhi 15: 795-799

Harabuchi Y, Takahara M, Kishibe K et al (2009) Nasal natural killer (NK) /T-cell lymphoma: clinical, histological, virological, and genetic features. Int J Clin Oncol 14:181-190

Heinrich EL, Walser TC, Krysan K et al (2012) The Inflammatory Tumor Microenvironment, Epithelial Mesenchymal Transition and Lung Carcinogenesis. Cancer Microenviron 4: 5-18

Hislop AD, Taylor GS, Sauce D et al (2007) Cellular responses to viral infection in humans: lessons from Epstein-Barr virus. Annu Rev Immunol 25: 587-617

Hjalgrim H, Askling J, Rostgaard K et al (2003) Characteristics of Hodgkin's lymphoma after infectious mononucleosis. N Engl J Med 349:1324-1332

Horikawa T, Sheen TS, Takeshita H et al (2001) Induction of c-Met proto-oncogene by Epstein-Barr virus latent membrane protein-1 and the correlation with cervical lymph node metastasis of nasopharyngeal carcinoma.Am J Pathol 159: 27-33

Hsu CY, Yi YH, Chang KP et al (2014) The Epstein-Barr virus-encoded microRNA MiR-BART9 promotes tumor metastasis by targeting E-cadherin in nasopharyngeal carcinoma. PLoS Pathog 10: e1003974

Hutt-Fletcher LM (2007) Epstein-Barr virus entry. J Virol 81: 7825-7832

Iizasa H, Wulff BE, Alla NR et al (2010) Editing of Epstein-Barr virus-encoded BART6 microRNAs controls their dicer targeting and consequently affects viral latency. J Biol Chem 285: 33358-33370

Imai S, Nishikawa J, Takada K (1998) Cell-to-cell contact as an efficient mode of Epstein-Barr virus infection of diverse human epithelial cells. J Virol 72: 4371-4378

Iwakiri D, Sheen TS, Chen JY et al (2005) Epstein-Barr virus-encoded small RNA induces insulin-like growth factor 1 and supports growth of nasopharyngeal carcinoma-derived cell lines. Oncogene 24: 1767-1773

Jarrett RF, Stark GL, White J et al (2005) Impact of tumor Epstein-Barr virus status on presenting features and outcome in age-defined subgroups of patients with classic Hodgkin lymphoma: a population-based study. Blood 106:2444-2451

Joshi D, Buehring GC (2012) Are viruses associated with human breast cancer? Scrutinizing the molecular evidence. Breast Cancer Res Treat 135:1-15

Kang MS, Kieff E (2015) Epstein-Barr virus latent genes. Exp Mol Med 47: e131

Kang MS, Lu H, Yasui T et al (2005) Epstein-Barr virus nuclear antigen 1 does not induce lymphoma in transgenic FVB mice. Proc Natl Acad Sci 102: 820-825

Kelly G, Bell A, Rickinson A (2002) Epstein-Barr virus-associated Burkitt lymphomagenesis selects for downregulation of the nuclear antigen EBNA2. Nat Med 8:1098-1104

Kim H, Choi H, Lee SK (2015) . Epstein-Barr virus miR-BART20-5p regulates cell proliferation and apoptosis by targeting BAD. Cancer Lett 356: 733-742

Klinke O, Feederle R, Delecluse HJ (2014) Genetics of Epstein-Barr virus microRNAs. Semin Cancer Biol 26: 52-59

Labrecque LG, Barnes DM, Fentiman IS et al (1995) Epstein-Barr virus in epithelial cell tumors: a breast cancer study. Cancer Res 55:39-45

Landgren O, Gilbert ES, Rizzo JD et al (2009) Risk factors for lymphoproliferative disorders after allogeneic hematopoietic cell transplantation. Blood 113:4992-5001

Lee AW, Ng WT, Chan YH et al (2012) The battle against nasopharyngeal cancer. Radiother Oncol 104:272-278

Lee HL, Kim DC, Lee SP et al (2012) Treatment of Epstein-Barr virus-associated gastric carcinoma with endoscopic submucosal dissection. Gastrointest Endosc 76:913-915

Lee JH, Kim SH, Han SH et al (2009) Clinicopathological and molecular characteristics of Epstein-Barr virus-associated gastric carcinoma: a meta-analysis. J Gastroenterol Hepatol 24:354-365

Lei T, Yuen KS, Xu R et al (2013) Targeting of DICE1 tumor suppressor by Epstein-Barr virus-encoded miR-BART3* microRNA in nasopharyngeal carcinoma. Int J Cancer 133: 79-87

Li G, Wu Z, Peng Y et al (2010) MicroRNA-10b induced by Epstein-Barr virus-encoded latent membrane protein-1 promotes the metastasis of human nasopharyngeal carcinoma cells. Cancer Lett 299: 29-36

Li Z, Chen X, Li L et al (2012) EBV encoded miR-BHRF1-1 potentiates viral lytic replication by downregulating host p53 in nasopharyngeal carcinoma. Int J Biochem Cell Biol 44: 275-279

Liebowitz D (1998) Epstein-Barr virus and a cellular signaling pathway in lymphomas from immunosuppressed patients. N Engl J Med 338:1413-1421

Lin S, Nadeau PE, Mergia A (2015) HIV inhibits endothelial reverse cholesterol transport through Impacting subcellular Cavelin-1 trafficking.Retrovirology 12:62 doi: 10.1186/s12977-015-0188-y

Lisnic VJ, Krmpotic A, Jonjic S (2010) Modulation of natural killer cell activity by viruses. Curr Opin Microbiol 13: 530-539

Liu F, Asano N, Tatematsu A et al (2012) Plasmablastic lymphoma of the elderly: a clinicopathological comparison with age-related Epstein-Barr virus-associated B cell lymphoproliferative disorder. Histopathology 61:1183-1197

Liu X, Wang Y, Wang X et al (2013) Epigenetic silencing of WNT5A in Epstein-Barr virus-associated gastric carcinoma. Arch Virol 158:123-132

Lo AK, Huang DP, Lo KW et al (2004) Phenotypic alterations induced by the Hong Kong-prevalent Epstein-Barr virus-encoded LMP1 variant (2117-LMP1) in nasopharyngeal epithelial cells. Int J Cancer 109: 919-925

Lo AK, To KF, Lo KW et al (2007) Modulation of LMP1 protein expression by EBV-encoded microRNAs. Proc Natl Acad Sci 104: 16164-16169

Lu JH, Tang YL, Yu HB et al (2010) Epstein-Barr virus facilitates the malignant potential of immortalized epithelial cells: from latent genome to viral production and maintenance. Lab Invest 90: 196-209

Lu JJ, Chen DY, Hsieh CW et al (2007) Association of Epstein-Barr virus infection with systemic lupus erythematosus in Taiwan. Lupus 16 : 168-175

Lung RW, Tong JH, Sung YM et al (2009) Modulation of LMP2A expression by a newly identified Epstein-Barr virus-encoded microRNA miR-BART22.Neoplasia 11: 1174-1184

Mansouri S, Pan Q, Blencowe BJ et al (2014) Epstein-Barr virus EBNA1 protein regulates viral latency through effects on let-7 microRNA and dicer. J Virol 88: 11166-11177

Marechal V, Dehee A, Chikhi-Brachet R et al (1999) Mapping EBNA-1 domains involved in binding to metaphase chromosomes. J Virol 73: 4385-4392

Mazouni C, Fina F, Romain S et al (2011) Epstein-Barr virus as a marker of biological aggressiveness in breast cancer. Br J Cancer 104:332-337

Meckes DG Jr, Shair KH, Marquitz AR et al (2010) Human tumor virus utilizes exosomes for intercellular communication. Proc Natl Acad Sci 7: 20370-20375

Mesri EA, Feitelson MA, Munger K (2014) Human viral oncogenesis: a cancer hallmarks analysis. Cell Host Microbe 15:266-282

Miao BP, Zhang RS, Li M et al (2014) Nasopharyngeal cancer-derived microRNA-21 promotes immune suppressive B cells. Cell Mol Immunol 12 doi: 10.1038/cmi

Murphy G, Pfeiffer R, Camargo MC et al (2009a) Meta-analysis shows that prevalence of Epstein-Barr virus-positive gastric cancer differs based on sex and anatomic location. Gastroenterology 137:824-833

Nachmani D, Stern-Ginossar N, Sarid R et al (2009) Diverse herpesvirus microRNAs target the stress-induced immune ligand MICB to escape recognition by natural killer cells. Cell Host Microbe 5: 376-385

Nguyen-Van D, Keane C, Han E et al (2011) Epstein-Barr virus-positive diffuse large B-cell lymphoma of the elderly expresses EBNA3A with conserved CD8 T-cell epitopes. Am J Blood Res 1:146-159

Ni C, Chen Y, Zeng M et al (2015) In-cell infection: a novel pathway for Epstein-Barr virus infection mediated by cell-in-cell structures. Cell Res 25:785-800

Njie R, Bell AI, Jia H et al (2009) The effects of acute malaria on Epstein-Barr virus (EBV) load and EBV-specific T cell immunity in Gambian children. J Infect Dis 199:31-38

Nowakowska J, Stuehler C, Eqli A et al (2015) T cells specific for different latent and lytic viral proteins efficiently control Epstein-Barr virus-transformed B cells. Cytotherapy 17: 1280-1291

Ok CY, Papathomas TG, Medeiros LJ et al (2013) EBV-positive diffuse large B-cell lymphoma of the elderly. Blood 122:328-340

Okano M, Gross TG (2012) Acute or chronic life-threatening diseases associated with Epstein-Barr virus infection. Am J Med Sci 343:483-489

Onnis A, Navari M, Antonicelli G et al (2012) Epstein-Barr nuclear antigen 1 induces expression of the cellular microRNA hsa-miR-127 and impairing B-cell differentiation in EBV-infected memory B cells. New insights into the pathogenesis of Burkitt lymphoma. Blood Cancer J 2: e84

Park S, Lee J, Ko YH et al (2007) The impact of Epstein-Barr virus status on clinical outcome in diffuse large B-cell lymphoma. Blood 110:972-978

Parker A, Bowles K, Bradley JA et al (2010) Management of post-transplant lymphoproliferative disorder in adult solid organ transplant recipients - BCSH and BTS Guidelines. Br J Haematol 149:693-705

Patel SA, Gooderham NJ (2015) IL6 mediates immune and colorectal cancer cell crosstalk via miR-21 and miR-29b. Mol Cancer Res 16: 1541-7786

Pegtel DM, Cosmopoulos K, Thorley-Lawson DA et al (2010) Functional delivery of viral miRNAs via exosomes. Proc Natl Acad Sci 107:6328-6333

Pegtel DM, Subramanian A, Meritt D et al (2007) IFN-alpha-stimulated genes and Epstein-Barr virus gene expression distinguish WHO type II and III nasopharyngeal carcinomas. Cancer Res 67:474-481

Petrara MR, Giunco S, Serraino D et al (2015) Post-transplant lymphoproliferative disorders: from epidemiology to pathogenesis-driven treatment. Cancer Lett doi: 10.1016/j.canlet

Poole BD, Templeton AK, Guthridge JM et al (2009) Aberrant Epstein-Barr viral infection in systemic lupus erythematosus. Autoimmun Rev 8: 337-342

Portal D, Zhou H, Zhao B et al (2013) Epstein-Barr virus nuclear antigen leader protein localizes to promoters and enhancers with cell transcription factors and EBNA2. Proc Natl Acad Sci U S A 110: 18537-18542

Raab-Traub N (2002) Epstein-Barr virus in the pathogenesis of NPC. Semin Cancer Biol 12 (6):431-441

Ramakrishnan R, Donahue H, Garcia D et al (2011) Epstein-Barr virus BART9 miRNA modulates LMP1 levels and affects growth rate of nasal NK T cell lymphomas. PLoS One 6: e27271

Reddy N, Rezvani K, Barrett AJ et al (2011) Strategies to prevent EBV reactivation and posttransplant lymphoproliferative disorders (PTLD) after allogeneic stem cell transplantation in high-risk patients. Biol Blood Marrow Transplant 17:591-597

Rickinson AB (1998) Epstein-Barr virus in action in vivo. N Engl J Med 338:1461-1463

Riley KJ, Rabinowitz GS, Yario TA et al (2012) EBV and human microRNAs co-target oncogenic and apoptotic viral and human genes during latency. EMBO J 31: 2207-2221

Rohner E, Wyss N, Heg Z et al (2015) HIV and human herpesvirus 8 co-infection across the globe: Systematic review and meta-analysis. Int J Cancer doi: 10.1002/ijc.29687

Rosato P, Anastasiadou E, Garg N et al (2012) Differential regulation of miR-21 and miR-146a by Epstein-Barr virus-encoded EBNA2. Leukemia 26: 2343-2352

Rovedo M, Longnecker R (2007) Epstein-barr virus latent membrane protein 2B (LMP2B) modulates LMP2A activity. J Virol 81: 84-94

Ruf IK, Rhyne PW, Yang C et al (2000) Epstein-Barr virus small RNAs potentiate tumorigenicity of Burkitt lymphoma cells independently of an effect on apoptosis. J Virol 74: 10223-10228

Rymo L (1979) Identification of transcribed regions of Epstein-Barr virus DNA in Burkitt lymphoma-derived cells. J Virol 32: 8-18

Saki N, Abroun S, Soleimani M et al (2015) Involvement of MicroRNA in T-Cell Differentiation and Malignancy. Int J Hematol Oncol Stem Cell Res 9: 33-49

Sam CK, Brooks LA, Niedobitek G et al (1993) Analysis of Epstein-Barr virus infection in nasopharyngeal biopsies from a group at high risk of nasopharyngeal carcinoma. Int J Cancer 53:957-962

Schiller JT, Lowy DR (2010) Vaccines to prevent infections by oncoviruses. Annu Rev Microbiol 64:23-41

Scholle F, Bendt KM, Raab-Traub N (2000) Epstein-Barr virus LMP2A transforms epithelial cells, inhibits cell differentiation, and activates Akt. J Virol 74: 10681-10689

Sheedy FJ (2015) Turning 21: Induction of miR-21 as a Key Switch in the Inflammatory Response. Front Immunol 6:19 doi: 10.3389/fimmu

Shin HJ, Kim DN, Lee SK (2011) Association between Epstein-Barr virus infection and chemoresistance to docetaxel in gastric carcinoma. Mol Cells 32:173-179

Sivachandran N, Wang X, Frappier L (2012) Functions of the Epstein-Barr virus EBNA1 protein in viral reactivation and lytic infection. J Virol 86: 6146-6158

Smets F, Bodeus M, Goubau P et al (2000) Characteristics of Epstein-Barr virus primary infection in pediatric liver transplant recipients. J Hepatol 32:100-104

Smets F, Sokal EM (2002) Lymphoproliferation in children after liver transplantation. J Pediatr Gastroenterol Nutr 34:499-505

Smits KM, Paranjape T, Nallur S et al (2011) A let-7 microRNA SNP in the KRAS 3'UTR is prognostic in early-stage colorectal cancer. Clin Cancer Res 17: 7723-7731

Song LB, Zeng MS, Liao WT et al (2006) Bmi-1 is a novel molecular marker of nasopharyngeal carcinoma progression and immortalizes primary human nasopharyngeal epithelial cells. Cancer Res 66:6225-6232

Steven NM (1997) Epstein-Barr virus latent infection in vivo. Rev Med Virol 7:97-106

Straathof KC, Leen AM, Buza EL et al (2005) Characterization of latent membrane protein 2 specificity in CTL lines from patients with EBV-positive nasopharyngeal carcinoma and lymphoma. J Immunol 175: 4137-4147

Sun X, Zhang J, Hou Z et al (2015) miR-146a is directly regulated by STAT3 in human hepatocellular carcinoma cells and involved in anti-tumor immune suppression. Cell Cycle 14: 243-252

Sun Y, Cai J, Ma F et al (2012) . miR-155 mediates suppressive effect of progesterone on TLR3, TLR4-triggered immune response. Immunol Lett 146: 25-30

Temple RM, Zhu J, Budgeon L et al (2014) Efficient replication of Epstein-Barr virus in stratified epithelium in vitro.Proc Natl Acad Sci 111: 16544-16549

Thorley-Lawson DA, Hawkins JB, Tracy SI et al (2013) The pathogenesis of Epstein-Barr virus persistent infection. Curr Opin Virol 3: 227-232

Trang P, Medina PP, Wiggins JF et al (2010) Regression of murine lung tumors by the let-7 microRNA. Oncogene 29: 1580-1587

Truong CD, Feng W, Li W et al (2009) Characteristics of Epstein-Barr virus-associated gastric cancer: a study of 235 cases at a comprehensive cancer center in U.S.A. J Exp Clin Cancer Res 28:14

Tsachouridou O, Skoura L, Zebekakis P et al (2015) The controversial impact of B cells subsets on immune response to pneumococcal vaccine in HIV-1 patients. Int J Infect Dis doi: 10.1016/j.ijid

Tsai JH, Hsu CS, Tsai CH et al (2007) Relationship between viral factors, axillary lymph node status and survival in breast cancer. J Cancer Res Clin Oncol 133:13-21

Tsao SW, Tsang CM, To KF et al (2015) The role of Epstein-Barr virus in epithelial malignancies. J Pathol 235: 323-333

Walling DM, Ray AJ, Nichols JE et al (2007) Epstein-Barr virus infection of Langerhans cell precursors as a mechanism of oral epithelial entry, persistence, and reactivation. J Virol 81: 7249-7268

Wang HB, Zhang H, Zhang JP et al (2015) Neuropilin 1 is an entry factor that promotes EBV infection of nasopharyngeal epithelial cells.Nat Commun 6:6240. doi: 10.1038/ncomms7240

Wang JY, Gao YB, Zhang N et al (2014) miR-21 overexpression enhances TGF-beta1-induced epithelial-to-mesenchymal transition by target smad7 and aggravates renal damage in diabetic nephropathy. Mol Cell Endocrinol 392: 163-172

Wang Y, Zhang X, Li H et al (2013) The role of miRNA-29 family in cancer. Eur J Cell Biol 92: 123-128

Wilson JB, Bell JL, Levine AJ (1996) Expression of Epstein-Barr virus nuclear antigen-1 induces B cell neoplasia in transgenic mice. EMBO J 15: 3117-3126

Xiong D, Du Y, Wang HB et al (2015) Nonmuscle myosin heavy chain IIA mediates Epstein-Barr virus infection of nasopharyngeal epithelial cells. Proc Natl Acad Sci 112:11036-41. doi: 10.1073/pnas.1513359112

Yang GD, Huang TJ, Peng LX et al (2013) Epstein-Barr Virus Encoded LMP1 upregulates microRNA-21 to promote the resistance of nasopharyngeal carcinoma cells to cisplatin-induced Apoptosis by suppressing PDCD4 and Fas-L. PLoS One 8: e78355

Young LS, Dawson CW, Clark D et al (1988) Epstein-Barr virus gene expression in nasopharyngeal carcinoma. J Gen Virol 69:1051-1065

Young LS, Rickinson AB (2004) Epstein-Barr virus: 40 years on. Nat Rev Cancer 4:757-768

Yu H, Lu J, Zuo L et al (2012) Epstein-Barr virus downregulates microRNA 203 through the oncoprotein latent membrane protein 1: a contribution to increased tumor incidence in epithelial cells. J Virol 86: 3088-3099

Yu SF, Wu HC, Tsai WC et al (2005) Detecting Epstein-Barr virus DNA from peripheral blood mononuclear cells in adult patients with systemic lupus erythematosus in Taiwan. Med Microbiol Immunol 194: 115-120

Zeng ZY, Zhou YH, Zhang WL et al (2007) Gene expression profiling of nasopharyngeal carcinoma reveals the abnormally regulated Wnt signaling pathway. Hum Pathol 38:120-133

Zhang G, Zong J, Lin S et al (2015) Circulating Epstein-Barr virus microRNAs miR-BART7 and miR-BART13 as biomarkers for nasopharyngeal carcinoma diagnosis and treatment. Int J Cancer136: 301-312

Zhang Y, Yang P, Wang XF (2014) Microenvironmental regulation of cancer metastasis by miRNAs.Trends Cell Biol 24: 153-160

Zhang Z, Zhang B, Li W et al (2011) Epigenetic Silencing of miR-203 Upregulates SNAI2 and Contributes to the Invasiveness of Malignant Breast Cancer Cells. Genes Cancer 2: 782-791

Zhao Y, Wang Y, Zeng S et al (2012) LMP1 expression is positively associated with metastasis of nasopharyngeal carcinoma: evidence from a meta-analysis. J Clin Pathol 65 : 41-45

Zhu X, Wang Y, Sun Y et al (2014) MiR-155 up-regulation by LMP1 DNA contributes to increased nasopharyngeal carcinoma cell proliferation and migration. Eur Arch Otorhinolaryngol 271: 1939-1945

Zuo LL, Zhu MJ, Du SJ et al (2014) The entry of Epstein-Barr virus into B lymphocytes and epithelial cells during infection. Bing Du Xue Bao 30 : 476-482

第 6 章 EB 病毒感染及相关性疾病的预防

摘　要　全球每年发生超过 20 万例 EBV 相关性肿瘤病例，因而疫苗接种和预防已成为世界性的公共卫生问题。由于 EBV 潜伏感染的特殊性和复杂性，目前的疫苗研究结果仍不理想。在治疗方面，也仍然需要学者们积极研究。EBV 感染导致的增生性疾病或淋巴瘤也是当前移植和艾滋病患者中的重要问题，寻求有效的预防方法非常重要。在目前取得的一些进展中，减少免疫抑制和加强对 EBV 感染的监测是重要手段。总之，早期的监测和诊断是目前预防 EBV 感染相关性疾病或肿瘤的最主要的方法。

关键词　EB 病毒，淋巴瘤，鼻咽癌，监测，治疗

1　引言

EB 病毒在全球的感染人数达 50 多亿，每年新发的 EBV 相关性肿瘤患者也达 20 万以上，因此 EBV 感染及其相关性癌症或疾病的预防和治疗已成为全世界范围的公共卫生问题。EBV 的潜伏感染会引起机体免疫反应，血清学抗体滴度的监测与疾病有相关性。疫苗的研究仍没有突破性进展，不能像对乙型肝炎病毒等一样使用疫苗有效预防感染和相关疾病。对于 EBV 相关性疾病的治疗方面，本章将重点讨论移植后增生性疾病（PTLD）的治疗。

2　EBV 感染的血清学检测

对 EB 病毒的特异性抗体的血清学检测可用来界定感染状态。通常情况下，只用病毒衣壳蛋白抗原（VCA）IgG、VCA IgM 和 EB 病毒核抗原 EBNA-1 IgG 这三个指标就可以区分急性感染（acute infection）与既往感染（past infection）。若存在 VCA IgM 和 VCA IgG 而无 EBNA-1 IgG，则表明为急性感染；若有 VCA IgG 和 EBNA-1 IgG 存在而无 VCA IgM，则为典型的既往感染（De Paschale and Clerici 2012）。在 EBV 表达的抗原中，只有很少的一部分进行了广泛研究并应用于诊断目的。抗早期抗原（EA）IgG（anti-EA antibody）有两种模式：弥散型 EA（D）IgG 和限制型 EA（R）IgG。EA（D）IgG 在感染后的 3~4 周内增加，但在 3~4 个月后便检测不出了，虽然在一些情况下，原发感染数年后仍可检测到 EA（D）

IgG（Bauer 2001）。EA（R）IgG 的水平可维持至两年，在 EBV 活化或免疫力低下患者中可见 EA（D）IgG 和/或 EA（R）IgG 的高水平表达。当急性感染出现临床症状时，VCA IgG 便开始出现并且终生存在，而 VCA IgM 通常与 VCA IgG 同时出现，且一般会在几周后消失。原发感染的儿童和成年人不一定是 VCA IgM 阳性（Sumaya and Ench 1985）。

血清流行病学已经证明 VCA IgA 和 EA IgA 在鼻咽癌（NPC）患者血清中高表达，VCA IgA 可作为预测 NPC 发生风险的一个生物分子标志（Henle and Henle 1976）。在很多实验中，还在用传统的方法如免疫荧光（IF）或免疫酶法（IEA）来测定 VCA IgA 等抗体，然而传统的方法有一些不足之处，它是半定量的并且很难标准化（Chen et al. 2014）。新兴的酶联免疫吸附测定（ELISA）是一种在不降低敏感性和特异性前提下，能够避免传统方法的一些固有主观性的方法，目前已有商品化试剂盒。然而血清 EBV 抗体测定对于疾病（如 NPC）诊断的特异性不是很高，会有假阳性或假阴性结果的出现，因为大多数人在幼年时期就感染了 EBV，而免疫力低下人群产生的抗体水平低。如果有一种或几种不受免疫力影响的蛋白质检测方法可以补充这种检测的不足，将提高检测的特异性和敏感性，有利于对疾病发生或进程的判断。

EBV DNA 载量与 EBV 的致瘤作用严重性有关，这在前一章中已讨论。随着实时荧光定量 PCR 检测技术的普及，很多实验室都将 EBV DNA 的定量检测作为 EBV 感染的一个分子生物标记，并且通过实验阐明 EBV DNA 检测相比 VCA IgA 和 EA IgA 检测，对 NPC 的诊断具有灵敏度高和特异性强的特点。EB 病毒血清学检测可以帮助疾病的诊断，但是，单靠临床检查往往不能确诊疾病。

3 EBV 疫苗

每年发生超过 20 万例 EBV 相关性肿瘤病例，因此，EBV 疫苗接种将会是预防和公共卫生领域的一个重大进步（Cohen et al. 2011；Schiller and Lowy 2010）。规模最大的一项 EBV 疫苗研究是，使用矾/单磷酰酯 A 作为佐剂的重组 gp350 疫苗（Sokal et al. 2007）。在这项涉及 181 名处于 EBV 感染初期的成年人并受安慰剂控制下的研究中，疫苗并不能阻止感染，但是显著地降低了 78%的 IM 发生率。在一项小型的针对健康受试者的研究中，显示了使用破伤风菌疫苗和油水型佐剂可产生 EBNA-3 肽的免疫原性，并具有病毒特异性 T 细胞反应，但是这项研究没有进行下去（Elliott et al. 2008）。治疗性免疫也在研究之中，一种 EBNA-1/LMP-2 疫苗可以在 NPC 患者中诱导免疫反应（Long et al. 2011）。到目前为止，还没有发现任何疫苗会产生对 EBV 的消除性免疫以完全预防 EBV 感染。然而，对于预防 EBV 相关的肿瘤而言，研制具备这种效果的疫苗并没有必要，因为 EBV 相关性肿瘤通常和高滴度 EBV 病毒有关。以减低 IM 发生率和/或减少病毒数量为目的的疫苗本身就对预防后续肿瘤的发生有效，建议在此领域进一步加强研究（Cohen et al. 2011；Schiller and Lowy 2010）。

4 PTLD 的治疗

有报道显示，移植后增生性疾病（PTLD）的病死率通常在 30%~60%（Bakker et al. 2007）。为了降低 PTLD 相关的发病率及死亡率，早期诊断和治疗是必需的。由于初始症状的非特异性，有必要在有症状时即高度怀疑。不明原因的发热、腺病、肝脾肿大、类似败血症的综合征，以及有另外的结节肿大（移植处、胃肠道、鼻腔鼻窦），都是 PTLD 常见的症状。移植局部病状在早期 PTLD 中常有报道。有研究表示，氟脱氧葡萄糖正电子发射计算机断层扫描术（FDG-PET）在疾病分期和后续治疗阶段显现出一定效果，但是在早期诊断方面发挥的作用还需要进一步鉴定。未能被识别的 PTLD 能快速导致移植、多个器官功能严重失调乃至死亡。

在实体器官移植之后的早期 PTLD 中，减轻免疫抑制（IS）是治疗的第一步，其目的是为了恢复特异性免疫功能及控制 EBV 感染的增殖细胞，报道显示，反应率可高达 75%（Heslop 2009）。在骨髓或干细胞移植之后，尽管逐步减少 IS 可以作为晚期 PTLD 的一个选择，但是在早期病例中通常是没有必要的，因为此阶段患者已经发生严重的免疫抑制。对于这些病例，未经过处理的捐献细胞输入或体外扩增的 EBV-CTL 接受性转移将是更佳的治疗选择。研究显示，在对 49 位 PTLD 患者进行造血干细胞移植后，对该治疗方案的持续性反应率大于 70%（Doubroniva et al. 2012；Heslop 2012），在捐献的未筛选淋巴细胞、捐献的 EBV-CTL 或第三方 EBV-CTL 中也观察到同样的结果。症状经过 5~15 天后有所改善，经过 3 周和 3 个月后，分别得到对放射性和完全治疗的反应。细胞疗法对中枢神经系统局部化 PTLD 也是有效的。研究表明，治疗失败与不匹配的病毒抗原、EBV-CTL 及肿瘤之间的 HLA 呈现关联，这也解释了为什么靶增殖细胞没有被识别即被消除。在一个 PTLD SCID 小鼠模型中，输入 EBV-CTL 导致延迟的肿瘤生长，肿瘤在 40% 的病例中可以预防（$P=0.001$）。通过预选 $CD8^+$ 细胞或通过组合 IL-2、IL-7 和 IL-15 来培养 CTLS 的适应性，结果有所改善（Johannessen et al. 2011）。除了 EBV-CTL 的输入外，每天注射 IL-2 在 78% 的动物中可以预防 PTLD 的发生。在 13 名高风险儿童接受部分匹配的干细胞移植病例中，细胞疗法也显示了是一个有效的先发策略（Leen et al. 2009）。移植发生的 30 天后，通过注射一剂 EBV-CTL，没有观察到 PTLD 和 GVHD。细胞疗法的局限性有：GVHD 风险性（主要和未经过处理的捐献 T 细胞有关），需要特殊的设施来扩增 EBV-CTL，并需要为进展迅速的疾病随时做好准备，因为扩增的时间需要 2~3 个月（Heslop

2009；Bollard et al. 2012）。

在 CD20$^+$肿瘤病例中，使用抗 CD20 抗体（利妥昔单抗，每周注射 375mg/m^2，共使用 4 周）靶向增殖细胞常常是作为初期治疗的一种措施，反应率大约是 50%。在 80 个实体器官移植后发生的 PTLD 成年人病例中，除了减少 IS 之外，74%首先接受了利妥昔单抗治疗，后续则使用或不使用化疗（Evens et al. 2010）。在接受利妥昔单抗的患者中，3 年之内病情无进一步恶化的存活率及整体存活率分别是 70%和 73%，而在未接受单抗治疗病例中分别是 21%和 33%（$P < 0.0001$ 和 $P = 0.0001$）。多变量分析显示有 3 个风险因素与疾病进展和低存活率有关：中枢神经系统、骨髓干预和低白蛋白血症。针对 0 个、1 个或多于 2 个风险因素的整体存活率分别是 93%、68%和 11%。在 8 周之内 PTLD 对 IS 减少和利妥昔单抗不发生反应的病例中，现在都推荐迅速开始化疗（Montserrat 2012）。在实体器官移植之后，有 70 位成年人患者发生了 B 细胞 PTLD，这些病例可望包括在第二阶段的国际性研究中（Trappe et al. 2012）。对 IS 减少无反应的受试者在进行 4 周化疗（环磷酰胺、阿霉素、长春新碱和氢化波尼松）之后，接受 4 个疗程的利妥昔单抗治疗。PTLD 在 76%的病例中属于晚期型，其中 96%属于单一型分类，只有 44%的患者与 EBV 相关。59 位患者接受完全的治疗，分别在 90%和 68%的病例中显示部分或全部的反应。存活的中位数是 6.6 年。主要的不良作用是严重白细胞减少（68%）或感染（41%），还有在 11%的病例中发生 CHOP 相关的死亡率（5/7 对利妥昔单抗无反应）。EBV 相关性 PTLD 发生更早、患者更年轻、更多地涉及移植和肾脏及较少见的淋巴结反应，会产生更低的行为反应，并发生更严重感染。在 40 例具有完全反应的患者中，8 例复发并死于 PTLD（有 5 例在 6 个月内死亡）。总体而言，在 EBV 相关性 PTLD 中观察到疾病发展的风险更低（HR=0.007），在连续治疗后部分缓解的患者中具有较高的风险（HR=20.83）。在接受肝脏移植的儿童患者中，低剂量化疗也有一定效果（Gross et al. 2005）。患有 EBV 相关性 PTLD 的患者在试验减轻 IS 之后，接受了 6 轮低剂量环磷酰胺和强的松治疗[每 3 周为一轮，第一天服用环磷酰胺 600mg/m^2（体表面积），在第 1~5 天每天两次口服强的松 1mg/kg 体重]。两年内无疾病的存活率和整体存活率分别是 67%和 73%。该研究组还报道了将利妥昔单抗与低剂量化疗并用的结果（前两轮中的第 1、第 8 和第 15 天使用 375mg/m^2）（Gross et al. 2012）。两年内无疾病的存活率和整体存活率分别是 71%和 83%。副作用与前一个研究类似。在 55 名儿童中，10 名死亡，7 名患 PTLD，3 名受到感染。

抗病毒药物（更昔洛韦、阿昔洛韦）对症状明显的 PTLD 并不是一种有效的治疗方法，因为它们对这些疾病中的潜伏 EBV 周期无能为力。手术或放疗在局部疾病或中枢神经相关的疾病中有作用，但经常需要辅助其他的治疗（Heslop 2009）。

造血干细胞移植接受者中 EBV-PTLD 的各种治疗方法所产生的结果被广泛

讨论过（Styczynski et al. 2009a），这说明了使用 EBV-CTL 的利妥昔单抗优先治疗法可以大大减少死亡的风险（存活率为 89.7%和 94.1%）。同样的治疗用于公开的 PTLD 也能改善存活率（分别为 63%和 88.2%）。减少 IS 的存活率大约为 56.6%。化疗和抗病毒药剂不会影响患者的存活。

根据以上描述的所有结果，给在实体器官或干细胞移植后的 PTLD 治疗方法确定了指导方针（Styczynski et al. 2009b；Parker et al. 2010）。在实体器官移植之后，提供以下一些建议：减少 IS 应该在所有患者中启用（针对局限期疾病，减少 25%；针对广泛期疾病，减少 50%钙调神经磷酸酶抑制剂，停止咪唑硫嘌呤/霉酚酸酯，强的松每天最多 10mg；对广泛期疾病和重症患者，除了强的松之外停止所有用药）。移植功能应该密切监测。对于具有低风险 PTLD 的患者（年龄大于 60 周岁，正常 LDH，行为状态 ECOG 0~1），以及虽减少 IS 但疾病仍然发展的患者，建议使用利妥昔单抗单一治疗。对于使用这种治疗方法的患者，如果疾病仍然发展，或者在临床上具有严重的 PTLD 的患者，应该立即增加使用化疗（基于 CHOP 的方案）。在应用化疗时，应该使用预防性粒细胞集落刺激因子和抗感染制剂。在感染中枢神经系统的情况下，应该在减少 IS 之后使用局部放疗和类固醇。年轻患者中可以考虑使用高剂量氨甲蝶呤。对于局部性疾病，手术治疗或放疗是适当的。其他的方法如使用 EBV-CTL 输入的治疗、抗病毒药物、丁酸精氨酸、干扰素或静脉注射免疫球蛋白，目前只限于临床试验。在移植失败或者被移除的病例中，如有可能，应该考虑 PTLD 治愈至少一年之后重新移植。在骨髓/干细胞移植之后，提供如下建议：考虑到预防 EBV 重新活化，异体移植的接受者和移植捐献者应该做 EBV 血清学检测，抗病毒制剂和免疫球蛋白没有作用，因此不建议使用。对于 PTLD 优选治疗方法，接受异体移植的高风险患者应该密切监测 EBV 病毒滴度和 PTLD 症状，对使用利妥昔单抗（1~2 剂）的优选者，应该在病毒数量较多的患者中考虑使用 IS 减轻或 EBV-CTL 治疗。在没有 T 细胞耗竭或自体移植的 HLA 一致的患者中，没有必要进行监测。对于 PTLD 治疗，推荐利妥昔单抗（4~8 剂）、IS 减轻或 EBV-CTL 作为一线治疗方案，化疗作为第二线治疗方案，不推荐使用抗病毒药物。

5 小结

EBV 在人类感染率非常高，而对于 EBV 相关性肿瘤的预防和治疗还没有特异性的有效方法，仍需要深入研究。PTLD 仍然是实体器官或干细胞移植后的常见并发症，具有很高的患病率和死亡率。优先治疗和治愈疗法在过去的十年间取得了明显的进步，形成了如图 6-1 中所总结出的指导策略。为进一步探索这些策略对 PTLD 发病和患者/移植存活的确切影响，还有待于进行多中心前瞻性研究。

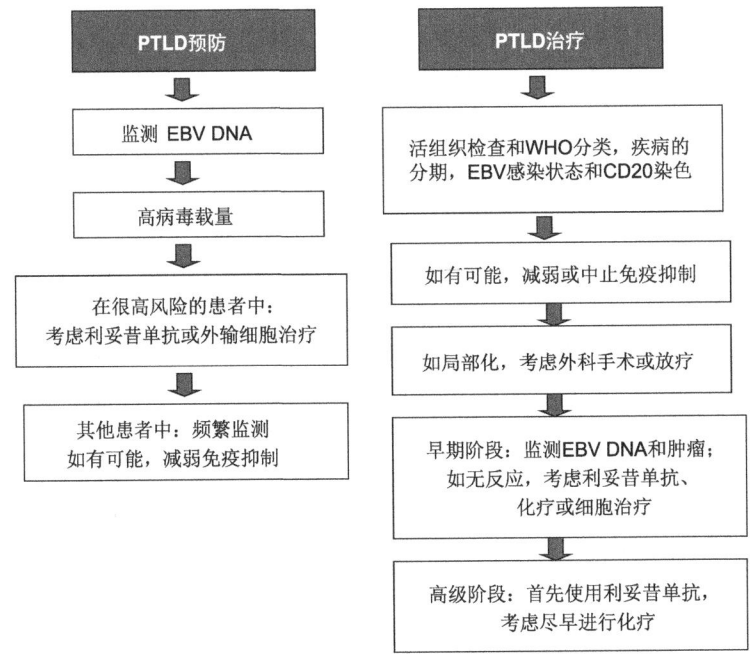

图 6-1　根据特定的指导方针，在实体器官或骨髓/干细胞移植之后，针对在患者体内产生的与 EBV 相关的 PTLD，本图提供了一套关于 EBV 监测和预防、治疗以及后续跟踪的流程（改编自 Heslop 2009 和 Parker et al. 2010）。

（卢建红，周中林　编译）

参 考 文 献

Bakker NA, van Imhoff GW, Verschuuren EA et al (2007) Presentation and early detection of post-transplant lymphoproliferative disorder after solid transplantation. Transpl Int 20:207–218

Bauer G (2001) Simplicity through complexity: immunoblot with recombinant antigens as the new gold standard in Epstein Barr virus serology. Clin Lab 47: 223–230

Bollard CM, Rooney CM, Heslop HE (2012) T-cell therapy in the treatment of post-transplant lymphoproliferative disease. Nat Rev Clin Oncol 9:510–519

Chen H, Chi P, Wang W et al (2014) Evaluation of a semi-quantitative ELISA for IgA antibody against Epstein-Barr virus capsid antigen in the serological diagnosis of nasopharyngeal carcinoma. Int J Infect Dis 25: 110–115

Cohen JI, Fauci AS, Varmus H et al (2011) Epstein-Barr virus: an important vaccine target for cancer prevention. Sci Transl Med 3:107fs7

De Paschale M, Clerici P (2012) Serological diagnosis of Epstein-Barr virus infection: Problems and solutions. World J Virol 1: 31–43

Doubroniva E, Oflaz-Sozmen B, Prockop SE et al (2012) Adoptive immunotherapy with unselected or EBV-specific T cells for biopsy-proven EBV+ lymphomas after allogeneic hematopoietic cell transplantation. Blood 119:2644–2656

Elliott SL, Suhrbier A, Miles JJ et al (2008) Phase I trial of a CD8+ T-cell peptide epitope-based vaccine for infectious mononucleosis. J Virol 82:1448–1457

Evens AM, David KA, Helenowski I et al (2010) Multicenter analysis of 80 solid organ transplantation recipients with post-transplant lymphoproliferative disease: outcomes and prognostic factors in the modern era. J Clin Oncol 28:1038–1046

Gross TG, Bucavals JC, Park JR et al (2005) Low-dose chemotherapy for Epstein-Barr virus positive post-transplantation lymphoproliferative disease in children after solid organ transplantation. J Clin Oncol 23:6481–6488

Gross TG, Orjuela MA, Perkins SL et al (2012) Low-dose chemotherapy and rituximab for posttransplant lymphoproliferative disease (PTLD):a children's oncology group report. Am J Transplant 12:3069–3075

Henle G, Henle W (1976) Epstein-Barr virus-specific IgA serum antibodies as an outstanding feature of nasopharyngeal carcinoma. Int J Cancer 17: 1–7

Heslop HE (2009) How I treat EBV lymphoproliferation. Blood 114:4002–4008

Heslop HE (2012) Equal-opportunity treatment of EBV–PTLD. Blood 119:2436–2438

Johannessen I, Bieleski L, Urquhart G et al (2011) Epstein-Barr virus, B cell lymphoproliferative disease, and SCID mice: modeling T cell immunotherapy in vivo. J Med Virol 83:1585–1596

Leen AM, Christin A, Myers GD et al (2009) Cytotoxic T lymphocyte therapy with donor T cells prevents and treats adenovirus and Epstein-Barr virus infections after haploidentical and matched unrelated stem cell transplantation. Blood 114:4283–4292

Long HM, Taylor GS, Rickinson AB (2011) Immune defence against EBV and EBV-associated disease. Curr Opin Immunol 23:258–264

Montserrat E (2012) PTLD treatment: a step forward, a long way to go. Lancet Oncol 13:120–121

Parker A, Bowles K, Bradley JA et al (2010) Management of post-transplant lymphoproliferative disorder in adult solid organ transplant recipients-BCSH and BTS guidelines. Br J Haematol 149:693–705

Schiller JT, Lowy DR (2010) Vaccines to prevent infections by oncoviruses. Annu Rev Microbiol 64:23–41

Sokal EM, Hoppenbrouwers K, Vandermeulen C et al (2007) Recombinant gp350 vaccine for infectious mononucleosis: a phase 2, randomized, double-blind, placebo-controlled trial to evaluate the safety, immunogenicity and efficacy of an Epstein-Barr virus vaccine in healthy young adults. J Infect Dis 196:1749–1753

Styczynski J, Einsele H, Gil L et al (2009a) Outcome of treatment of Epstein-Barr virus-related post-transplant lymphoproliferative disorder in hematopoietic stem cell recipients: a comprehensive review of reported cases. Transpl Infect Dis 11:383–392

Styczynski J, Reusser P, Einsele H et al (2009b) Management of HSV, VZV and EBV infections in patients with hematological malignancies and after SCT: guidelines from the second European conference on infections in leukemia. Bone Marrow Transplant 43:757–770

Sumaya CV, Ench Y (1985) Epstein-Barr virus infectious mononucleosis in children. II. Heterophil antibody and viral-specific responses. Pediatrics 75: 1011–1019

Trappe R, Oertel S, Leblond V et al (2012) Sequential treatment with rituximab followed by CHOP chemotherapy in adult B-cell post-transplant lymphoproliferative disorder (PTLD): the prospective international multicentre phase 2 PTLD-1 trial. Lancet Oncol 13:196–206

第7章 乙型肝炎病毒的致癌作用

Lise Rivière, Aurélie Ducroux 和 Marie Annick Buendia

摘 要 乙型肝炎病毒（HBV）是一种小的有包膜 DNA 病毒，感染后能引起人的急、慢性肝炎。HBV 感染是一个世界性的公共健康问题，全球约有 3.5 亿 HBV 慢性感染者面临着发展成肝病和肝细胞癌（HCC）的风险。慢性 HBV 携带者与肝癌（HCC）的发生存在确凿的流行病学相关性，因此 HBV 也被界定为人类肿瘤病毒。由于 HBV 感染并不会引起细胞病变，其致癌效应可能是 HBV 在肝脏癌变复杂步骤中直接和间接作用于细胞分子的综合结果。HBV 感染后宿主免疫反应引起的肝脏炎症与肝细胞增殖可能是细胞转化癌变的主要原因，病毒 DNA 整合到宿主染色体持续表达病毒相关产物能引起基因及表观遗传学的改变。值得注意的是，HBV 的 X 基因编码的转录调节蛋白 HBx 已被确认具有明显的促癌作用，HBx 有多重功能活性，在 HBV 致病性及肝癌形成中发挥重要作用。由于 HCC 预后差，迫切需要开发 HCC 早期诊断标志物及有效的抗慢性 HBV 感染的治疗方法。综上，阐明 HBV 相关的致癌机制将非常有助于制定合适、有效的治疗策略。

关键词 炎症，肝病，肝细胞癌，HBx，转录，遗传学，表观遗传学

1 引言

HBV 属小的有包膜 DNA 病毒，有明显的嗜肝性。HBV 有高度传染性，使用表面抗原 HBsAg 作为血清标记物进行检测，可以很容易地发现 HBV 在世界各国都有传播（El-Serag 2012）。流行病学研究证实慢性 HBV 携带者与 HCC 的产生密切

M. A. Buendia (✉)

Inserm U785, University Paris-Sud, 12 Avenue Paul Vaillant Couturier, 94800, Villejuif, France

e-mail: marie-annick.buendia@inserm.fr; marie-annick.buendia@pasteur.fr

L. Rivière _ A. Ducroux

Institut Pasteur, Hepacivirus and Innate Immunity Unit, 28 rue du Dr Roux, 75015, Paris, France

e-mail: lise.riviere@pasteur.fr

A. Ducroux

e-mail: aurelie.ducroux@pasteur.fr

相关，例如，HBV 暴发流行地区肝癌发病率明显偏高，在肝癌患者中，HBV 感染率明显高于普通人群，HBV 携带者肝癌发生明显增高，提示 HBV 感染可显著增加肝癌发生的风险（Beasley et al. 1981；Pagano et al. 2004）。与 HBV 同种属的其他哺乳动物嗜肝病毒，如土拨鼠肝炎病毒（WHV）和地松鼠肝炎病毒（GSHV），均能在其宿主中引起宿主肝肿瘤的产生（Benhenda et al. 2009b）。HCC 发生的风险不仅与 HBV 慢性感染相关，疾病转归还取决于宿主的自身状况及病毒参数和特性，如男性、早期感染、感染合并黄曲霉素 B1、酒精、糖尿病、过度肥胖、HBV 高病毒载量、HBeAg 阳性及 HBV 病毒基因型别（Fallot et al. 2012），均可增加 HCC 发生。对 11 582 名 HBV 感染者的 meta 荟萃分析结果显示，慢性肝炎患者从健康携带状态向 HCC 发展过程中，HBV 基因特定位置存在突变积累。值得注意的是，前 S 区功能域突变、基底核心启动子与 X 基因 3′端重叠区域的 C1653T、T1753V 和 A1762T/G1764A 突变相结合，与肝癌的发生高度相关（Liu et al. 2009）。

目前全球超过一半的 HCC 与慢性 HBV 感染有关，然而西方国家和日本只有 15%~20%的肿瘤发生在 HBsAg 阳性的患者中（Parkin 2006）。流行病学研究发现，HBsAg 阴性的 HCC 患者中 HBs 抗体和 HBc 抗体的检出较高，并且未经过肝硬化的 HBsAg 阴性患者体内仍然可以检测到 HBV DNA（Matsuzaki et al. 1997）。因此，无论 HBV 感染是否恢复均具有癌变风险。"隐匿性"HBV 感染发展为肿瘤的特点是：虽然缺乏 HBV 血清学标记，但是在血清和/或肝中仍可以通过聚合酶链反应（PCR）检测到低水平的 HBV DNA（Brechot 2004；Raimondo et al. 2008）。

慢性 HBV 感染的治疗方式主要有：聚乙二醇干扰素 α（IFN-α）；口服核苷或核苷类似物拉米夫定和阿德福韦。其中，聚乙二醇干扰素具有抗病毒、免疫调节和可能的抗肿瘤活性（Scaglione and Lok 2012）。虽然这些治疗方案不能完全清除病毒，但可以阻止进一步的肝损伤，甚至逆转治疗之前的肝损伤。值得注意的是，接受治疗持续 2 年的慢性乙型肝炎患者 HCC 发生率较没有治疗的患者明显降低（Papatheodoridis et al. 2010）。

乙型肝炎疫苗可以阻止慢性 HBV 感染及相关肝疾病的产生，在绝大多数的国家现被纳入儿童基础免疫计划。有地方性 HBV 流行的国家已充分证明乙型肝炎疫苗的普及能有效降低 HBV 感染及肝癌的发生（特别是在儿童）(Ott et al. 2012）。但是世界范围内慢性 HBV 携带者的总人数仍在持续增加，占全球人口的 6%。

2　HBV 基因组及复制

HBV 基因组大小 3.2kb，是最小的人类 DNA 病毒，现分为 8 个型别（A~H 型），不同型别间有超过 8%的核酸序列不一致，各型别可以进一步分成不同的亚型（Schaefer 2005）。HBV 病毒基因组高度紧凑，由 4 个重叠的开放阅读框（ORF）

覆盖整个基因组，编码衣壳蛋白、表面蛋白、聚合酶和 HBx 反式激活因子（图 7-1）。另外，通过聚合酶基因的一个框移剪切 mRNA 可以翻译一种称为 HBSP 的蛋白质（Soussan et al. 2000）。综上，整个调节区域（包括启动子、增强子、转录起始区、多聚 A 尾信号）都嵌入到编码序列中。

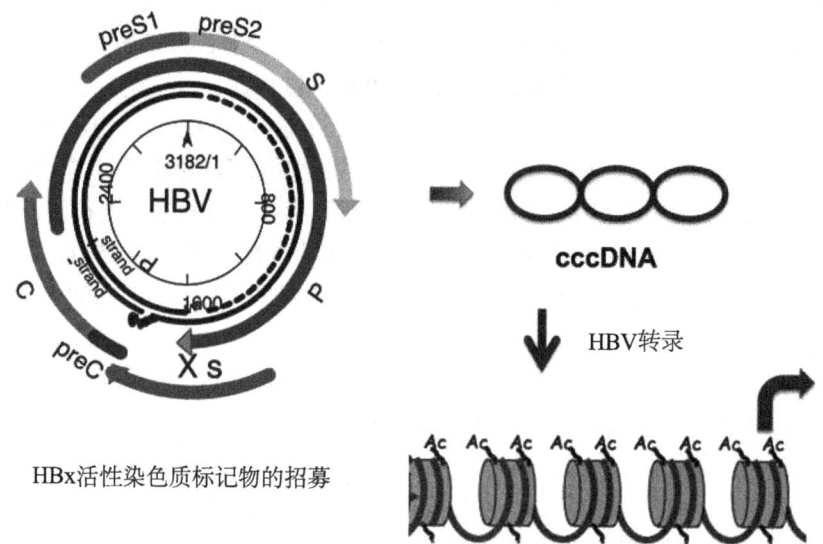

图 7-1　乙型肝炎病毒基因组合和共价闭合环状 DNA（cccDNA）。病毒基因组（图 7-1 左）由两段线性 DNA 链通过连贯的末端首尾连接成环状结构。负链长度大约为 3.182kb，正链长度可变，其具有固定位置的 5′端和可变位置的 3′端。环绕病毒基因组的粗箭头表示 4 个编码病毒蛋白的开放阅读框。病毒入侵后，HBV 基因组被释放到细胞核中，在那里通过细胞机制转变成 cccDNA。cccDNA 被组织成微小染色体，结合在组蛋白、非组蛋白（如 HBx 和核心蛋白）上。通过招募不同的染色质修饰因子（如 CBP/p300），HBx 在表观遗传标志物（如组蛋白末端乙酰化和甲基化）的调节中起到核心作用，从而导致活性 HBV 转录。

　　HBV 感染时，部分双链 DNA 基因组运送至细胞核，转变为共价闭合环状 DNA（cccDNA）。cccDNA 作为转录模板，通过宿主的 RNA 聚合酶 II 进行整个病毒 RNA 转录（图 7-1）。HBV 主要的转录产物（3.5kb、2.4kb、2.1kb、0.7kb）由 4 个不同的病毒启动子及 2 个增强子（Enh I 和 Enh II）进行调控（Doitsh and Shaul 2004；Moolla et al. 2002）。在 HBV 转录启动子和增强子顺式序列上已鉴定出几个普遍存在的、肝特异性的转录因子结合位点，它们可能调节 HBV 在体内的转录（Fallot et al. 2012；Moolla et al. 2002）。而且，HBV cccDNA 转录是通过 DNA 甲基化和组蛋白乙酰化等表观遗传机制进行调节的（Pollicino et al. 2006；Vivekanandan et al. 2009）。并且，由于 cccDNA 持续存在，导致大部分抗病毒治疗不能完全清除病毒而失败。因此，cccDNA 可作为抗慢性乙肝感染有效治疗的重要靶点。

HBV RNA 被运输到细胞质并转录为病毒蛋白后，前基因组 RNA 选择性地与聚合酶一起包装为子代衣壳，然后被病毒聚合酶逆转录为 RC-DNA。HBV 聚合酶具有 RNA 依赖的 DNA 聚合酶活性，与逆转录酶病毒及花椰菜花叶病毒（CaMV）的 RT 序列同源（Toh et al. 1983）。HBV 复制启动是通过病毒 RT 结合到前基因组 RNA 的 5'端衣壳化包装信号上引起病毒衣壳化（Bartenschlager and Schaller 1992）。在两条 HBV DNA 链不对称复制后，包含成熟 RC-DNA 的衣壳在内质网被包装进病毒包膜，一般认为随后的病毒出芽是发生在细胞内膜（Bruss 2007）。此外，上述包装会产生大量过剩的空包膜粒子，可能是病毒诱导宿主免疫产生无效免疫反应（从而产生免疫逃逸）。一小部分成熟的衣壳能循环运送 RC-DNA 到细胞核，有利于核内的 cccDNA 池扩增。包膜蛋白的数量和包装成核衣壳的效率对于病毒形态形成及 cccDNA 累积是非常重要的（Summers et al. 1991）。由于无症状 HBV 携带者的健康肝脏也能产生大量的病毒粒子，肝损伤也可能是正常的病毒复制过程受到破坏，肝内大量的大包膜蛋白积累或过量的 cccDNA 累积导致（Wang et al. 2006）。

3 HBx——一个具有复杂结构和功能的反式激活因子

X 基因编码的 HBx（或 pX）蛋白是一个只有 154 个氨基酸的多肽（16.5kDa），在急性和慢性感染时呈低水平表达，可以诱导机体产生体液和细胞免疫反应（Su et al. 1998）。X 基因在哺乳动物嗜肝病毒中保留，但是在禽类嗜肝病毒基因组中缺失。HBx 这个小蛋白中与特异功能相关的不同功能域已经被鉴定（图 7-2）。然而，由于目前还不能生产出足够数量的可溶性蛋白，所以对于 HBx 的三维结构知之甚少。HBx 是一个非结构蛋白，通过与伴侣蛋白相互作用并被折叠获得二级结构（Rui et al. 2005），这种结构灵活性导致 HBx 活性非常广泛多样。

HBx 在体内的一个重要作用是进行病毒复制，但是这种作用机制还未完全阐明，可能是多因子的作用途径。HBx 蛋白的确天生具有多重活性，作为一种有多重活性的反式激活因子在细胞质和细胞核中对病毒与细胞基因起作用。HBx 能激活细胞和病毒启动子的转录，包括 HBV 的启动子，通过调节胞浆钙、细胞增殖及凋亡来破坏多种细胞功能和细胞转导通路。虽然 HBx 调节的这些细胞活动有助于增加病毒复制，细胞与小鼠动物模型的研究提示 HBx 其实是直接刺激 HBV 转录。在 HBV 转基因小鼠和注射质粒编码 HBV 基因组小鼠中，HBx 表达能显著活化 HBV 复制，但是这种作用在肝癌细胞系中并不明显（Keasler et al. 2007；Leupin et al. 2005；Tang et al. 2005）。在 HBV 感染中，HBx 通常会作为一个重要的调节因子在自然感染 HBV 的过程中启动和维持 HBV 复制（Lucifora et al. 2011）。最近研究发现，HBx 通过增加活性染色质标志物、拮抗抑制性因子，与 HBV 微小染色体的表观遗传调节相互作用（Belloni et al. 2009；Cougot et al. 2012）。

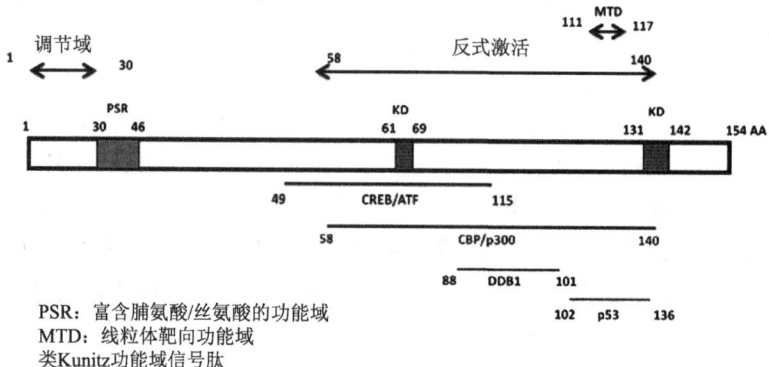

图 7-2 具有重要功能域的小蛋白 HBx 模式图。N 端结构域编码一个调节域（Murakami 1999）和一个富含脯氨酸/丝氨酸的功能域。Kumar 和同事们绘制了 HBx 大多数执行转录反式激活的功能域图谱（Kumar et al. 1996），包含线粒体靶向功能域（Li et al. 2008）。分子伴侣结合域（图中下面部分）包括 CREB/ATF（Maguire et al. 1991）、CBP/p300（Cougot et al. 2007）、DDB1（Becker et al. 1998；Lin-Marq et al. 2001）和 p53（Lin et al. 1997）。

　　HBx 通过与大量位于细胞质或细胞核的细胞伴侣相互作用来发挥作用，这种现象与 HBx 的核质双重定位是一致的。已经表明，HBx 可以与基底的转录复合物（RPB5、TFIIB、TBP、TFIIH）、转录因子（ATF/CREB、c/EBP、NF-1L6、RXR 受体）、共刺激物（CBP/P300、ASC-2）及抑制剂（DNMT）发生相互作用，这与它在转录中的作用一致（Benhenda et al. 2009a）。我们的研究发现，HBx 被募集到 CREB 靶基因的启动子区域，进一步增加 CBP/P300 在 CREB 上的募集，从而激活转录（Cougot et al. 2007）。这样，HBx 还可以直接参与到增强子转录因子复合物的组装中。综上，HBx 在大分子蛋白复合体中通过调节转录调控因子网络，在 HBV 转录的表观遗传学调控中发挥直接作用（Belloni et al. 2009；Cougot et al. 2012）。

4　HBx 与 E3 泛素连接酶：不仅仅是蛋白稳定性的一种联系？

　　调控蛋白降解机制是病毒利于自身复制并逃逸宿主细胞保护机制的一种常见策略（Barry and Fruh 2006）。损伤特异 DNA 结合蛋白 1（DDB1）是以 Cul4A 为基础的泛素蛋白 E3 连接酶复合体的转接亚单位。大量文献报道，HBx 可以与损伤特异 DNA 结合蛋白 1（DDB1）（Cul4A 泛素 E3 连接酶复合物的转接亚单位）相互作用（Lee et al. 1995；Leupin et al. 2003；Sitterlin et al. 1997）。DDB1 是一个高度保守的蛋白质，通过多个 WD40 蛋白连接到 CUL4-ROC1-E2 催化中心，并与 DDB2 共同参与 DNA 修复（Jackson and Xiong 2009）。HBx 上最小的 DDB1 结合域（氨基酸 88~100）包含有一个可以诱发 DDB1 结合 WD40（DWD）的结构基序序列，这个基序序列也存在于细胞 DCAF 上（He et al. 2006）。这个区域的几个点突变能阻止 HBx 结合 DDB1（Bergametti et al. 2002；Hodgson et al. 2012）（表 7-1）。高分辨率的 HBx 晶体结构显示 HBx 上第 88~100 肽能直接结合到 DDB1 上（Li et al. 2010）。而且，在 DDB1 上与 HBx 结合的特殊区域是大多数 DCAF 上常见的结合位点。这些数据表明，HBx 与细胞的 DCAF 有某些相似的特点，可能取代其他的 DCAF，从而改变 Cul4A 复合物底物的特征。到目前为止，还没有鉴定出 HBx 在调节这些底物的稳定性和定位方面的作用。

表 7-1 肝细胞癌中常见 HBx 突变的检测及用来显示 HBx 特异性功能的合成变异体。对于每一个 HBx 突变体，表中列出了它们已知的特异性活性，如转录反式激活、细胞周期、存活能力和转化的异常。与野生型 HBx 相比，突变体增强活性用+表示，相同活性用=表示，减弱的活性用-表示。来自两篇不同论文的不同数据用两个符号表示（=/+或=/-）。相应的信息可以在参考文献中找到

	流行病学	反式激活	生长抑制/凋亡/G_1 阻滞	细胞转化对 HBx WT	其他	参考文献
HBx wt (1-154)		是	是	看具体情况		
HCC 中的常见变异	增加 HCC 发生风险	−	+		T 细胞活性低效	Takahashi et al. 1998
K130M + V131I	与重型肝炎和肝硬化的相关					Malmassari et al. 2007
L30F S144A	32%肿瘤中检测到	=/−	=/−			Liu et al. 2009
V88I	27%HCC 和肝硬化患者中检测到					Wang et al. 2012
S31A						Wang et al. 2012
	常在 HCC 中检测到（整合 HBV 序列）					Yeh et al. 2000
C 端删除			−	+		Poussin et al. 1999
1-101			−	+		Sirma et al. 1999
1-114						
1-120			−	=		Tu et al. 2001
1-124			−	=		Ma et al. 2008
1-128			−	+	不大稳定	Lizzano et al. 2011
1-131			−	=/+		
1-134			−	+		Luo et al. 2012
1-136						
1-140						Fujimoto et al. 2012
1-143						
1-144						Sung et al. 2012
1-146						

续表

	流行病学	反式激活	生长抑制/凋亡/G_1阻滞	细胞转化对HBx WT	其他	参考文献
其他突变/删除		=/−	=	+	不大稳定	Cheong et al. 1995
1—50		=	=	=		Luo et al. 2012
43—154		=	=	=		
51—154				=		
58—140						
106—154						
R35E		−				
C61L						
C69L		=/−	=	=	与RPB5没有相互作用	Gottlob et al. 1998
P90V/K91L		=				Kumar et al. 1996
C115A		−				Gottlob et al. 1998
		−			和DDB1相互作用减弱	Leupin et al. 2003
		−				Becker et al. 1998
					线粒体靶向破坏	Lin-Marq et al. 2001
						Li et al. 2008

研究显示,HBx/DDB1 相互作用是存在于哺乳动物嗜肝病毒中,并在病毒复制,以及在 HBx 的稳定性和功能中起重要作用(Bontron et al. 2002;Sitterlin et al. 2000a)。特别是 HBx 的转录和促凋亡特征依赖于其与 DDB1 的相互作用(Lin-Marq et al. 2001;Sitterlin et al. 2000b)。突变的 HBx 一旦失去与 DDB1 的结合能力,其相应的细胞毒性作用也会丧失,但是直接与 DDB1 融合时又会恢复活性。这些研究提示 HBx 不抑制正常的 DDB1 功能,但是将凋亡的潜能传递给 DDB1(Bontron et al. 2002)。然而,利用不能结合 DDB1 的 HBx 突变体进行试验表明,HBx 的转录活性与其是否结合 DDB1 无关(Wentz et al. 2000)(表 7-1)。近来关于 HBx 介导 HBV 转录和复制的激活确定了 HBx-DDB1 相互作用的重要性,但也指出了最大限度地刺激 HBV 的转录需要 HBx 羧基末端区域的参与(Hodgson et al. 2012;Luo et al. 2012)。

DDB1 也属于 UV-DDB 复合物,参与紫外损伤 DNA 的修复,而 HBx 抑制核苷酸切除修复(NER)(Mathonnet et al. 2004)。关于 HBx-DDB1 相互作用对 DNA 修复影响的深入研究发现,HBx 通过干扰 S 期,间接诱导不正常的细胞有丝分裂,S 期的改变能导致异常的中心体复制。有正常双极纺锤体的细胞分裂中,HBx 能诱导延迟的染色体,接着形成异常数量的中心体和多极纺锤体的多核细胞

（Martin-Lluesma et al. 2008）。因此，这种相互作用对于乙肝慢性化病理机制至关重要。

5 HBx 与肝细胞恶性转化

可调节性乙型肝炎病毒X蛋白被认为参与肝脏癌变过程。HBx 本身并不致癌，小鼠实验发现 HBx 可以转化 SV40-永生化的小鼠肝细胞，在 HBx 转基因小鼠中通过致癌物质或通过 c-Myc 能诱导肝肿瘤或加速致癌作用（Höhne et al. 1990；Kim et al. 1991；Madden et al. 2001；Terradillos et al. 1997）。细胞癌基因和生长因子的反式激活及细胞周期失调是构成这个病毒蛋白弱致癌性的两个机制（Bouchard and Schneider 2004）。其他的人类肿瘤病毒如人类 T 细胞白血病病毒（HTLV-1）、EB 病毒（EBV）、人类乳头瘤病毒 16 和 18（HPV-16 和-18），转化能力与病毒基因产物的转录反式激活相关。比较分析不同病毒反式激活方式，有助于指导病毒与癌症相关领域未来的研究。此外，HBx 可诱导几种信号通路的异常激活，包括 Src、Ras、MAP 激酶和 CREB 通路，从而引起细胞功能失调的积累，促成恶性转化（Andrisani and Barnabas 1999）。

HBx 的另一个促癌活性是攻击细胞有丝分裂周期。HBx 和不同细胞伴侣相互作用参与中心体形成，可能导致中心体动力学及有丝分裂纺锤体形成的缺陷。HBx 可能结合并部分灭活 BubR1（一种有丝分裂激酶效应器，能特异地结合微管，发挥关卡功能）（Kim et al. 2008）。HBx 也可以结合 HBXIP（HBXIP 是中心体复制的一个主要调节物，是双极纺锤体形成和细胞质分裂所必需的）（Wen et al. 2008）。值得注意的是，HBx 诱导的 DNA 再复制通常被认为与部分多倍体相关，多倍体是一种与癌症相关的状态（Rakotomalala et al. 2008）。HBx 还参与染色体不稳定性（CIN，癌症的一种标志）的诱导。具有额外中心体的 CIN 细胞在细胞分裂后期显示出延迟染色体增多，导致染色质杂合并错误分离。在表达 HBx 的细胞中，异常的中心体复制、多极纺锤体形成、染色体分离缺陷及多核细胞的形成都与 S 期延长有关（Studach et al. 2009，2010）。HBx 表达的多极细胞倾向于癌变，这种癌变是由有丝分裂进入因子 polo 样激酶 1（Plk1）介导的。反过来，Plk1 通过表观遗传机制下调 ZNF198 和 SUZ12 来调节 HBV 转录与复制（Wang et al. 2011）。另一些研究提示了 HBx 与 DDB1 相互作用可增加基因不稳定性（Li et al. 2010；Martin-Lluesma et al. 2008）。总之，上述研究都说明 HBx 活性与染色体不稳定性之间有很强的联系，与其他风险因素相比，在 HBV 感染相关肿瘤中 HBx 活性大大增加了染色体缺陷发生的比例（Boyault et al. 2007）。

作者观察到 HBx 表达在人类 HCC 中经常是保留的，HBV 甲基化研究显示除了 X 基因，HCC 中 HBV 基因组普遍出现高度甲基化修饰，因此 HBx 是否参与到癌症的进展需要进一步的研究（Fernandez et al. 2009）。

6 HCC 中 HBV DNA 整合及突变的 X 基因

绝大多数 HBV 相关的 HCC 中都可以检测到整合的 HBV DNA（Bréchot et al. 1980；Bonilla Guerrero and Roberts 2005）。近年来用多种 PCR 方法分析病毒插入位点，结果显示整合位点不仅出现在重复序列和脆性位点，在活性转录区域（紧靠或在细胞内基因）出现的频率也很高（Murakami et al. 2005）。有少量研究发现嵌合的 HBV/细胞转录子产生的病毒/细胞蛋白具有致癌作用，证实重排的病毒、宿主序列有致癌潜能。除了"传统"靶点，如视黄酸受体 α（RARα）和细胞周期蛋白 A2，还有许多 HBV 嵌合物是调节细胞增殖和死亡的靶向关键调节子。HBx 融合蛋白相关报道已经很多，包括与 *SERCA1* 基因，以及 *MLL2*、*MLL3* 和 *MLL4* 基因的融合（Chami et al. 2000；Saigo et al. 2008；Tamori et al. 2005）。

另一方面，整合的 HBx 序列经常发生突变，具有一些特殊的特性，导致"反式作用"致癌机制的发生。因为 X 基因的 3′端与位于 HBV 基因组正向 DR1 和 DR2 中易于重组的区域序列一致，所以在 HCC 中可经常检测到 C 端截短的 X 基因（Luo et al. 2012）（表 7-1）。功能性研究已经总结出肿瘤来源的 HBx 蛋白与野生型 HBx 的不同特征。在一些情况下，这些序列保留着反式激活潜能及结合 p53 并阻滞 p53 介导的凋亡能力，这可能有利于肿瘤细胞的生长（Huo et al. 2001）。而且，体内外研究截短而不是全长的 HBx 能更有效转化肝细胞永生化，调节那些与细胞周期和凋亡相关基因的表达（Ma et al. 2008）。最近的研究表明，HBx 的 C 端影响整个蛋白质的稳定性、反式激活性能和增加 HBV 复制（Lizzano et al. 2011）。相反，在另一些报道中，截短的 X 序列可以引起一些错义突变，降低转录的反式激活、凋亡诱导和 HBV 复制效率（Sirma et al. 1999）。综上所述，对 HBx 蛋白功能的研究将有助于更好地理解 X 基因产物对于持续 HBV 感染引起恶性转化不同阶段的重要性。

7 结论与展望

HCC 在很多国家已成为最常见的肿瘤，并且其发生率在过去几年里一直呈上升趋势（Ferlay et al. 2010）。和其他的人类肿瘤一样，HBV 相关的肿瘤是通过多重步骤引起遗传和表观遗传学损伤累积的结果（图 7-3）。由于细胞系和转基因小鼠中 HBV 病毒缺乏直接转化能力，并且从 HBV 首次感染到发展为 HCC 后需经历一段很长的潜伏期，因此 HBV 是否致癌还存在疑问。简单地看，免疫系统对病毒感染的肝细胞产生免疫反应触发与持续坏死和细胞再生相关的促癌炎症过程，导致遗传与表观遗传学缺陷的累积。在这个模型中，HBV 感染时病毒基因产物的长期毒性效应可能增强外源致癌因素的致癌作用，如黄曲霉素 B1 和酒精。值得注意的是，越来越多的流行病学研究和证据表明，野生型或突变型的 HBx 蛋白及表面糖蛋白具有潜在致癌性，提示 HBV 感染是一个独立的致癌因素。因此，HBV 与其他的人类致瘤病毒有相似的基本策略。可以推测，HBV 整合决定着 HCC 的潜伏期，并促进基因不稳定或导致相关基因的顺式或反式激活。鉴定与 HBV 感染和肝细胞转化相关的细胞效应是非常重要的。

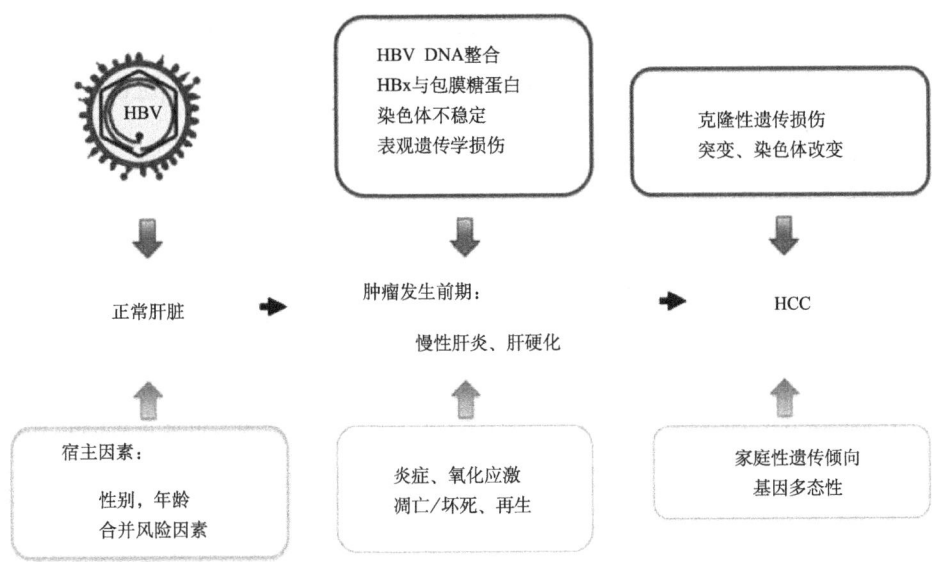

图 7-3 HBV 诱导肝癌发生的多步骤过程。慢性 HBV 感染，无论是单独或是和其他因素共同作用，会触发级联反应，最终导致转化。在肿瘤出现前期，免疫响应诱导一种炎性组织疾病，从而为基因和表观遗传损伤创造一个合适的环境。整合 HBV DNA 到宿主基因组，以及长期产生病毒性 HBx 和表面蛋白会通过多种机制促进肿瘤发生。

现在可以通过对全基因组表达、遗传和表观遗传改变及蛋白质组学等的全基因扫描新技术明确 HBV 是否触发与其他风险因素不同的致癌通路。因此，根据肿瘤发生的途径及 HBV 相关的肿瘤被分为不同亚类，这些亚类表现出染色体高度不稳定、干细胞表型、p53 突变频率增加，以及 β-连环蛋白低突变（Boyault et al. 2007；Guichard et al. 2012）。运用现有技术分析不同阶段的慢性乙肝以发现合适的预后指标和治疗靶点是很重要的，另外，有必要进一步明确 HBV 在甲基化相关的基因沉默和 microRNA 异常表达等表观遗传改变方面对于肿瘤恶性转化的作用。对这个领域研究的不断发展无疑会对控制慢性乙型肝炎病毒感染及相关肝癌治疗提供新的途径。

(瞿小旺,刘文培 译)

参 考 文 献

Andrisani OM, Barnabas S (1999) The transcriptional function of the hepatitis B virus X protein and its role in hepatocarcinogenesis. Int J Oncol 15:373–379

Barry M, Fruh K (2006) Viral modulators of cullin RING ubiquitin ligases: culling the host defense. Sci STKE 335:21

Bartenschlager R, Schaller H (1992) Hepadnaviral assembly is initiated by polymerase binding to the encapsidation signal in the viral genome. EMBO J 11:3413–3420

Beasley RP, Lin CC, Hwang LY et al (1981) Hepatocellular carcinoma and hepatitis B virus: a prospective study of 22,707 men in Taiwan. Lancet 2:1129–1133

Becker SA, Lee TH, Butel JS et al (1998) Hepatitis B virus X protein interferes with cellular DNA repair. J Virol 72:266–272

Belloni L, Pollicino T, De Nicola F et al (2009) Nuclear HBx binds the HBV minichromosome and modifies the epigenetic regulation of cccDNA function. Proc Natl Acad Sci U S A 106:19975–19979

Benhenda S, Cougot D, Buendia MA et al (2009a) Hepatitis B virus X protein molecular functions and its role in virus life cycle and pathogenesis. Adv Cancer Res 103:75–109

Benhenda S, Cougot D, Neuveut C et al (2009b) Liver cell transformation in chronic HBV infection. Viruses 1:630–646

Bergametti F, Sitterlin D, Transy C (2002) Turnover of hepatitis B virus X protein is regulated by damaged DNA-binding complex. J Virol 76:6495–6501

Bonilla Guerrero R, Roberts LR (2005) The role of hepatitis B virus integrations in the pathogenesis of human hepatocellular carcinoma. J Hepatol 42:760–777

Bontron S, Lin-Marq N, Strubin M (2002) Hepatitis B virus X protein associated with UV-DDB1 induces cell death in the nucleus and is functionally antagonized by UV-DDB2. J Biol Chem 277:38847–38854

Bouchard MJ, Schneider RJ (2004) The enigmatic X gene of hepatitis B virus. J Virol 78:12725–12734

Boyault S, Rickman DS, de Reynies A et al (2007) Transcriptome classification of HCC is related to gene alterations and to new therapeutic targets. Hepatology 45:42–52

Brechot C (2004) Pathogenesis of hepatitis B virus-related hepatocellular carcinoma: old and new paradigms. Gastroenterology 127:S56–S61

Bréchot C, Pourcel C, Louise A et al (1980) Presence of integrated hepatitis B virus DNA sequences in cellular DNA of human hepatocellular carcinoma. Nature 286:533–535

Bruss V (2007) Hepatitis B virus morphogenesis. World J Gastroenterol 13:65–73

Chami M, Gozuacik D, Saigo K et al (2000) Hepatitis B virus-related insertional mutagenesis implicates SERCA1 gene in the control of apoptosis. Oncogene 19:2877–2886

Cheong J, Yi M, Lin Y et al (1995) Human RPB5, a subunit shared by eukaryotic nuclear RNA polymerases, binds human hepatitis B virus X protein and may play a role in X transactivation. EMBO J 14:143–150

Cougot D, Allemand E, Riviere L et al (2012) Inhibition of PP1 phosphatase activity by HBx: a mechanism for the activation of hepatitis B virus transcription. Sci Signal 5(250):ra1

Cougot D, Wu Y, Cairo S et al (2007) The hepatitis B virus X protein functionally interacts with CREB-binding protein/p300 in the regulation of CREB-mediated transcription. J Biol Chem 282:4277–4287

Doitsh G, Shaul Y (2004) Enhancer I predominance in hepatitis B virus gene expression. Mol Cell Biol 24:1799–1808

El-Serag HB (2012) Epidemiology of viral hepatitis and hepatocellular carcinoma. Gastroenterology 142(1264–1273):e1261

Fallot G, Neuveut C, Buendia MA (2012) Diverse roles of hepatitis B virus in liver cancer. Curr Opin Virol available online (in press)

Ferlay J, Shin HR, Bray F et al (2010) Estimates of worldwide burden of cancer in 2008: GLOBOCAN 2008. Int J Cancer 127:2893–2917

Fernandez AF, Rosales C, Lopez-Nieva P et al (2009) The dynamic DNA methylomes of double-stranded DNA viruses associated with human cancer. Genome Res 19:438–451

Fujimoto A, Totoki Y, Abe T et al (2012) Whole-genome sequencing of liver cancers identifies etiological influences on mutation patterns and recurrent mutations in chromatin regulators. Nat Genet 44:760–764

Gottlob K, Pagano S, Levrero M et al (1998) Hepatitis B virus X protein transcription activation domains are neither required nor sufficient for cell transformation. Cancer Res 58:3566–3570

Guichard C, Amaddeo G, Imbeaud S et al (2012) Integrated analysis of somatic mutations and focal copy-number changes identifies key genes and pathways in hepatocellular carcinoma. Nat Genet 44:694–698

He YJ, McCall CM, Hu J et al (2006) DDB1 functions as a linker to recruit receptor WD40 proteins to CUL4-ROC1 ubiquitin ligases. Genes Dev 20:2949–2954

Hodgson AJ, Hyser JM, Keasler VV et al (2012) Hepatitis B virus regulatory HBx protein binding to DDB1 is required but is not sufficient for maximal HBV replication. Virology 426:73–82

Höhne M, Schaefer S, Seifer M et al (1990) Malignant transformation of immortalized transgenic hepatocytes after transfection with hepatitis B virus DNA. EMBO J 9:1137–1145

Huo TI, Wang XW, Forgues M et al (2001) Hepatitis B virus X mutants derived from human hepatocellular carcinoma retain the ability to abrogate p53-induced apoptosis. Oncogene 20:3620–3628

Jackson S, Xiong Y (2009) CRL4 s: the CUL4-RING E3 ubiquitin ligases. Trends Biochem Sci 34:562–570

Keasler VV, Hodgson AJ, Madden CR et al (2007) Enhancement of hepatitis B virus replication by the regulatory X protein in vitro and in vivo. J Virol 81:2656–2662

Kim CM, Koike K, Saito I et al (1991) HBx gene of hepatitis B virus induces liver cancer in transgenic mice. Nature 351:317–320

Kim S, Park SY, Yong H et al (2008) HBV X protein targets hBubR1, which induces dysregulation of the mitotic checkpoint. Oncogene 27:3457–3464

Kumar V, Jayasuryan N, Kumar R (1996) A truncated mutant (residues 58–140) of the hepatitis B virus X protein retains transactivation function. Proc Natl Acad Sci USA 93:5647–5652

Lee TH, Elledge SJ, Butel JS (1995) Hepatitis B virus X protein interacts with a probable DNA repair protein. J Virol 69:1107–1114

Leupin O, Bontron S, Schaeffer C et al (2005) Hepatitis B virus X protein stimulates viral genome replication via a DDB1-dependent pathway distinct from that leading to cell death. J Virol 79:4238–4245

Leupin O, Bontron S, Strubin M (2003) Hepatitis B virus X protein and simian virus 5 V protein exhibit similar UV-DDB1 binding properties to mediate distinct activities. J Virol 77:6274–6283

Li SK, Ho SF, Tsui KW et al (2008) Identification of functionally important amino acid residues in the mitochondria targeting sequence of hepatitis B virus X protein. Virology 381:81–88

Li T, Robert EI, van Breugel PC et al (2010) A promiscuous alpha-helical motif anchors viral hijackers and substrate receptors to the CUL4-DDB1 ubiquitin ligase machinery. Nat Struct Mol Biol 17:105–111

Lin Y, Nomura T, Yamashita T et al (1997) The transactivation and p53-interacting functions of hepatitis B virus X protein are mutually interfering but distinct. Cancer Res 57:5137–5142

Lin-Marq N, Bontron S, Leupin O et al (2001) Hepatitis B virus X protein interferes with cell viability through interaction with the p127-kDa UV-damaged DNA-binding protein. Virology 287:266–274

Liu S, Zhang H, Gu C et al (2009) Associations between hepatitis B virus mutations and the risk of hepatocellular carcinoma: a meta-analysis. J Natl Cancer Inst 101:1066–1082

Lizzano RA, Yang B, Clippinger AJ et al (2011) The C-terminal region of the hepatitis B virus X protein is essential for its stability and function. Virus Res 155:231–239

Lucifora J, Arzberger S, Durantel D et al (2011) Hepatitis B virus X protein is essential to initiate and maintain virus replication after infection. J Hepatol 55:996–1003

Luo N, Cai Y, Zhang J et al (2012) The C-terminal region of the hepatitis B virus X protein is required for its stimulation of HBV replication in primary mouse hepatocytes. Virus Res 165:170–178

Ma NF, Lau SH, Hu L et al (2008) COOH-terminal truncated HBV X protein plays key role in hepatocarcinogenesis. Clin Cancer Res 14:5061–5068

Madden CR, Finegold MJ, Slagle BL (2001) Hepatitis B virus X protein acts as a tumor promoter in development of diethylnitrosamine-induced preneoplastic lesions. J Virol 75:3851–3858

Maguire HF, Hoeffler JP, Siddiqui A (1991) HBV X protein alters the DNA binding specificity of CREB and ATF-2 by protein-protein interactions. Science 252:842–844

Malmassari SL, Deng Q, Fontaine H et al (2007) Impact of hepatitis B virus basic core promoter mutations on T cell response to an immunodominant HBx-derived epitope. Hepatology 45:1199–1209

Martin-Lluesma S, Schaeffer C, Robert EI et al (2008) Hepatitis B virus X protein affects S phase progression leading to chromosome segregation defects by binding to damaged DNA binding protein 1. Hepatology 48:1467–1476

Mathonnet G, Lachance S, Alaoui-Jamali M et al (2004) Expression of hepatitis B virus X oncoprotein inhibits transcription-coupled nucleotide excision repair in human cells. Mutat Res 554:305–318

Matsuzaki Y, Chiba T, Hadama T et al (1997) HBV genome integration and genetic instability in HBsAg-negative and anti-HCV-positive hepatocellular carcinoma in Japan. Cancer Lett 119:53–61

Moolla N, Kew M, Arbuthnot P (2002) Regulatory elements of hepatitis B virus transcription. J Viral Hepat 9:323–331

Murakami S (1999) Hepatitis B virus X protein: structure, function and biology. Intervirology 42:81–99

Murakami Y, Saigo K, Takashima H et al (2005) Large scaled analysis of hepatitis B virus (HBV) DNA integration in HBV related hepatocellular carcinomas. Gut 54:1162–1168

Ott JJ, Stevens GA, Groeger J et al (2012) Global epidemiology of hepatitis B virus infection: new estimates of age-specific HBsAg seroprevalence and endemicity. Vaccine 30:2212–2219
Pagano JS, Blaser M, Buendia MA et al (2004) Infectious agents and cancer: criteria for a causal relation. Sem Cancer Biol 14:453–471

Papatheodoridis GV, Lampertico P, Manolakopoulos S et al (2010) Incidence of hepatocellular carcinoma in chronic hepatitis B patients receiving nucleos(t)ide therapy: a systematic review. J Hepatol 53:348–356

Parkin DM (2006) The global health burden of infection-associated cancers in the year 2002. Int J Cancer 118:3030–3044

Pollicino T, Belloni L, Raffa G et al (2006) Hepatitis B virus replication is regulated by the acetylation status of hepatitis B virus cccDNA-bound H3 and H4 histones. Gastroenterology 130:823–837

Poussin K, Dienes H, Sirma H et al (1999) Expression of mutated hepatitis B virus X genes in human hepatocellular carcinomas. Int J Cancer 80:497–505

Raimondo G, Allain JP, Brunetto MR et al (2008) Statements from the Taormina expert meeting on occult hepatitis B virus infection. J Hepatol 49:652–657

Rakotomalala L, Studach L, Wang WH et al (2008) Hepatitis B virus X protein increases the Cdt1-to-geminin ratio inducing DNA re-replication and polyploidy. J Biol Chem 283:28729–28740

Rui E, Moura PR, Goncalves Kde A et al (2005) Expression and spectroscopic analysis of a mutant hepatitis B virus onco-protein HBx without cysteine residues. J Virol Methods 126:65–74

Saigo K, Yoshida K, Ikeda R et al (2008) Integration of hepatitis B virus DNA into the myeloid/lymphoid or mixed-lineage leukemia (MLL4) gene and rearrangements of MLL4 in human hepatocellular carcinoma. Hum Mutat 29:703–708

Scaglione SJ, Lok AS (2012) Effectiveness of hepatitis B treatment in clinical practice. Gastroenterology 142(1360–1368):e1361

Schaefer S (2005) Hepatitis B virus: significance of genotypes. J Viral Hepat 12:111–124 Sirma H, Giannini C, Poussin K et al (1999) Hepatitis B virus X mutants, present in hepatocellular carcinoma tissue abrogate both the antiproliferative and transactivation effects of HBx. Oncogene 18:4848–4859

Sitterlin D, Bergametti F, Tiollais P et al (2000a) Correct binding of viral X protein to UVDDB-p127 cellular protein is critical for efficient infection by hepatitis B viruses. Oncogene 19:4427–4431

Sitterlin D, Bergametti F, Transy C (2000b) UVDDB p127-binding modulates activities and intracellular distribution of hepatitis B virus X protein. Oncogene 19:4417–4426

Sitterlin D, Lee TH, Prigent S et al (1997) Interaction of the UV-damaged DNA-binding protein with hepatitis B virus X protein is conserved among mammalian hepadnaviruses and restricted to transactivation-proficient X-insertion mutants. J Virol 71:6194–6199

Soussan P, Garreau F, Zylberberg H et al (2000) In vivo expression of a new hepatitis B virus protein encoded by a spliced RNA. J Clin Invest 105:55–60

Studach L, Wang WH, Weber G et al (2010) Polo-like kinase 1 activated by the hepatitis B virus X protein attenuates both the DNA damage checkpoint and DNA repair resulting in partial polyploidy. J Biol Chem 285:30282–30293

Studach LL, Rakotomalala L, Wang WH et al (2009) Polo-like kinase 1 inhibition suppresses hepatitis B virus X protein-induced transformation in an in vitro model of liver cancer progression. Hepatology 50:414–423

Su Q, Schröder CH, Hofman WJ et al (1998) Expression of hepatitis B virus X protein in HBV-infected human livers and hepatocellular carcinoma. Hepatology 27:1109–1120

Summers J, Smith PM, Huang M et al (1991) Morphogenetic and regulatory effects of mutations in the envelope proteins of an avian hepadnavirus. J Virol 65:1310–1317

Sung WK, Zheng H, Li S et al (2012) Genome-wide survey of recurrent HBV integration in hepatocellular carcinoma. Nat Genet 44:765–769

Takahashi K, Akahane Y, Hino K et al (1998) Hepatitis B virus genomic sequence in the circulation of hepatocellular carcinoma patients: comparative analysis of 40 full-length isolates. Arch Virol 143:2313–2326

Tamori A, Yamanishi Y, Kawashima S et al (2005) Alteration of gene expression in human hepatocellular carcinoma with integrated hepatitis B virus DNA. Clin Cancer Res 11:5821–5826

Tang H, Delgermaa L, Huang F et al (2005) The transcriptional transactivation function of HBx protein is important for its augmentation role in hepatitis B virus replication. J Virol 79:5548–

5556

Terradillos O, Billet O, Renard CA et al (1997) The hepatitis B virus X gene potentiates c-myc-induced liver oncogenesis in transgenic mice. Oncogene 14:395–404

Toh H, Hyashida H, Miyata T (1983) Sequence homology between retroviral reverse transcriptase and putative polymerases of hepatitis B virus and cauliflower mosaic virus. Nature 305:827–829

Tu H, Bonura C, Giannini C et al (2001) Biological impact of natural COOH-terminal deletions of hepatitis B virus X protein in hepatocellular carcinoma tissues. Cancer Res 61:7803–7810

Vivekanandan P, Thomas D, Torbenson M (2009) Methylation regulates hepatitis B viral protein expression. J Infect Dis 199:1286–1291

Wang HC, Huang W, Lai MD et al (2006) Hepatitis B virus pre-S mutants, endoplasmic reticulum stress and hepatocarcinogenesis. Cancer Sci 97:683–688

Wang Q, Zhang T, Ye L et al (2012) Analysis of hepatitis B virus X gene (HBx) mutants in tissues of patients suffered from hepatocellular carcinoma in China. Cancer Epidemiol 36:369–374

Wang WH, Studach LL, Andrisani OM (2011) Proteins ZNF198 and SUZ12 are down-regulated in hepatitis B virus (HBV) X protein-mediated hepatocyte transformation and in HBV replication. Hepatology 53:1137–1147

Wen Y, Golubkov VS, Strongin AY et al (2008) Interaction of hepatitis B viral oncoprotein with cellular target HBXIP dysregulates centrosome dynamics and mitotic spindle formation. J Biol Chem 283:2793–2803

Wentz MJ, Becker SA, Slagle BL (2000) Dissociation of DDB1-binding and transactivation properties of the hepatitis B virus X protein. Virus Res 68:87–92

Yeh CT, Shen CH, Tai DI et al (2000) Identification and characterization of a prevalent hepatitis B virus X protein mutant in Taiwanese patients with hepatocellular carcinoma. Oncogene 19:5213–5220

第8章 乙型肝炎病毒感染与肝癌的预防

Mei-Hwei Chang

摘 要 肝细胞癌（HCC）是人类五大高死亡率肿瘤之一。在世界范围内，乙型肝炎病毒（HBV）是造成 HCC 最常见的病因，特别是在 HBV 感染广泛流行地区，如亚洲、非洲、中欧和东欧的南部，以及中东地区。HBV 相关性 HCC 的危险因素包括：①病毒因素，如持续高病毒载量、HBV 基因型 C 或者 D 亚型、前 S2 或核心启动子突变；②宿主因素，如较高年龄（>40 岁）、HBeAg 血清学转阳、男性；③母婴传播；④其他致癌性因素，如吸烟、嗜酒等。预防是控制癌症发生的最好方法。对 HCC 预防有三个级别：一级预防主要是对广大人群普及乙型肝炎疫苗接种；二级预防是针对已经有 HBV 慢性感染的高危人群使用抗病毒药物；三级预防是针对 HCC 成功治愈者使用抗病毒药物预防复发。通过普及乙肝疫苗接种的一级预防是最经济有效的，乙肝疫苗是人类迄今为止所有癌症预防性疫苗中最为成功的。这个经验可以借鉴到其他肿瘤预防性疫苗研发策略中进行相关疾病的预防。开发理想的保护性疫苗，需要进行细致的基础和临床研究。了解病原的主要传播途径和初始感染年龄有助于确定疫苗预防接种的最佳年龄，并启动新的肿瘤预防性疫苗计划。除及时接种疫苗之外，在出生之后立即注射乙型肝炎免疫球蛋白，甚至在妊娠晚期服用抗病毒药物阻断 HBV 母婴传播，可能是增强对 HBV 感染及其相关性肝癌预防效果的策略。

关键词 肝癌，乙肝病毒，母婴传播，乙型肝炎疫苗，初级癌症预防，癌症预防性疫苗

1 引言

肝细胞性肝癌（HCC）是全世界五大主要癌症之一（Parkin et al. 2001），由于它的高致死率（死亡率/发生率总比值为 0.93），肝癌是全世界癌症死亡的第三

M.-H. Chang (✉)

Department of Pediatrics, College of Medicine, National Taiwan University, Taipei, Taiwan

e-mail: changmh@ntu.edu.tw

大死因。在 2008 年，估计有 69.4 万人因 HCC 死亡（47.7 万为男性，21.7 万为女性）（资料来源：www.globocan.iarc.fr，获取于 2012 年 3 月 13 日）。大约 90%的 HCC 的发生与乙型肝炎病毒（HBV）或丙型肝炎病毒（HCV）感染有关。流行病学研究、病例对照研究、动物实验及分子生物学研究都表明，HBV 和 HCV 在 HCC 发生中起直接或间接的重要致癌作用。发展中国家人群感染 HBV 的大样本研究证实了 HBV 仍是人类 HCC 中最为流行的致瘤病毒。估计在全球范围内，大约 55%~70%的 HCC 与 HBV 感染有关，大约 25%的 HCC 与 HCV 感染有关（Bosch and Ribes 2002）。肝硬化是一种常见的癌前病变，这适应于包括儿童在内的 80%的 HCC 患者（Hsu et al. 1983）。而肝硬化通常是由 HBV 或 HCV 慢性感染造成严重肝损伤形成的。

乙型肝炎疫苗已被证实是第一个能成功预防人类癌症的肿瘤预防性疫苗。HBV 持续性感染的流行病学、传播途径、长期临床跟踪随访、临床预后、病毒学和 HBV 致癌机制等多方面的研究，将对开发控制感染相关性癌症的有效策略提供最有帮助的例证。

2　HCC 造成的疾病负担

在全球，估计有 57%的肝硬化和 78%的原发性 HCC 是因 HBV 或 HCV 感染引起的。全世界大约已有 20 亿人感染了 HBV，其中超过 3.5 亿人是慢性感染，每年大约有 50 万~70 万人死于 HBV 感染相关疾病（http://www.who.int/immunization/topics/hepatitis/en/）（资料获取于 2012 年 1 月 26 日）。HCC 高发病率地区主要分布在发展中国家的地区，如东亚和东南亚、非洲中部及西部（Ferlay et al. 2010）。死亡率的地理分布与可观察到的发病率相似，甚至在同一个国家，不同种族之间 HCC 的发生率也不相同。据统计，在美国的阿拉斯加州，爱斯基摩人男性中 HCC 发病率为 11.2/100 000，为白人男性的 5 倍（Heyward et al. 1981）。

在全球，HCC 的地理分布与慢性 HBV 感染的地理分布非常吻合（Beasley 1982）。HBV 感染高发地区，HCC 患病率也高。60%~80%的原发性 HCC 起因于 HBV 感染，占癌症死因的 1/3，特别是在 HBV 高流行地区如亚洲、太平洋周边和非洲（Boasch and Ribes 2002）。中欧和东欧的南部、亚马孙盆地、中东和印度次大陆也是 HBV 感染和 HCC 高发区（Lavanchy 2004）。

3　HBV 感染的传播途径

HBV 感染在亚洲、非洲、南欧及拉丁美洲流行最为广泛，其人群 HBsAg 阳性率波动在 2%~20%之间。HBV 初次感染的年龄和传染源是影响感染预后的重要因素。

产妇的血清 HBV 表面抗原（HBsAg）和 HBV 包膜抗原（HBeAg）的状态影响她们的下一代 HBV 感染的结局。在普及乙型肝炎疫苗前，亚洲和许多其他 HBV 流行地区，有 40%~50%的 HBsAg 阳性携带者是通过围产期 HBsAg 携带者传播。不论人群中 HBsAg 携带率的程度如何，HBeAg 阳性母亲的婴儿大约 85%~90%会成为 HBsAg 携带者（Stevens et al. 1975）。在流行地区，HBV 感染主要发生在婴儿期和幼儿期。与成人感染相比，幼儿期感染 HBV 导致持续感染和发生严重并发症（肝硬化和 HCC）的比例更高。以中国台湾流行区为例，2 岁以下感染人群 HBsAg 携带率在慢性 HBsAg 携带者是最高的（Hsu et al. 1986）。

在 HBV 疫苗使用之前，HBV 水平传播中有一半的传播途径是通过使用未消毒的针头或医疗设备、不安全的血液制品或输血、无保护措施的性行为、皮肤穿刺未消毒或其他家庭内密切接触而引起的。在非洲 HBV 流行区，HBV 在幼儿期主要以水平传播感染为主，例如，在塞内加尔的农村，2 岁儿童只有 25%感染 HBV，而到 15 岁时，HBV 感染率上升到 80%（Feret et al. 1987）。

4 慢性 HBV 感染与 HCC

慢性 HBV 感染造成的肝损伤是肝脏肿瘤发生中最重要的起始事件（Bruix et al. 2004）。HBV 在肿瘤形成中的作用机制较为复杂，可能涉及直接和间接的致癌机制（Grisham 2001；Villanueva et al. 2007）（详见第 7 章）。持续性 HBV 感染造成的结局则是来自于宿主、病毒及环境因素之间的相互作用（表 8-1）。

表 8-1　HBV 感染个体中发展成 HCC 的危险因素总结

风险因素	高风险/低风险	参考文献
病毒因素		
1. HBsAg	阳性/阴性=66/1	Beasley et al.（1981）
2. HBsAg 阳性个体中的 HBeAg	阳性/阴性=60/10	Yang et al.（2002）
3. HBV DNA 水平	高 $\{[>10^6]/10^5 \sim 10^6/[10^4 \sim 10^5]\}$/低 $[<10^4]$copies/ml = 11/9/3/1	Chen et al.（2006）
4. HBV 基因型	[C 或 D]/[A 或 B]	Tseng et al.（2012）
宿主因素		
1. 年龄	>40/<40 岁 = 2~12/1	Chen et al.（2008），Tseng et al.（2012）
2. HBeAg 血清转化者的年龄	高龄（>40 岁）/低龄（<30 岁）=5/1	Chen et al.（2010）

续表

风险因素	高风险/低风险	参考文献
3. 族群	亚裔或非洲裔/其他	Ferlay et al.（2010）
4. 性别	男性/女性=2~4/1	Ferlay et al.（2010），Ni et al.（1991），Schafer and Sorrell（1999）
5. 家族 HCC 历史	阳性/阴性=2~3/1	Turati et al.（2012）
6. 肝硬化	是/否=12/1	Yu et al.（1997）
7. 母体 HBsAg	阳性/阴性=30/1	Chang et al.（2009）
其他因素		
吸烟	是/否=1-2/1	Yu et al.（1997），Jee et al.（2004）
嗜酒	是/否=1-2/1	Yu et al.（1997），Jee et al.（2004）

4.1 发生 HCC 的病毒（HBV）风险因素

4.1.1 血清 HBsAg 阳性

慢性 HBV 感染并伴随血清 HBsAg 持续阳性是发生 HCC 最重要的决定因素。对 22 707 名中国台湾男性的前瞻性研究表明，在长期随访中，相比非 HBsAg 携带者，慢性 HBV 感染者的 HCC 发生率高很多，相对危险度为 66。这些结果支持 HBV 在 HCC 病因学中起首要作用这一假说（Beasley et al. 1981）。

4.1.2 活跃的病毒复制

HBeAg 是 HBV 复制活跃的标志。随访研究发现，30 岁以后 HBV 持续感染个体伴随 HBV 高水平复制或 HBeAg 阳性，则发展为 HCC 的风险明显增加。相比血清 HBeAg 阴性的乙型肝炎携带者，HBeAg 持续阳性的 HBsAg 携带者患 HCC 的风险要高 3~6 倍（Yang et al. 2002）（表 8-1）。在慢性 HBV 感染者中，HBV-DNA 水平更高者，HCC 的发生率也更高。在长期随访中发现，相比这些血清 HBVDNA 水平 $<10^4$ 拷贝/ml 患者，血清 HBV DNA 水平在 10^4~10^5、10^5~10^6 或 $>10^6$ 拷贝/ml 的患者发生 HCC 的风险更大 [2.7、8.9 或 10.7]（Chen et al. 2006）。

4.1.3 HBV 基因型

从不同地区已经鉴别出至少有 10 个 HBV 基因型。C 或 D 型 HBV 较 A 或 B 型 HBV 有更高的 HCC 发病风险（Tseng et al. 2012）。在阿拉斯加，感染 F 型 HBV 比感染其他基因型别 HBV 的患者发生 HCC 风险更高（Livingston et al. 2007）。

4.1.4 HBV 突变

HBV 携带者如出现前-S 突变体，则发生 HCC 风险增加，因此前-S 突变体被认为在 HBV 相关 HCC 发生中发挥潜在作用（Wang et al. 2006）。感染了有核心启动子突变的 HBV，据报道有更高的发生 HCC 的风险。

4.2 HCC 宿主因素（表 8-1）

4.2.1 年龄影响

年龄较大（>40 岁）是 HCC 发生的一个风险因素（Tseng et al. 2012；Chen et al. 2008）。可能是因为慢性乙肝感染中，随着时间推移会导致遗传改变（碱基增加或缺失）和 HBV 肝损伤的累积。大部分 HCC 患者（约 80%）可出现 HBe 抗体阳性（Chien et al. 1981），提示 HCC 发生于长期 HBV 感染和肝损伤，且存在 HBe 抗体血清学转阳。在慢性 HBV 感染者中，相比 30 岁之前就已经出现 HBeAg 血清学转换者，推迟到 40 岁之后才出现 HBeAg 血清学转换者发展为 HCC 的风险性显著增加（危险比 5.22）（Chen et al. 2010）。

4.2.2 男性多见

HBV 相关性 HCC 中，男性发病率更高，甚至在儿童中也类似，男女性别比率为 2~4:1（Ferlay et al. 2010，2010；Ni et al. 1991；Schafer and Sorrell 1999）。男性性别是 HCC 进展的一个危险因素，但其机制并不完全清楚。在男性肝癌形成过程中，作为促癌因素的雄激素信号通路活性更高；而在女性肝癌形成过程中，作为抑癌因素的雌激素信号通路活性更高。因为这两种因子作用机制都是以配体依赖性方式产生作用，因此这些性激素的配体和受体可用来评价各种性别 HCC 患者的相对风险（Yeh and Chen 2012）。此外，Y 染色体上的 RNA 结合基序（RRM）基因（RBMY），编码男性生殖细胞特异性 RNA 结合蛋白（与生精功能相关），被认为是一个男性 HCC 特异的候选癌基因（Tsuei et al. 2004）。

4.2.3 其他宿主因素

因肝炎病毒或其他病毒造成的慢性严重肝损伤，导致肝细胞转化最终发展为 HCC。肝硬化是 HCC 的一种癌前病变（Yu et al. 1997）。已经发展为肝硬化的 HBV 携带者每年有 3%~8% 的患者发展为 HCC。不同种族发生 HCC 的风险也不尽相同。以北美为例，亚裔、西班牙裔和非裔美国人比非西班牙裔白人患 HCC 风险更大（Ferlay et al. 2010）。

相比那些无 HCC 家族史患者，有 HCC 家族史患者发生 HCC 的风险更高。

HCC 家族聚集现象提示，除了家庭内密切接触造成的 HBV 传染外，HCC 具有遗传易感性（Chang et al. 1984）。基于 9 个病例-对照及 4 个群体列队研究共计 3600 例 HCC 患者的 meta 分析发现，具有 HCC 家族史患者的相对危险度为 2.50（95%CI，2.06~3.03）（Turati et al. 2012）（表 8-1）。

4.3 母体影响

母亲血清 HBsAg 阳性者，婴儿发生 HCC 风险是阴性者的 30 倍（Chang et al. 2009）。HBeAg 是由 HBV 产生的可溶性抗原，可以从母体穿过胎盘屏障传染到婴儿。若新生儿的母亲为 HBeAg 阳性的 HBsAg 携带者，从母亲经胎盘传播的 HBeAg 能诱导特异性辅助性 T 细胞缺失，不能应答 HBeAg 和 HBcAg（Hsu et al. 1992）。这可能有助于解释为什么母亲为 HBeAg 阳性者生产的婴儿 85%~90%发展为持续感染（Beasley et al. 1977），而母亲为 HBeAg 阴性者生产的婴儿仅约 5%发展为持续感染。新生儿感染 HBV 后，免疫耐受状态持续数年甚至数十年。

4.4 环境或生活方式因素

吸烟、嗜酒，以及暴露于黄曲霉毒素都是 HCC 发生的高风险因素（Yu et al. 1997；Jee et al. 2004；Chen et al. 2008）。

5　HCC 预防

除非经早期发现并完全切除，HCC 的预后很差。即使在 HCC 经完全切除的病例中，癌症复发仍然是个常见的问题。因此，预防是控制 HCC 的最佳途径。预防 HCC 有三个级别，即一级、二级和三级预防（图 8-1）。从新生儿开始阻断 HBV 感染、普及疫苗接种、阻断母婴传播和水平传播途径，是预防 HCC 最有效、最安全的方法。

乙型肝炎的抗病毒治疗是针对肝脏酶代谢和肝功能正常化、HBeAg 的清除、降低 HBVDNA 水平，以及减轻肝脏炎症和肝纤维化。研究提示，传统的、有限疗程的 IFN-α 治疗可能有利于机体获得应答反应累积、减轻肝纤维化进程及肝硬化和/或 HCC 发生。核苷类似物长期治疗也能改善纤维化或逆转晚期肝纤维化，缓解疾病进程甚至阻止 HCC 的发展。然而，现有抗病毒治疗和免疫调节剂并不能产生持续的高应答率，即使能对上述药物产生持续应答的患者，HBV 在大多数治疗的患者中也不能被完全清除，因为这些治疗方案很难清除 cccDNA。NUC 的长期使用产生耐药性是又一个问题。因此，抗病毒治疗在预防乙型肝炎相关并发症包括 HCC 时只能起到有限的治疗效果。

HBV 相关性肝硬化患者抗病毒治疗的前瞻性随机对照试验显示，在平均时长

32 个月的随访中，拉米夫定治疗组中有 3.9%患者被诊断为 HCC，安慰剂对照组有 7.4%患者被诊断为 HCC（P=0.047）（Liaw et al. 2004）。另一项长达 15 年（中位数为 6.8 年）的回顾性研究显示，233 名干扰素（IFN）治疗组的 HCC 累计发生率为 2.7%，明显低于 233 名对照组 12.5%的 HCC 发病率（P=0.011）。然而，HCC 发生显著减少仅是对于在已患肝硬化且 HBeAg 血清转阳者的观察（Lin et al. 2007）。聚乙二醇干扰素（PEG-IFN）和新一代核苷/核苷酸类似物治疗效果可能更好，因为其病毒抑制更有效，耐药风险更低。然而，这些治疗方案仍需要改进和完善，因此需要进一步研制更有效、安全、经济实惠的抗 HBV 病毒药物和策略（Liaw 2011）。

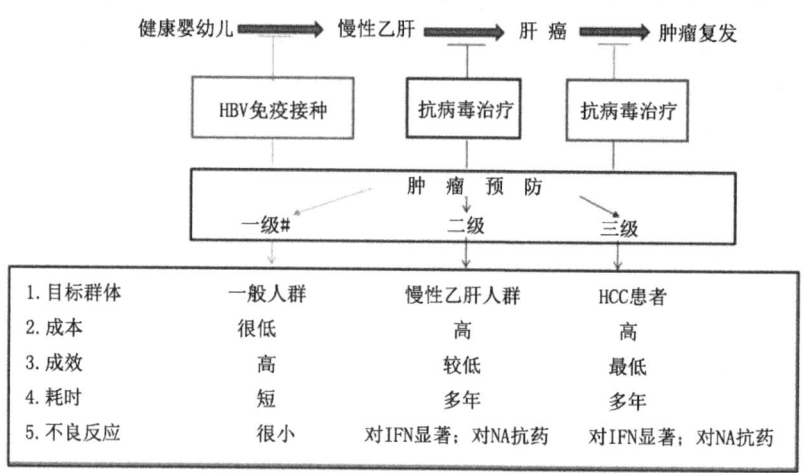

图 8-1 肝癌一级、二级和三级预防的策略。HBV 接种疫苗是最有效的方法。对于已经感染肝炎病毒的人群，抗病毒治疗可以在一定程度上推延或减少发生 HCC 的风险。其他策略（如化学预防和规避风险行为）的效果还未确定，正处于研究之中。HBV，乙型肝炎病毒；IFN，干扰素；NA，核苷类似物。

对于那些已经经过手术、肝移植或局部治疗成功的 HCC 患者，使用抗病毒治疗（抗 HBV 或 HCV）的 HCC 三级预防可预防晚期 HCC 复发（Braitenstein et al. 2009），但效果需进一步研究证实。

其他预防 HCC 的策略，如高危人群的化学预防（Jacobson et al. 1997；Egner et al. 2001）、高危险行为的预防、改变环境及饮食习惯、在癌变前进行肝移植（如肝硬化），也可能有助于预防 HCC，但是需要更多的证据支持其功效。

5.1 一级预防：通过免疫接种预防 HBV 感染

5.1.1 对幼儿普及乙型肝炎疫苗接种

目前，全世界计划免疫的普及主要有三大策略，取决于 HBV 感染的来源和流行状况（表 8-2）。在一些具有充足财力、物力的国家如美国，对孕妇筛查 HBsAg 而不是 HBeAg。每个婴儿出生后均接受三针乙型肝炎疫苗预防。此外，所有母亲为 HBsAg 阳性的婴儿，不管 HBeAg 状态，在出生后 24h 内注射 HBIG（Shepard et al. 2006）。这种策略可以节省和减少产妇 HBeAg 筛查的成本和程序，但会增加 HBIG 的使用，而 HBIG 非常昂贵。

表 8-2 不同国家当前孕妇筛查和婴儿乙肝病毒（HBV）普及疫苗接种预防策略，对特定的具有突破性感染的高风险儿童的监测

策略类型	孕妇筛查		新生儿接种疫苗[#]		
	HBsAg	HBeAg	HBV 疫苗	母亲 HBsAg 阳性/HBeAg 阴性，给新生儿 HBIG	母亲 HBsAg 阳性/HBeAg 阳性，给新生儿 HBIG
I	是	否	是	是	是
II*	是	是	是	否	是
III	否	否	是	否	否

[#]适用国家地区的例子：策略类型 I：美国，意大利，韩国；策略类型 II：中国台湾，新加坡；策略类型 III：泰国

*在策略类型 II 中，可以同时或者依序进行 HBsAg 和 HBeAg 测试。所有的孕妇同时筛查 HBsAg 和 HBeAg；或者，对所有孕妇先筛查 HBsAg，但是只在 HBsAg 为阳性的妇女中进行 HBeAg 测试；前一个方案比较耗时，后者可以节省开支

1984 年 7 月，中国台湾在全球率先启动乙型肝炎疫苗计划免疫（Chen et al. 1987），以及孕妇血清 HBsAg 和 HBeAg 筛查方案（战略 II）。

为了节省筛查和乙型肝炎免疫球蛋白的费用，一些 HBV 感染中/低流行国家或资源不足国家不进行孕妇筛查，所有婴儿都接受三次乙型肝炎疫苗接种（不包括 HBIG）。使用这种策略，可以节省产妇筛查和乙型肝炎免疫球蛋白的费用，降低成本，其预防婴儿 HBV 慢性感染的效果是令人满意的（Poovorawan et al. 1989）。

5.2 接种 HBV 疫苗有效地减少 HBV 感染及相关并发症

乙型肝炎疫苗一直是世界卫生组织全球免疫的一部分，导致全球的急性和慢性 HBV 感染大幅下降。在那些已经实施婴儿期乙型肝炎疫苗免疫普及的地区，

儿童慢性乙肝发病率大约可以明显减少90%。在普及婴儿乙肝疫苗计划免疫之后，世界各地的慢性HBV感染率减少到普及接种之前的1/10，暴发性和急性肝炎也明显减少。

在中国台湾进行了一系列关于血清HBV标志物的流行病学调查（Hsu et al. 1986；Chen et al. 1996；Ni et al. 2001，2007），发现在儿童期已经接种疫苗的年龄小于20岁的人群中，HBsAg携带率显著下降，从普及疫苗接种方案之前的10%左右下降为0.6%~0.7%。在已经实施普及乙型肝炎疫苗计划的许多其他国家也已观察到相似的效果（Whittle et al. 2002；Jang et al. 2001）。婴儿期普及乙型肝炎疫苗接种预防HBV感染比选择性地对高危人群免疫接种更为有效。

乙型肝炎疫苗接种计划的确可以减少全世界的HBV围产期感染和水平传播（Da Villa et al. 1995；Whittle et al. 2002）。许多国家如冈比亚、韩国，普及计划免疫接种方案也一样很成功，乙型肝炎携带率已经从5%~10%下降至1%，这进一步证实普及乙型肝炎疫苗计划免疫接种比选择性免疫接种高危人群更有效（Montesano 2011）。

6　通过免疫接种阻止HBV感染和预防HCC的效果

目前对HCC的治疗并不令人满意。即使早期发现和及时治疗，在长期随访中仍然会出现HCC复发或新发HCC的麻烦问题。到目前为止，疫苗接种是预防HBV感染和相关HCC的最好方法。在大多数情况下，HBV感染后需要40年甚至更长的时间才能发展为HCC，因此我们期望在普及乙型肝炎疫苗接种计划40年后减少成人HCC发生人数。如果儿童HCC发生与成人HCC相似，比较高发地区普及婴儿乙型肝炎疫苗免疫接种前后出生的儿童HCC发生率的变化，有利于我们了解HBV免疫接种预防HCC的效果。

表8-3　HCC在6~19周岁且在出生前后经过普及HBV疫苗接种计划的青少年中的发病率

诊断时的年龄	HBV免疫接种	年份	HCC		
			HCC发生病例数	发病率（每10^5人·年）	发生率比（95% CI）
台湾（中国）		出生年份			
6~19	无	1963~1984	444	0.57	1（基准值）
	有	1984~1998	64	0.17	0.30（0.18~0.42）
孔敬地区（泰国）		出生年份			
>5~18	无	1990年前	15	0.097	1（基准值）
	有	1990年后	3	0.024	0.25

续表

诊断时的年龄	HBV 免疫接种	年份	HCC 发生病例数	发病率（每 10^5 人·年）	发生率比率（95% CI）
阿拉斯加（美国）		诊断年份			
<20	无	1969~1984			0.7~2.6
	有	1984~1988			2.9
	有	1989~2008			0.0~1.4

参考文献：1. Taiwan-Chang 等（2009）；2. Thailand-Wichajarn 等（2008）；3. Alaska-McMahon 等（2011）

儿童 HCC 与 HBV 感染密切相关，其发生特点也与成人相似（Chang et al. 1989）。相比世界上其他部分地区，中国台湾儿童 HBV 感染及 HCC 发病率很高。中国台湾儿童 HCC 患者几乎 100%都是 HBsAg 阳性，大多数（86%）患者 HBeAg 为阴性，大多数儿童 HCC 病例（94%）都有母亲 HBsAg 阳性，80%非肿瘤部分都存在肝硬化。在儿童 HCC 组织中证实有 HBV 基因组整合到宿主基因组（Chang et al. 1991）。儿童 HCC 的组织学特征也与成人的非常相似。

自 1984 年 7 月中国台湾实施普及乙型肝炎疫苗计划免疫后，HBV 感染的下降导致 HCC 发生率显著减少。6~14 岁儿童的肝细胞性 HCC 的年发生率在 1984 年 7 月之前出生的人群中为 0.52~0.54/100 000，而在 1984 年 7 月之后出生的人群中为 0.13~0.20/100 000，年发生率减少到 1/4（Chang et al. 1997，2000，2005）。

HBsAg 阳性的 HCC 患儿的母亲大约 90%是 HBsAg 阳性，这有力地证明了在免疫时代之后，母源性 HBV 围产期传播是 HCC 患儿感染 HBV 的主要途径，且 HBV 垂直传播没有被乙型肝炎疫苗免疫接种计划完全清除（Chang et al. 2009）。在乙型肝炎疫苗计划普及 20 年后，其预防癌症的效果进一步扩展至儿童之外（表 8-3）。相比出生时未接种疫苗组，已接种疫苗的儿童和 6~19 岁青少年的 HCC 发病率显著降低，且有统计学意义。

在泰国，出生时（1990 年之后出生）接种乙型肝炎疫苗儿童比未接种疫苗儿童的 HCC 发生率显著降低。对 1985~2007 年间泰国孔敬地区 18 岁以下儿童诊断为肝肿瘤的病例进行分析，大于 10 岁的未接种疫苗和接种疫苗的 HCC 儿童的年龄标准化发病率（ASR）分别为 0.88/1 000 000 和 0.07/1 000 000（$P=0.039$）（Wichajarn et al. 2008）。

在美国阿拉斯加的本土居民中，急性和慢性乙型肝炎发病率曾经最高。在阿拉斯加施行了新生儿乙型肝炎疫苗普及和大规模 HBV 筛查可疑患者后，完全清除了当地儿童 HCC 的发生：小于 20 岁的人群中 HCC 发病率从 1984~1988 年的 3/100 000 下降到 1995~1999 年的 0，自 1999 年后 HCC 就再没有发生（McMahon et al. 2011）。

7 肝癌预防中亟待解决的问题

接种疫苗的人群患 HCC 的危险性与不完全的乙型肝炎疫苗接种、产前母体血清 HBsAg 或 HBeAg 阳性呈统计学显著相关性（Chang et al. 2005，2009）。HCC 预防失败常由于有高度传染性的母亲未能成功控制 HBV 感染给下一代。为消除 HBV 感染及其相关疾病，我们必须克服那些阻碍普及乙型肝炎疫苗接种的困难。

7.1 覆盖率低

7.1.1 发展中国家财力不足

东南亚和非洲一些国家，由于没有吸引国家政府资金耽误了乙型肝炎疫苗免疫接种进入 EPI 项目，即使有些国家参加了 EPI 项目，而乙型肝炎疫苗接种的覆盖率仍不够，一个主要原因是因为需自己支付乙型肝炎疫苗费用。

自 1991 年以来，WHO 要求所有国家将乙型肝炎疫苗纳入到国家基础免疫中。但是还有许多低收入的贫穷国家并未采纳疫苗。1992 年，WHO 进一步要求所有 HBV 相关疾病高负担国家应该在 1995 年将乙型肝炎疫苗纳入其常规婴儿免疫接种中，在 1997 年之前全球都将乙肝疫苗纳入基础免疫（Kane 1996）。1996 年，WHO 将目标定为：到 2001 年，全球儿童新发乙型肝炎携带者的发病率减少 80%（Kane and Brooke 2002）。在 HBV 感染和 HCC 高流行地区任务尤为紧迫。

如何降低疫苗的费用，并增加乙型肝炎疫苗基金帮助贫困流行地区儿童，对解决消灭 HBV 感染及其相关 HCC 非常重要。疫苗和免疫全球联盟（GAVI）于 1999 年成立，在帮助发展中国家扩大乙型肝炎疫苗的覆盖率方面做出了巨大贡献。

全球使用乙型肝炎疫苗次数逐年增长。世界卫生组织最新报告显示，193 个成员国中已经有 179 个国家（包括印度和苏丹部分地区）在 2010 年底全国全面实施婴儿乙型肝炎疫苗基础免疫。到目前为止，全球乙型肝炎疫苗接种覆盖率估计在 75%，西太平洋高达 91%，美洲有 89%。然而，2010 年在东南亚地区的覆盖率只达到 52%（World Health Organization 2012）。

7.1.2 对疫苗不良反应的焦虑或无知造成疫苗接种的依从性差

在财力充足的国家，由于家长/监护人的无知或对疫苗接种的敌对心态促使一部分人拒绝接种疫苗。阐明疫苗相关的副作用可以减少疫苗接种的敌对心态。举例来说，怀疑中枢神经系统脱髓鞘疾病和乙型肝炎疫苗相关是缺乏证据的，澄清这个问题将有助于消除对疫苗接种的抵触心态，消除这些阻碍全球 HBV 感染和相关肝疾病清除的因素（Halsey et al. 1999）。教育和宣传乙型肝炎疫苗的益处将有利于推动包括低流行地区的公众和政府采纳乙型肝炎疫苗接种计划。

7.2 疫苗接种后的突破性感染（免疫失败）

HBV突破性感染（breakthrough infection）或机体对疫苗无应答，包括产妇体内存在高病毒载量HBV（Lee et al. 1986）、宫内感染（Tang et al. 1998；Lin et al. 1987）、表面抗原基因突变（Hsu et al. 1999，2004，2010）、依从性差、遗传低反应性和免疫缺损状态等原因都可引起。中国台湾启动乙型肝炎疫苗基础免疫后出生的人群中，89%血清HBsAg阳性患者的母亲血清中HBsAg阳性（Ni et al. 2007）。母体传播是HBV突破性感染的主要原因，也是未来疫苗接种方案中需要解决的挑战性问题。

7.2.1 母婴传播：母体内高病毒载量和血清HBeAg、HBsAg阳性

乙型肝炎疫苗免疫预防失败的危险因素包括母体内HBV DNA水平过高、分娩过程中子宫收缩和胎盘渗漏、HBc抗体水平过低（Lin et al. 1991；Chang et al. 1996）。

母婴传播是已接受免疫接种儿童感染HBV的主要原因。在2356名经产前筛查鉴定母亲为HBsAg阳性的中国台湾儿童中，尽管出生后24h内接种乙型肝炎免疫球蛋白及婴儿期定时接种全部疫苗，母亲为HBeAg阳性的儿童感染HBV（9.26%）的风险仍然很大（Chen et al. 2012）。宫内HBV感染虽然罕见，但也是母婴传播的一种可能的原因。

虽然免疫接种预防HBV感染是非常成功的，但仍然存在2.4%HBeAg阳性母亲的婴儿在出生时或出生后不久在血清中就检测到乙型肝炎表面抗原（Tang et al. 1998），并持续到12个月或更长时间。尽管进行严格、完全的免疫预防，他们仍有可能成为HBsAg携带者。

7.2.2 乙型肝炎表面抗原基因突变

在乙型肝炎疫苗接种规划启动后，HBsAg携带者乙型肝炎表面抗原基因突变率随着时间增加。在乙型肝炎疫苗接种计划启动之前，以及启动之后5年、10年和15年，HBV DNA阳性者乙型肝炎表面基因突变率分别为7.8%、17.8%、28.1%和23.8%（Hsu et al. 1999，2010）。幸运的是，在疫苗接种规划实施20年后，HBsAg的突变率一直保持在22.6%左右。目前，虽然乙型肝炎疫苗表面基因突变蛋白不是常规HBV免疫接种所急需，但详细和连续监测的表面基因突变是有必要的。

7.2.3 宿主免疫力低下、低或无免疫应答反应

接受免疫抑制剂或器官移植之前，需常规检测乙型肝炎标志物和抗 HB 抗体，那些抗 HB 抗体水平不足的患者常被建议进行乙型肝炎疫苗接种。弱应答者可给予双倍剂量的乙型肝炎疫苗接种，以增强疫苗免疫反应效果。针对传统乙型肝炎疫苗无应答者，应进一步研发更好的疫苗。

8 有效控制 HBV 相关性 HCC 的策略

通过普及疫苗接种这样的一级预防策略能有效控制 HBV 感染及其相关并发症。然而，目前仍有几个亟待解决的问题。其中最重要的是如何为每一个婴儿提供有效的一级预防以便更好地控制全球 HBV 感染，包括进一步提高乙型肝炎疫苗的全球覆盖率，以及更有效地应对 HBV 突破性感染和疫苗无应答的方法。最为重要的是寻找降低乙型肝炎疫苗成本的方法并增加发展中国家 HBV 感染流行区儿童的乙型肝炎疫苗免疫的资金扶持。这些需求在 HBV 感染与 HCC 流行区是特别紧迫的。

消除急性和慢性乙型肝炎需更加进一步的努力，由于其他新疫苗的竞争，HBV 还没有得到政策制定者、宣传团体及公众的足够重视，这些在未来是一个主要的挑战（van Herck et al. 2008）。说服和支持那些还没有普及 HBV 免疫接种国家的政策制定者制定乙肝疫苗接种计划，鼓励已将乙型肝炎疫苗纳入基础免疫的国家扩大疫苗接种覆盖率是非常重要的。综合的公共健康预防规划方案应该包括预防、检测、控制 HBV 感染及其相关并发症和预防效果评价（Lavanchy 2008）。

8.1 预防 HBV 突破性感染

深入研究 HBV 突破性感染或疫苗无应答的机制对制定预防 HBV 突破性感染的有效策略至关重要。目前现有乙型肝炎疫苗能诱导良好的免疫应答，能预防大部分的 HBV 感染。然而，HBsAg 携带的母亲有 HBeAg 阳性和/或高病毒载量，其高危儿童的 HBV 突破性感染率仍有大约 10%。

8.1.1 更好的疫苗

开发出的新乙肝疫苗是否能抵抗乙型肝炎表面抗原基因突变，从而进一步针对免疫缺陷者减少新发 HBV 感染，这些需要进一步研发更好的疫苗。

8.1.2 治疗高风险孕妇

怀孕期间使用核苷类似物治疗 HBV 防止 HBV 的围产期传播。在临床实验初

步研究中，8 例高病毒血症（HBV DNA≥$1.2×10^9$拷贝/ml）母亲在怀孕的最后一个月每天服用拉米夫定，在婴儿 12 个月大时，拉米夫定组只有 12.5%的婴儿为 HBsAg 和 HBVDNA 阳性，对照组则为 28%（van Zonneveld et al. 2003）。另一个临床试验中 HBsAg 阳性高病毒载量孕妇自怀孕 34 周至生产后 4 周每天服用拉米夫定 100mg（Xu et al. 2009），结果显示，在出生后第 52 周，相比对照组（39%），治疗组婴儿 HBsAg 阳性率明显降低（18%）。

最近的一项研究中，募集了 HBeAg 阳性和 HBV DNA＞$1.0×10^7$拷贝/ml 的孕妇。随访发现，相比对照组，定期使用替比夫定治疗的孕妇围产期 HBV 传播发生率较低（0 和 8%；P=0.002）（Han et al. 2011）。有必要进一步阐明核苷/核苷酸类似物在预防宫内/围产期感染方面的优势和功效。

8.2 高危人群筛查和 HBV 相关 HCC 的二级预防

HBsAg 携带者患 HCC 的风险增加。筛查血清中的 HBsAg 可以作为早期筛查 HCC 高危人群的第一步。由于资源有限，可按图 8-2 的筛选策略进行 HBV 优先人群筛查。母亲或 HBsAg 携带的家庭成员皆为慢性 HBV 感染和 HCC 的高危人群。应首先筛查 HBsAg，如果为阳性，再进一步筛查 HCC。在孕妇中筛查 HBsAg

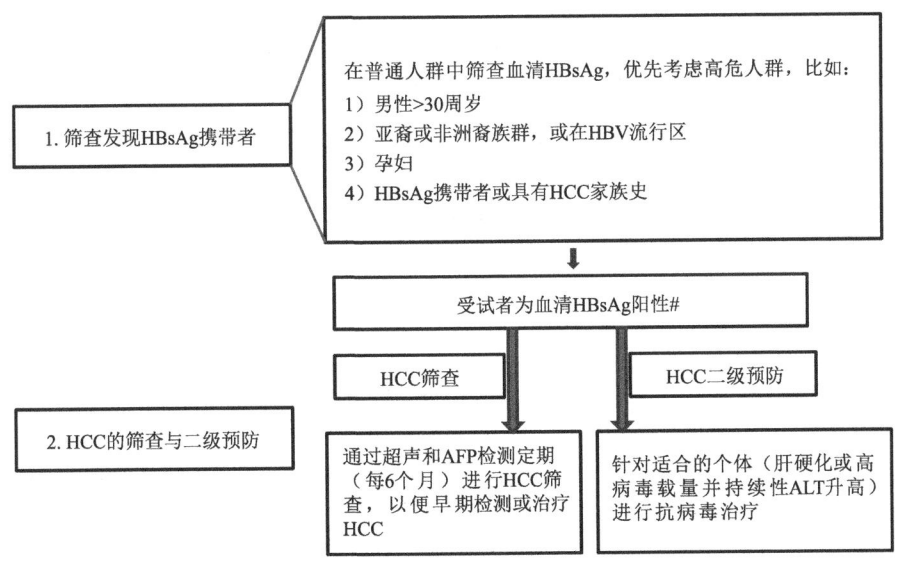

图 8-2 HBV 相关性肝癌的筛查和二级预防。HBsAg 携带者处于是发生 HCC 的高危险人群。因此，第一步是通过筛查找出 HBsAg 阳性的个体。#对于 HBsAg 阳性的个体，特别是具有高危险发生 HCC 的个体，即年龄大于 40 岁的男性、HCC 阳性家族史、肝硬化、高病毒载量并持续性异常 ALT 水平的人群，需要优先考虑接受定期 HCC 筛查和二级预防 HCC 的群体。

有助于阻断母婴传播。并且，这些 HBsAg 阳性的女性可以定期随访进行 HCC 二级预防。

HBsAg 阳性携带的男性、年龄大于 40 岁、亚洲或非洲族群且患有肝硬化、有 HCC 家族史，以及 HBV DNA＞10 000 拷贝/ml（表 8-1）的感染者患 HCC 的风险更高。由于 HBV 携带者是患 HCC 高危人群，建议定期（每 6 个月）进行超声和甲胎蛋白（AFP）检查来筛查 HCC。对于不能进行超声检查的地区，可以考虑定期检测甲胎蛋白（AFP）（Bruix and Sherman 2005）。

慢性 HBV 感染如同时存在肝硬化，或 HBV DNA 高水平（＞10 000 拷贝/ml），以及持续性、间歇性异常 ALT 水平的 HCC 高危人群，可以考虑进行 HCC 的二级预防。

9　其他癌症预防的未来前景和意义

预防是控制癌症的最好方法。乙肝疫苗预防肝癌是人类迄今为止所有癌症预防性疫苗中第一个成功的例子。如果世界各国能将乙型肝炎疫苗从新生儿期纳入儿童基础免疫，HBV 感染及其并发症在这个世纪将会进一步减少。成人 HCC 发生率在不久的将来能得到有效的控制。此外，乙型肝炎疫苗对控制 HBV 感染及相关疾病的预防作用可以推广到其他感染病原相关性癌症的控制上，如人乳头瘤病毒和宫颈癌、EB 病毒和伯基特淋巴瘤、鼻咽癌、人体 T 细胞白血病病毒（HTLV-1）和成人 T 细胞白血病/淋巴瘤（ATL）、幽门螺旋杆菌和黏膜相关淋巴组织淋巴瘤或胃癌。除接种常规疫苗之外，在出生后立刻注射乙型肝炎免疫球蛋白，乃至在妊娠晚期抗病毒治疗以阻断 HBV 母婴传播也是目前可能正在兴起的、预防 HBV 感染及其相关性肝癌的策略。

（瞿小旺，刘文培 译）

参 考 文 献

Beasley RP (1982) Hepatitis B virus as the etiologic agent in hepatocellular carcinoma: epidemiologic considerations. Hepatology 2:21s–26s

Beasley RP, Hwang LY, Lin CC et al (1981) Hepatocellular carcinoma and hepatitis B virus. A prospective study of 22707 men in Taiwan. Lancet 2:1129–1133

Beasley RP, Trepo C, Stevens CE et al (1977) The e antigen and vertical transmission of hepatitis B surface antigen. Amer J Epidemiol 105:94–98

Bosch FX, Ribes J (2002) The epidemiology of primary liver cancer: global epidemiology. In: Tabor E (ed) Viruses and liver cancer. Elsevier, Amsterdam, pp 1–16

Braitenstein S, Dimitroulis D, Petrowsky H et al (2009) Systematic review and meta-analysis of interferon after curative treatment of hepatocellular carcinoma in patients with viral hepatitis. Br J Surg 96:975–981

Bruix J, Boix L, Sala M et al (2004) Focus on hepatocellular carcinoma. Cancer Cell 5:215–219

Bruix J, Sherman M (2005) Management of hepatocellular carcinoma AASLD Guideline recommendations for HCC screening. Hepatology 42:1208–1236

Chang MH, Chen CJ, Lai MS et al (1997) Universal hepatitis B vaccination in Taiwan and the incidence of hepatocellular carcinoma in children. N Engl J Med 336:1855–1859

Chang MH, Chen DS, Hsu HC et al (1989) Maternal transmission of hepatitis B virus in childhood hepatocellular carcinoma. Cancer 64:2377–2380

Chang MH, Chen PJ, Chen JY et al (1991) Hepatitis B virus integration in hepatitis B virus- related hepatocellular carcinoma in childhood. Heptology 13:316–320

Chang MH, Chen TH, Hsu HM et al (2005) Problems in the prevention of childhood hepatocellular carcinoma in the era of universal hepatitis B immunization. Clin Cancer Res 11:7953–7957

Chang MH, Hsu HC, Lee CY et al (1984) Fraternal hepatocellular carcinoma in young children in two families. Cancer 53:1807–1810

Chang MH, Hsu HY, Huang LM et al (1996) The role of transplacental hepatitis B core antibody in the mother-to-infant transmission of hepatitis B virus. J Hepatol 24:674–679

Chang MH, Shau WY, Chen CJ et al (2000) The effect of universal hepatitis B vaccination on hepatocellular carcinoma rates in boys and girls. JAMA 284:3040–3042

Chang MH, You SL, Chen CJ et al (2009) Decreased incidence of hepatocellular carcinoma in hepatitis B vaccinees: a 20-year follow-up study. J Natl Cancer Inst 101:1348–1355

Chen CJ, Yang HI, Su J et al (2006) Risk of hepatocellular carcinoma across a biological gradient of serum hepatitis B virus DNA level. JAMA 295:65–73

Chen CL, Yang HI, Yang WS et al (2008) Metabolic factors and risk of hepatocellular carcinoma by chronic hepatitis B/C infection: a follow-up study in Taiwan. Gastroenterology 135:111–121

Chen DS, Hsu NHM, Sung JL et al (1987) A mass vaccination program in Taiwan against hepatitis B virus infection in infants of hepatitis B surface antigen-carrier mothers. JAMA 257:2597–2603

Chen HL, Chang MH, Ni YH et al (1996) Seroepidemiology of hepatitis B virus infection in children: ten years after a hepatitis B mass vaccination program in Taiwan. JAMA 276:906–908

Chen HL, Lin LH, Hu FC et al (2012) Effects of maternal screening and universal immunization to prevent mother- to-infant transmission of HBV. Gastroenterology 142:773–781

Chen YC, Chu CM, Liaw YF (2010) Age- specific prognosis following spontaneous hepatitis B e antigen seroconversion in chronic hepatitis B. Hepatology 51:435–444

Chien MC, Tong MJ, Lo KJ et al (1981) Hepatitis B viral markers in patients with primary hepatocellular carcinoma in Taiwan. J Natl Cancer Inst 66:475–479

Da Villa G, Picciottoc L, Elia S et al (1995) Hepatitis B vaccination: universal vaccination of newborn babies and children at 12 years of age versus high risk groups: a comparison in the field. Vaccine 13:1240–1243

Egner PA, Wang JB, Shu YR et al (2001) Chlorophyline intervention reduces aflatoxin-DNA adducts in individuals at high risk for liver cancer. Proc Natl Acad Sci USA 98:14601–14606

Feret E, Larouze B, Diop B et al (1987) Epidemiology of hepatitis B virus infection in the rural community of tip, Senegal. Am J Epidemiol 125:140–149

Ferlay J, Parkin DM, Curado MP, et al (2010) Cancer incidence in five continents, Volumes I to IX: IARC CancerBase No. 9 [Internet]. Lyon, France: International Agency for Research on Cancer; 2010. [http://ci5.iarc.fr, accessed 26 Jan 2012]

Grisham JW (2001) Molecular genetic alterations in primary hepatocellular neoplasms. In: Coleman WB, Tsongalis GJ (eds) The molecular basis of human cancer. Humana Press, Totowa, pp 269–346

Han GR, Cao MK, Zhao W et al (2011) A prospective and open-label study for the efficacy and safety of telbivudine in pregnancy for the prevention of perinatal transmission of hepatitis B virus infection. J Hepatol 55:1215–1221

Halsey NA, Duclos P, van Damme P et al (1999) Hepatitis B vaccine and central nervous system demyelinating diseases. Pediatrc Infect Dis J 18:23–24

Heyward WL, Lanier AP, Bender TR et al (1981) Primary hepatocellular carcinoma in Alaskan natives, 1969–1979. Int J Cancer 28:47–50

Hsu HC, Lin WS, Tsai MJ (1983) Hepatitis B surface antigen and hepatocellular carcinoma in Taiwan. With special reference to types and localization of HBsAg in the tumor cells. Cancer 52:1825–1832

Hsu HY, Chang MH, Ni YH, Chen HL (2004) Survey of hepatitis B surface variant infection in children 15 years after nationwide vaccination program in Taiwan. Gut 53:1499–503

Hsu HY, Chang MH, Chen DS et al (1986) Baseline seroepidemiology of hepatitis B virus infection in children in Taipei, 1984: a study just before mass hepatitis B vaccination program in Taiwan. J Med Virol 18:301–307

Hsu HY, Chang MH, Hsieh KH et al (1992) Cellular immune response to hepatitis B core antigen in maternal-infant transmission of hepatitis B virus. Hepatology 15:770–776

Hsu HY, Chang MH, Liaw SH et al (1999) Changes of hepatitis B surface variants in carrier children before and after universal vaccination in Taiwan. Hepatology 30:1312–1317

Hsu HY, Chang MH, Ni YH et al (2010) Twenty-year trends in the emergence of hepatitis B surface antigen variants in children and adolescents after universal vaccination in Taiwan. J

Infect Dis 201:1192–1200

Jacobson LP, Zhang BC, Shu YR et al (1997) Oltipratz chemoprevention trial in Qidong, People's Republic of China: study design and clinical outcomes. Cancer Epidemiol Biomarkers Prev 6:257–265

Jang MK, Lee JY, Lee JH et al (2001) Seroepidemiology of HBV infection in South Korea, 1995 through 1999. Korean J Intern Med 16:153–159

Jee SH, Ohrr H, Sull JW et al (2004) Cigarette smoking, alcohol drinking, hepatitis B, and risk for hepatocellular carcinoma in Korea. J Natl Cancer Inst 96:1851–1855

Kane MA (1996) Global status of hepatitis B immunization. Lancet 348:696

Kane MA, Brooks A (2002) New immunization initiatives and progress toward the global control of hepatitis B. Curr Opin Infect Dis 15:465–469

Lavanchy D (2004) Hepatitis B virus epidemiology, disease burden, treatment, and current and emerging prevention and control measures. J Viral Hepatitis 11:97–107

Lavanchy D (2008) Chronic viral hepatitis as a public health issue in the world. Best Pract Res Clin Gastroenterol 22:991–1008

Lee SD, Lo KJ, Wu JC et al (1986) Prevention of maternal-infant hepatitis B virus transmission by immunization: the role of serum hepatitis B virus DNA. Hepatology 6(3):369–373

Liaw YF (2011) Impact of hepatitis B therapy on the long-term outcome of liver disease. Liver Int Suppl 1:117–121

Liaw YF, Sung JJ, Chow WC et al (2004) Lamivudine for patients with chronic hepatitis B and advanced liver disease. N Engl J Med 351:1521–1531

Lin HH, Chang MH, Chen DS et al (1991) Early predictor of the efficacy of immunoprophylaxis against perinatal hepatitis B transmission: analysis of prophylaxis failure. Vaccine 9:457–460

Lin HH, Lee TY, Chen DS et al (1987) Transplacental leakage of HBeAg-positive maternal blood as the most likely route in causing intrauterine infection with hepatitis intrauterine infection with hepatitis B virus. J Pediatr 111:877–881

Lin SM, Yu ML, Lee CM et al (2007) Interferon therapy in HBeAg positive chronic hepatitis reduces progression to cirrhosis and hepatocellular carcinoma. J Hepatol 46:45–52

Livingston SE, Simonetti J, McMahon B et al (2007) Hepatitis B virus genotypes in Alaska Native people with hepatocellular carcinoma: preponderance of genotype F. J Infect Dis 195(5–11):1

McMahon BJ, Bulkow LR, Singleton RJ et al (2011) Elimination of hepatocellular carcinoma and acute hepatitis B in children 25 years after a hepatitis B newborn and catch-up immunization program. Hepatology 54:801–807

Montesano R (2011) Preventing primary liver cancer: the HBV vaccination project in the Gambia (West Africa). Environ Health 10(Suppl 1):S6

Ni YH, Chang MH, Hsu HY et al (1991) Hepatocellular carcinoma in childhood. Clinical manifestations and prognosis. Cancer 68:1737–1741

Ni YH, Chang MH, Huang LM et al (2001) Hepatitis B virus infection in children and adolescents in an hyperendemic area: 15 years after universal hepatitis B vaccination. Ann Intern Med 135:796–800

Ni YH, Huang LM, Chang MH et al (2007) Two decades of universal hepatitis B vaccination in Taiwan: impact and implication for future strategies. Gastroenterology 132:1287–1293

Parkin DM, Bray F, Ferlay J et al (2001) Estimating the world cancer burden: Globocan 2000. Int J Cancer 94:153–156

Poovorawan Y, Sanpavat S, Pongpunlert W et al (1989) Protective efficacy of a recombinant DNA hepatitis B vaccine in neonates of HBe antigen-positive mothers. JAMA 261:3278–3281

Schafer DF, Sorrell MF (1999) Hepatocellular carcinoma. Lancet 353:1253–1257

Shepard CW, Simard EP, Finelli L et al (2006) Hepatitis B virus infection: epidemiology and vaccination. Epidemiol Rev 28:112–125

Stevens CE, Beasley RP, Tsui J et al (1975) Vertical transmission of hepatitis B antigen in Taiwan. N Engl J Med 292:771–774

Tang JR, Hsu HY, Lin HH et al (1998) Hepatitis B surface antigenemia at birth: a long-term follow-up study. J Pediatr 133:374–377

Tseng TC, Liu CJ, Yang HC et al (2012) High levels of hepatitis B surface antigen increase risk of hepatocellular carcinoma in patients with low HBV load. Gastroenterology 142:1140–1149

Tsuei DJ, Hsu HC, Lee PH et al (2004) RBMY, a male germ cell-specific RNA-binding protein, activated in human liver cancers and transforms rodent fibroblasts. Oncogene 29(23):5815–5822

Turati F, Edefonti V, Talamini R et al (2012) Family history of liver cancer and hepatocellular carcinoma. Hepatology 55:1416–1425

van Herck K, Vorsters A, Van Damme P (2008) Prevention of viral hepatitis (B and C) reassessed. Best Pract Res Clin Gastroenterol 22:1009–1029

van Zonneveld M, van Nunen AB, Niesters HG et al (2003) Lamivudine treatment during pregnancy to prevent perinatal transmission of hepatitis B virus infection. J Viral Hepat 10:294–297

Villanueva A, Newell P, Chiang DY et al (2007) Genomics and signaling pathways in hepatocellular carcinoma. Semin Liver Dis 27:55–76

Wang HC, Huang W, Lai MD et al (2006) Hepatitis B virus pre-S mutants, endoplasmic reticulum stress and hepatocarcinogenesis. Cancer Sci 97:683–688

Whittle H, Jaffar S, Wansbrough M et al (2002) Observational study of vaccine efficacy 14 years after trial of hepatitis B vaccination in Gambian children. BMJ 325:569–573

Wichajarn K, Kosalaraksa P, Wiangnon S (2008) Incidence of hepatocellular carcinoma in children in Khon Kaen before and after national hepatitis B vaccine program. Asian Pac J Cancer Prev 9:507–509

World Health Organization (2012) Data, statistics and graphics. Global routine vaccination coverage, (http://www.who.int/immunization_monitoring/data/en/, accessed Mar 2012)

Xu WM, Cui YT, Wang L et al (2009) Lamivudine in late pregnancy to prevent perinatal transmission of hepatitis B virus infection: a multicentre, randomized, double-blind, placebo-controlled study. J Viral Hepat 16:94–103

Yang HI, Lu SN, Liaw YF et al (2002) Hepatitis B e antigen and the risks of hepatocellular carcinoma. N Engl J Med 347:168–174

Yeh SH, Chen PJ (2012) Gender disparity of hepatocellular carcinoma: the roles of sex hormones. Oncology 78(suppl 1):172–179

Yu MW, Hsu FC, Sheen IS et al (1997) Prospective study of hepatocellular carcinoma and liver cirrhosis in asymptomatic chronic hepatitis B virus carriers. Am J Epidemiol 145:1039–1047

第 9 章 丙型肝炎病毒的致癌作用

Kazuhiko Koike

摘 要 丙型肝炎病毒（HCV）持续感染是发生肝细胞癌（HCC）的主要风险因素之一。然而，对于 HCV 相关的 HCC 发病机理，病毒在这个过程中起直接作用还是间接作用，仍存在争议。研究发现，有持续高水平血清丙氨酸转氨酶的慢性丙型肝炎患者更容易发生 HCC，提示炎症在丙肝肝细胞癌发生中起重要作用。但是，并发强烈炎症的自身免疫性肝炎患者，即使发生了肝硬化，也很少发展成 HCC。这种现象暗示 HCV 在 HCC 发生中起直接作用。然而，HCV 是单股正链 RNA 病毒，其基因组从不被整合到宿主基因组中，它在肝癌发生中到底起了什么作用？表达 HCV 蛋白的转基因小鼠和体外细胞培养模型的研究结果显示，HCV 有直接致病性和致癌活性。特别是 HCV 的核心蛋白，通过抑制分子伴侣抑制素的作用，弱化线粒体的电子传递系统，诱导过度的氧化应激。HCV 也调节细胞内信号通路，包括分裂素激活的蛋白激酶，使肝细胞获得生长优势。此外，HCV 导致葡萄糖代谢紊乱，从而加速肝纤维化进程和 HCC 发展。这些结果为我们进一步了解包括肝癌发生在内的 HCV 持续感染的致病机理提供了线索。

关键词 丙肝，肝细胞癌，核心蛋白，氧化应激，脂代谢，胰岛素抗性

1 引言

全世界大约有 1.7 亿人持续感染 HCV，感染引起一系列慢性肝脏疾病，包括慢性肝炎、肝硬化，最后发展为肝细胞癌（HCC）（Saito et al. 1990）。由于 HCC 对社会广泛而深入的影响，以及 HCC 发病率在 HCV 持续感染的患者中居高不下，HCV 正日益受到人们的关注。一旦丙肝患者发生肝硬化，HCC 的年发病率为 7%（Ikeda et al. 1998）。依此推算，将近 90% 的 HCV 相关的肝硬化患者在 15 年内

K. Koike (✉)
Department of Gastroenterology, Graduate School of Medicine,
The University of Tokyo, Tokyo, Japan
e-mail: kkoike-tky@umin.ac.jp

发展为HCC。此外，与HCV感染有关的肝癌的突出特征，如HCC的多中心性和高发性，除在家族性结肠息肉瘤等遗传性癌症中较常见外，在其他的恶性肿瘤中并不常见。因此，为了预防HCC的发生，迫切需要了解在HCV持续感染中发生HCC的机制。

2　HCV和病毒蛋白

HCV是一种有包膜的RNA病毒，属于黄病毒科，其基因组是单链正义RNA，由大约9600个核苷酸组成（Houghton et al. 1991）。基因组包含一个大的开放阅读框（ORF），编码一个大约3010个氨基酸的多聚蛋白，这个开放阅读框紧连5'端和3'端的非编码区。5'端非编码区包含341个核苷酸，作为内部核糖体进入位点。这种结构特征使RNA基因组使用一种帽子非依赖型的翻译机制，不需要核糖体从带帽子的5'端进行扫描。

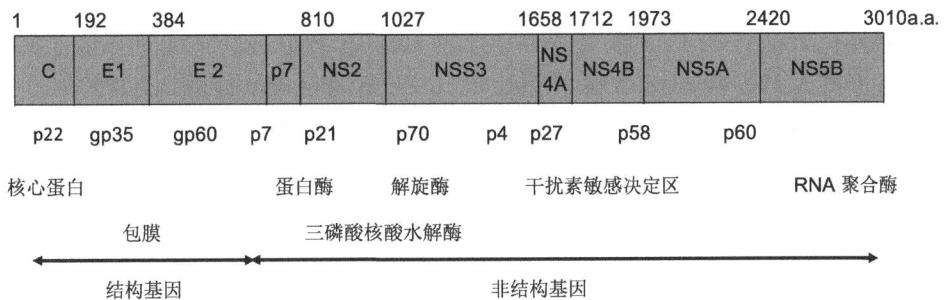

图9-1　HCV的基因组结构。HCV的基因组RNA编码一个大约3010个氨基酸的多聚蛋白，经细胞和病毒蛋白酶处理为结构蛋白和非结构蛋白。其中一个结构蛋白——核心蛋白，在体内和体外实验中表现了多种不一样的特性。ISDR，干扰素敏感决定区域。

HCV多聚蛋白由细胞和病毒蛋白酶处理，产生病毒基因产物，可分为结构蛋白和非结构蛋白。结构蛋白由NH_2端约占基因组1/4长度的序列编码，包括核心蛋白和包膜蛋白E1、E2。虽然还不清楚p7是否是病毒粒子的组成部分，E2可与p7形成E2-p7形式。NS2、NS3、NS4A、NS4B、NS5A和NS5B是非结构蛋白，由结构蛋白基因之外的编码序列编码，其中包括丝氨酸蛋白酶（NS3/4A）、三磷酸核苷水解酶/解旋酶(NTPase/helicase)(NS3)和RNA依赖的RNA聚合酶(NS5B)。

HCV核心蛋白位于多聚蛋白前体的1~191位残基，它由宿主信号肽酶在核心蛋白和E1之间切割分开而产生。核心蛋白的C端膜锚定区被宿主信号肽酶进一步加工处理（Moradpour et al. 2007）。成熟的核心蛋白大约由177~179个氨基酸构成，在多种HCV基因型中具有极高的同源性。HCV核心蛋白包含亲水的N端区,称"区域(domain) I"(1~117位残基),紧接其后是一个称为"区域 II"的疏水性区域(118~170位残基)。区域 I 富含碱性氨基酸,参与 RNA 结合和蛋白质的同源寡聚反应。两性螺旋(AH) I 和 II 分别包括区域 II 中的 119~136 和 148~164 位残基,参与 HCV 核心蛋白与脂类的联系(Boulant et al. 2006)。另外,112~152 位残基区域与内质网膜和线粒体膜相关联(Suzuki et al. 2005)。核心蛋白也定位于细胞核中(Miyamoto et al. 2007;Shirakura et al. 2007),与细胞核蛋白酶体激活子 PA28γ/REGγ 结合,导致核心蛋白的 PA28γ 依赖性降解(Moriishi et al. 2003)。自噬涉及细胞器的降解和入侵微生物的清除。破坏自噬作用常常导致几种蛋白沉积病。最近,研究表明,HCV RNA 复制诱导的自噬有毒株特异性,这提示 HCV 可利用自噬来逃避细胞死亡,自噬通量紊乱可能参与 HCV 基因型特异性的致病机制(Taguwa et al. 2011)。

3 HCV 在肝癌发生中的可能作用

虽然在日本约 80%、世界范围内 30%的 HCC 患者是 HCV 持续感染者(Perz et al. 2006;Kiyosawa et al. 1990;Saito et al. 1990;Yotsuyanagi et al. 2000),但是我们仍不清楚 HCV 感染中的肝癌的发生机制。因此,我们仍需寻找和鉴定 HCV 在肝癌形成中的作用。在肝炎病毒感染中,应该考虑 HCV 感染导致的炎症。慢性炎症后的肝细胞坏死和随后的再生,加剧了宿主细胞内基因的变异,这种变异的累积在 HCC 中达到高峰。该理论预设了 HCV 通过引发肝脏炎症,间接参与 HCC 的形成。然而,这个理论却给我们留下一下重要问题:只有炎症能导致如此高的 HCC 发病率(15 年内达 90%)或 HCC 发生的多中心性吗?

HCV 的另一个作用也需要被权衡考虑:在持续重度肝脏炎症的自身免疫肝炎患者中,即使在肝硬化之后,很少发生 HCC。根据这些基础推理,病毒蛋白可能有致瘤活性。利用引入 HCV 基因的方法,在培养的肝细胞中对这种可能性进行评估,但收效甚微。如果 HCV 有致癌能力,这种能力可能很弱,因此,利用细胞培养进行致癌性研究的一个困难就是,可能需要很长时间才能表现出其致癌作用。事实上,HCV 感染的个体发展成 HCC 也需要 30~40 年时间。正是由于以上这些观点,现在已经开始利用转基因小鼠技术,在活体内研究慢性 HCV 的致癌作用。

4 HCV 在小鼠体内表现致癌作用

关于 HCV 相关的肝脏病变的一个主要问题是病毒蛋白对病理学表型是否有直接作用。虽然已经利用几种不同的方法对 HCV 蛋白进行了研究,但还未能阐明蛋白表达与疾病表型之间的关系。针对这个问题，已经建立了几个不同品系的 HCV 转基因小鼠模型（表 9-1）。这些模型包括携带 HCV 基因组的整个编码区（Lerat et al. 2002）、核心蛋白区（Machida et al. 2006；Moriya et al. 1997）、包膜蛋白区（Koike et al. 1995；Pasquinelli et al. 1997）、核心蛋白区与包膜蛋白区（Lerat et al. 2002；Naas et al. 2005），或者从核心蛋白区到 NS2 区（Wakita et al. 1998）。在这些转基因小鼠模型中，虽然有报道称可检测到非结构蛋白基因 mRNA（Honda et al. 1999；Lerat et al. 2002），但是在小鼠肝脏中未能检测到非结构蛋白，其原因还不清楚。有可能是表达的非结构蛋白表现出的酶活性对小鼠发育不利，因此，只能建立低水平表达非结构蛋白的转基因小鼠模型。

表 9-1 小鼠中 HCV 蛋白的表达结果

HCV 基因	基因型	启动子	蛋白表达	表型	参考文献
核心蛋白	1b	HBV	与患者相似	脂肪变性，肝癌，胰岛素抗性，氧化应激	Moriya et al.（1997，1998）Moriishi et al.（2003，2007）Shintani et al.（2004）Miyamoto et al.（2007）
核心蛋白	1b	延伸因子-1a	与患者相似	脂肪变性，肿瘤，肝癌，氧化应激	Machida et al.（2006）
E1-E2	1b	HBV	丰富的	肝中什么也没发生	Koike et al.（1995，1997）
核心蛋白-E1-E2	1b	白蛋白	与患者相似	脂肪变性，肝癌，氧化应激	Lerat（2003）
核心蛋白-E1-E2	1a	巨细胞病毒	与患者相似	脂肪变性，肝癌	Naas et al.（2005）
结构蛋白	1b	主要组织相容性复合体	在肝中很低	肝炎	Honda et al.（1999）
全部的多聚蛋白	1b	白蛋白	只检测到 mRNA	脂肪变性，肝癌	Lerat（2003）
全部的多聚蛋白	1a	抗胰蛋白酶		脂肪变性，肝内的 T-细胞招募	Alonzi et al.（2004）
NS3/4A	1a	主要尿蛋白		没有（免疫调节）	Frelin et al.（2006）
NS5A	1a	载脂蛋白 E		没有（抵制坏死因子）	Majumder et al.（2002）

HBV，乙型肝炎病毒；EF，延伸因子；MUP，主要尿蛋白；Alb，白蛋白；CMV，巨细胞病毒；MHC，主要组织相容性复合体；AT，抗胰蛋白酶；ApoE，载脂蛋白 E

我们建立了携带 HCV 1b 型基因组 cDNA 的 4 种转基因小鼠（Moriya et al. 1997，1998）。这 4 种小鼠都利用相同的转录调控元件，分别携带核心蛋白基因、包膜蛋白基因、整个非结构区域的基因、NS5A 基因。在这些小鼠系中，只有携带核心蛋白基因的两个独立谱系的小鼠发生 HCC（Moriya et al. 1998）。虽然高水平表达 E1 和 E2 蛋白,但是携带包膜蛋白基因的小鼠却不发生 HCC(Koike et al. 1995,1997)。携带完整 NS 基因或 NS5A 基因的转基因小鼠也不发生 HCC。

核心蛋白转基因小鼠在早期就发生脂肪肝,并伴随淋巴卵泡的形成和胆管损伤,而脂肪肝是慢性丙型肝炎的组织学特征之一。因此,核心蛋白转基因小鼠模型能较好地重现慢性丙型肝炎的特点。但是,需要注意的是,这些动物肝脏中没有发现任何反映炎症的特征。这些转基因小鼠在生命晚期发展成 HCC。特别是携带全部 HCV 基因的小鼠,或者是携带包括核心蛋白在内的结构基因的小鼠,都发生脂肪肝和 HCC（Lerat et al. 2002；Machida et al. 2006；Naas et al. 2005）。这些证据显示,核心蛋白通过 HCV 自身在活体内表达时,具有潜在致癌性。

5 HCV 增强产生氧化应激作用和调节胞内信号

核心蛋白在肝细胞中的显著特点是,主要定位于与脂滴关联的细胞质中,同时也出现在线粒体和细胞核内（Moriya et al. 1998）。正因为如此,对线粒体和细胞核相关的路径也研究得比较全面。

核心蛋白的一个作用是增强肝脏中氧化应激作用。特别值得注意的是,在没有发生炎症的肝脏中,核心蛋白转基因小鼠中的氧化应激作用是增强的。过强的氧化应激作用会导致线粒体和核 DNA 的缺失,这指示引起了遗传损伤（Moriya et al. 2001a）。

不少临床和基础研究显示,氧化应激的增强与 HCV 引起的肝脏发病有关联（Farinati et al. 1995）。活性氧类（ROS）是内源性氧,包含氧化代谢中形成的正常产物分子。ROS 能诱导遗传突变和线粒体改变,利于多步癌变过程中的癌症发展（Fujita et al. 2008；Kato et al. 2001）。丙肝中氧化应激的增强,比在其他类型的肝炎中更为突出,如 HBV（Farinati et al. 1995）。增强氧化应激作用是 HCV 相关的肝病发病的一个因素,但是对其增强的机制还知之甚少。因此,从 ROS 的产生和清除方面去理解氧化应激作用的机制,可能会使我们开发出新的 HCV 治疗方法。

肝癌发生的其他途径可能是细胞基因的表达和胞内信号通路的调控改变。例如,已经发现肝癌中肿瘤坏死因子（TNF）-α 和白细胞介素-1β 的转录激活（Tsutsumi et al. 2002）。细胞分裂素激活蛋白激酶（MAPK）级联反应在核心蛋白转基因小鼠模型中被激活。MAPK 通路由三条路径组成,包括 c-Jun N 端激酶（JNK）、p38 和细胞外信号调节激酶（ERK）,涉及包括细胞增殖在内的许多细胞事件。在核心蛋白转基因小鼠发生肝癌前的肝脏中,只有 JNK 路径被激活。JNK 激活的下游,转录因子激活蛋白（AP）-1 的激活被显著增强（Tsutsumi et al. 2003）。在远下游,周期蛋白 D1 和周期依赖性激酶（CDK）4 的水平也被增加。

因此，HCV 核心蛋白调节细胞内的信号途径，有利于肝细胞增殖。此外，HCV 核心蛋白还抑制细胞因子信号抑制子（SOCS）-1 的表达。SOCS-1 是细胞因子信号通路的负调节因子，可能作为一种抑瘤基因起作用（Miyoshi et al. 2005）。

这种核心蛋白在 MAPK 通路中的作用，结合氧化应激作用，可能是慢性丙型肝炎患者中高发 HCC 的原因（图 9-2）。

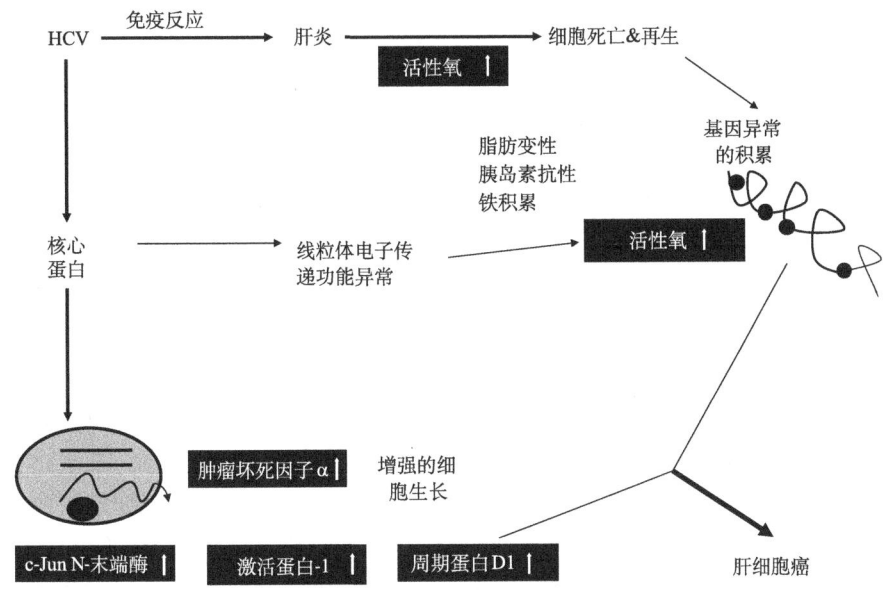

图 9-2　HCV 感染相关的肝癌发病的分子机制。HCV 核心蛋白引起的氧化应激作用和脂肪肝对肝癌的形成起关键作用。细胞内基因表达的改变，如肿瘤坏死因子（TNF）-α，还有细胞内其他的信号途径，包括 J-Jun N 端激酶（JNK），都会共同加快 HCV 感染中的肝癌的形成。

6　HCV 感染中的 ROS 来自线粒体

丙肝患者肝脏中氧化应激增强的源头是什么？核心蛋白主要定位于内质网，但也存在于细胞培养物和转基因小鼠的线粒体内（Moriya et al. 1998；Suzuki et al. 2005）。另外，在核心蛋白转基因小鼠肝细胞中，线粒体膜的双层结构被破坏。事实证明，核心蛋白调节线粒体的一些功能，包括脂肪酸 β-氧化。脂肪酸 β-氧化的减弱可能导致脂代谢异常和脂肪肝。另外，线粒体是 ROS 的重要来源。在核心蛋白转基因小鼠的肝脏中，可观察到 ROS 产量的增加（Moriya et al. 2001a）。利用活检样品的蛋白质组学方法，最近的研究表明，包括脂肪酸氧化和氧化磷酸化作用在内的关键线粒体过程，以及氧化应激作用，都在 HCV 感染的高级纤维化的肝脏中发生（Diamond et al. 2007）。因此，HCV 核心蛋白有可能影响线粒体的功能，因为这种病理表现在 HCV 核心蛋白转基因小鼠、表达核心蛋白的体外培养细胞中（Korenaga et al. 2005），以及 HCV 患者中，都能观察到。

蛋白质组学的新发展为发现疾病相关的生物标记物开辟了新途径。我们从稳定表达 HCV 核心蛋白的 HepG2 细胞中分离线粒体，然后进行二维聚丙烯酰胺凝胶电泳（2D-PAGE），鉴定得到与对照 HepG2 细胞有表达差异的几种蛋白质。在表达核心蛋白的细胞内表达上调的蛋白质中，我们集中研究抑制素。抑制素是一个线粒体蛋白伴侣。研究发现，核心蛋白和抑制素相互作用，并阻断抑制素和细胞色素 C 氧化酶（COX）亚单位蛋白之间的相互作用，导致蛋白质表达水平和 COX 活性的下降。

作为线粒体蛋白伴侣的抑制素在稳定表达核心蛋白的细胞中是一种上调蛋白。抑制素是一种广泛表达和高度保守的蛋白质。最早发现，它通过减少 DNA 合成，在抑制细胞周期进程和细胞增殖中起主导作用（Mishra et al. 2005）。它存在于细胞核，与细胞周期进程中的关键转录因子相互作用。在表达核心蛋白的细胞中，细胞核内也检测到抑制素，并且它的表达水平高于对照细胞。线粒体的抑制素作为分子伴侣，通过直接作用稳定新合成的线粒体翻译产物（Nijtmans et al. 2000）。我们研究抑制素和线粒体编码的 COX 亚基Ⅱ之间的相互作用发现，在表达核心蛋白的细胞中，这些蛋白质之间的相互作用被抑制了。另外，一些研究表明，抑制素与线粒体呼吸复合体Ⅰ和细胞色素氧化酶Ⅳ（COX）的装配有关（Nijtmans et al. 2000）。复合体Ⅰ也包含核和线粒体 DNA 编码的亚基，因此，复合体Ⅰ的装配和功能可能被核心蛋白减弱。关于复合体Ⅰ的功能，作者发现在表达核心蛋白的细胞中，复合体Ⅰ活性下降。其他研究组也发现，在细胞培养中，复合体Ⅰ活性也下降（Piccoli et al. 2007）。从这些发现来看，抑制素和核心蛋白的相互作用可能会减弱复合体Ⅰ和复合体Ⅳ的功能，导致 ROS 含量增加。实际上，抑制素的压制作用引起 ROS 含量增加（Theiss et al. 2007），这种现象在本实验使用的表达核心蛋白的细胞中，以及核心蛋白转基因小鼠中，都可观察到（Moriya et al. 2001a）。非常有意思的是，特异性删除肝脏抑制素会导致形态学异常和 HCC（Ko et al. 2010）。

HCV 通过抑制线粒体内分子伴侣的功能，诱发线粒体功能紊乱，这是病毒感染造成 ROS 过量产生的一种新机制（Tsutsumi et al. 2009）。

7　HCV 在诱导 ROS 的同时减弱某种抗氧化系统

如上所述，慢性丙型肝炎有氧化应激作用显著增强的特征。与此相关，肝中铁的富集会加剧氧化应激，同时肝中 DNA 加合物的含量也会增加（Farinati et al.

1995）。铁富集在表达核心蛋白的小鼠肝脏中（Moriya et al. 2010）。在正常喂食的核心蛋白转基因小鼠的肝脏中有铁的累积，这很好地印证了在慢性丙肝患者中观察到的现象（Farinati et al. 1995；Fujita et al. 2008）。之后，这种小鼠模型和细胞培养被用于研究铁过量对氧化/抗氧化系统的影响。铁过量会诱导产生 ROS 和抗氧化物质。但是，一些重要的抗氧化酶却没有因此而升高，如血红素加氧酶（HO）-1、NADH 脱氢酶和醌（NDQ）-1。其他的抗氧化酶，如过氧化氢酶和谷胱甘肽-S-转移酶（GST），在铁过量的核心蛋白转基因小鼠中的增强作用，比只有铁过量的正常小鼠或者没有铁过量的核心蛋白转基因小鼠的对照组更为强烈。铁诱导的 HO-1 增强作用的减弱，也在表达核心蛋白的 HepG2 细胞中得到证实。HO-1 催化分解代谢中起始和限速反应，并分解促氧化血红素，形成胆绿素。胆绿素在哺乳动物中形成胆红素，两者都具有强烈的抗氧化活性（Stocker et al. 1987）。另外，当谷胱甘肽耗竭时，HO-1 被认为是一个中心抗氧化物。因此，HO-1 是抵抗氧化应激作用的一个必需的内源性保护机制，特别是在铁过量的情况下。因此，HO-1 和 NDQ-1 的减弱有可能阻碍抗氧化系统，导致 HCV 感染中的氧化应激作用明显增强。

因此，HCV 感染不仅诱导产生 ROS，也阻碍肝中的抗氧化物激活，从而加剧氧化应激，促进肝癌形成。在携带 HCV 基因组的其他转基因小鼠中也发现，铁过量加剧氧化应激作用（Nishinaet al. 2008）。

8　HCV 感染的代谢改变：肝病发展的共同因素

脂肪变性（steatosis）常见于慢性丙型肝炎患者，与肝纤维化的加速发展有明显关系（Powell et al. 2005）。核心蛋白转基因小鼠肝脏中积累的脂肪酸组成，不同于单纯肥胖形成的脂肪肝。C18 单不饱和脂肪酸（C18:1）的含量显著上升，如促进癌细胞增殖的油酸或异油酸（Kudo et al. 2011）。丙型肝炎患者的肝脏组织与肥胖导致脂肪肝患者的肝脏组织也不一样（Moriya et al. 2001b）。

可以使用核心蛋白转基因小鼠模型研究丙型肝炎的脂肪生成机理。至少有三种途径与脂肪变性有关。第一种途径是丙肝患者和核心蛋白转基因小鼠中频繁出现的胰岛素抗性，这种现象是通过抑制胰岛素受体底物（IRS）-1 的酪氨酸磷酸化作用而产生的（Shintani et al. 2004）。胰岛素抗性增加了脂肪酸的外周释放和肝脏摄取，致使脂在肝脏中积累。第二种途径是，HCV 核心蛋白抑制微粒体甘油三酯转移蛋白（MTP）活性（Perlemuter et al. 2002）。这种作用阻抑肝脏分泌极低密度脂蛋白（VLDL），增加肝脏中的甘油三酯。第三种途径包含调节甘油三酯和磷脂产量的胆固醇调节元件结合蛋白（SREBP）-1c。在 HCV 核心蛋白转基因小鼠中，SREBP-1c 被上调，但是 SREBP-2 和 SREBP-1a 却没有被上调（Moriishi et al. 2007）。来自体外研究（Kim et al. 2007；Waris et al. 2007）和黑猩猩研究（Su et al. 2002）的结果也印证了这一现象。因此，这三种途径的参与可能很容易导致丙肝患者发生肝脏的脂肪变性（图9-3）。脂肪变性加剧ROS的产生，并加快丙型肝炎的肝病进程。

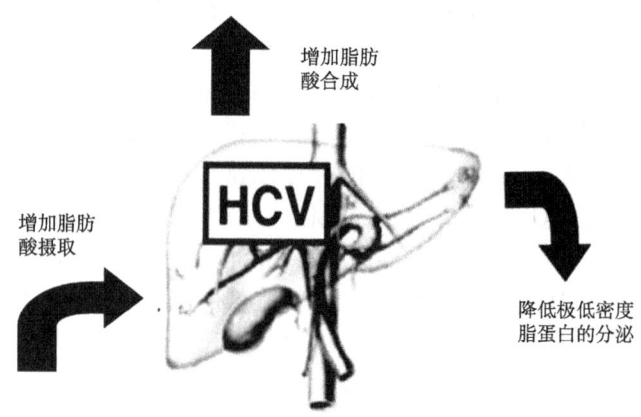

图9-3　HCV通过脂肪代谢的三种途径诱导肝脏脂肪变性。第一，HCV核心蛋白诱导胰岛素抗性，增加脂肪酸的外周释放和肝脏摄取。第二，HCV核心蛋白抑制微粒体甘油三酯转移蛋白（MTP）活性，这种作用阻抑肝脏分泌极低密度脂蛋白（VLDL），从而增加肝脏中的甘油三酯。第三，HCV核心蛋白诱导转录因子SREBP-1c上调，导致甘油三酯含量增加。因此，三种途径都很容易导致丙肝患者的肝脏中脂肪变性。MTP，微粒体甘油三酯转移蛋白；VLDL，极低密度脂蛋白；SREBP，胆固醇调节元件结合蛋白。

9　小结

HCV小鼠模型的研究结果显示，HCV核心蛋白在体内有致癌活性，因此，HCV在肝脏中有潜在的致癌作用。癌症发生方面的研究表明，一整套细胞遗传变异的积累是发展成肿瘤的必需条件,如结肠直肠癌（Kinzler and Vogelstein 1996）。那些导致APC基因失活、K-ras基因激活和p53基因失活的突变的积累，共同促进大肠癌的发生。这种理论已经用于其他癌症的癌变，称为"沃格尔斯坦型（Vogelstein-type）"癌变。

根据HCV核心蛋白诱导形成HCC的这个结果，我们可用一种不同的机制来解释HCV感染中的肝癌发生。我们仍然遵循所有癌症发生的多阶段性，但大量突变在肝细胞中积累将迫使肝癌发生。然而，在HCV感染的HCC发展过程中，可能会跳过一些癌变阶段，这些阶段可能由 HCV 核心蛋白的作用弥补。病毒蛋白表达导致的普遍结果应是诱发 HCC，即使缺少对癌症发生所需要的一整套遗传变异（图 9-4）。考虑到"非沃格尔斯坦型（non-Vogelstein-type）"诱导 HCC 发生，就可能更合理地解释 HCV 携带者中发生的一些非常规事件（Koike 2005）。现在，我们似乎不难理解，为什么在 HCV 持续感染的患者中，HCC 发病率显著增高。我们的理论还可能解释，由于 HCV 持续感染而引发 HCC 的非转移性和多中心性的原始发生特性。

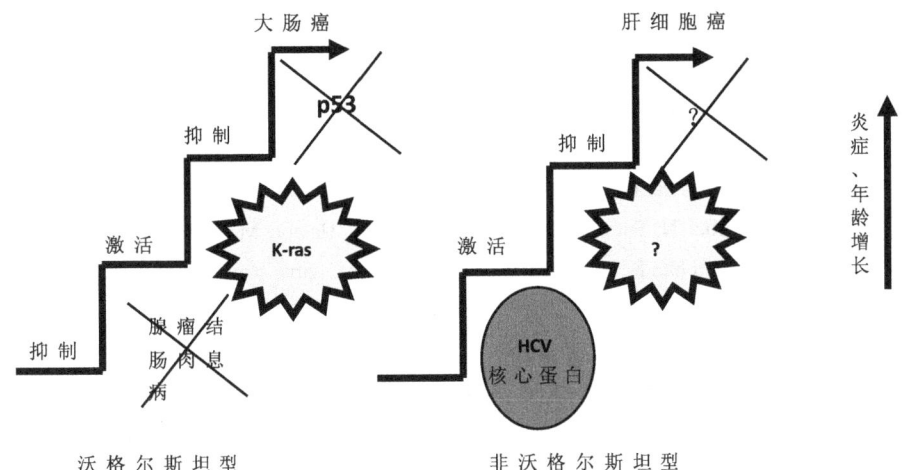

图 9-4 HCV 在肝癌发生中的作用。所有癌症的诱发都需要很多步骤；大量遗传突变积累在肝细胞中迫使肝癌发生。然而，在 HCV 感染的 HCC 发展过程中，由于 HCV 核心蛋白的作用，可能会跳过一些癌变阶段。即使没有癌症发生所需要的一整套遗传变异，核心蛋白的作用可能加强 HCC 的发生。结合"非沃格尔斯坦型（non-Vogelstein-type）"的肝癌发生过程，就可能更合理的解释 HCV 携带者中发生的一些非常规事件，比如 HCC 的高发病率和多中心性的特点。CRC，大肠癌。

（李义平，郑福祥，徐占雪 译）

参 考 文 献

Alonzi T, Agrati C, Costabile B, Cicchini C, Amicone L, Cavallari C, Rocca CD, Folgori A, Fipaldini C, Poccia F, Monica NL, Tripodi M (2004) Steatosis and intrahepatic lymphocyte recruitment in hepatitis C virus transgenic mice. J Gen Virol 85:1509–1520

Boulant S, Montserret R, Hope RG, Ratinier M, Targett-Adams P, Lavergne JP et al (2006) Structural determinants that target the hepatitis C virus core protein to lipid droplets. J Biol Chem 281:22236–22247

Diamond DL, Jacobs JM, Paeper B, Proll SC, Gritsenko MA, Carithers RL Jr et al (2007) Proteomic profiling of human liver biopsies: hepatitis C virus-induced fibrosis and mitochondrial dysfunction. Hepatology 46:649–657

Farinati F, Cardin R, De Maria N, Della Libera G, Marafin C, Lecis E, Burra P, Floreani A, Cecchetto A, Naccarato R (1995) Iron storage, lipid peroxidation and glutathione turnover in chronic anti-HCV positive hepatitis. J Hepatol 22:449–456

Frelin L, Brenndörfer ED, Ahlén G, Weiland M, Hultgren C, Alheim M, Glaumann H, Rozell B, Milich DR, Bode JG, Sällberg M (2006) The hepatitis C virus and immune evasion: nonstructural 3/4A transgenic mice are resistant to lethal tumour necrosis factor alpha mediated liver disease. Gut 55:1475–1483

Fujita N, Sugimoto R, Ma N, Tanaka H, Iwasa M, Kobayashi Y, Kawanishi S, Watanabe S, Kaito M, Takei Y (2008) Comparison of hepatic oxidative DNA damage in patients with chronic hepatitis B and C. J Viral Hepat 15:498–507

Honda A, Arai Y, Hirota N, Sato T, Ikegaki J, Koizumi T, Hatano M, Kohara M, Moriyama T, Imawari M, Shimotohno K, Tokuhisa T (1999) Hepatitis C virus structural proteins induce liver cell injury in transgenic mice. J Med Virol 59:281–289

Houghton M, Weiner A, Han J, Kuo G, Choo QL (1991) Molecular biology of hepatitis C viruses. Implications for diagnosis, development and control of viral diseases. Hepatology 14:381–388

Ikeda K, Saitoh S, Suzuki Y, Kobayashi M, Tsubota A, Koida I et al (1998) Disease progression and hepatocellular carcinogenesis in patients with chronic viral hepatitis: a prospective observation of 2215 patients. J Hepatol 28:930–938

Kato J, Kobune M, Nakamura T, Kuroiwa G, Takada K, Takimoto R, Sato Y, Fujikawa K, Takahashi M, Takayama T, Ikeda T, Niitsu Y (2001) Normalization of elevated hepatic 8-hydroxy-2'-deoxyguanosine levels in chronic hepatitis C patients by phlebotomy and low iron diet. Cancer Res 61:8697–8702

Kim KH, Hong SP, Kim K, Park MJ, Kim KJ, Cheong J (2007) HCV core protein induces hepatic lipid accumulation by activating SREBP1 and PPARgamma. Biochem Biophys Res Commun 55:883–888

Kinzler KW, Vogelstein B (1996) Lessons from hereditary colorectal cancer. Cell 87:159–170

Kiyosawa K, Sodeyama T, Tanaka E, Gibo Y, Yoshizawa K, Nakano Y et al (1990) Interrelationship of blood transfusion, non-A, non-B hepatitis and hepatocellular carcinoma: analysis by detection of antibody to hepatitis C virus. Hepatology 12:671–675

Ko KS, Tomasi ML, Iglesias-Ara A, French BA, French SW, Ramani K, Lozano JJ, Oh P, He L, Stiles BL, Li TW, Yang H, Martínez-Chantar ML, Mato JM, Lu SC (2010) Liver-specific deletion of prohibitin 1 results in spontaneous liver injury, fibrosis, and hepatocellular carcinoma in mice. Hepatology 52:2096–2108

Koike K (2005) Molecular basis of hepatitis C virus-associated hepatocarcinogenesis: lessons from animal model studies. Clin Gastroenterol Hepatol 3:S132–S135

Koike K, Moriya K, Ishibashi K, Matsuura Y, Suzuki T, Saito I et al (1995) Expression of hepatitis C virus envelope proteins in transgenic mice. J Gen Virol 76:3031–3038

Koike K, Moriya K, Yotsuyanagi H, Shintani Y, Fujie H, Ishibashi K et al (1997) Sialadenitis resembling Sjögren's syndrome in mice transgenic for hepatitis C virus envelope genes. Proc Natl Acad Sci USA 94:233–236

Korenaga M, Wang T, Li Y, Showalter LA, Chan T, Sun J, Weinman SA (2005) Hepatitis C virus core protein inhibits mitochondrial electron transport and increases reactive oxygen species (ROS) production. J Biol Chem 280:37481–37488

Kudo Y, Tanaka Y, Tateishi K, Yamamoto K, Yamamoto S, Mohri D, Isomura Y, Seto M, Nakagawa H, Asaoka Y, Tada M, Ohta M, Ijichi H, Hirata Y, Otsuka M, Ikenoue T, Maeda S, Shiina S, Yoshida H, Nakajima O, Kanai F, Omata M, Koike K (2011) Altered composition of fatty acids exacerbates hepatotumorigenesis during activation of the phosphatidylinositol 3-kinase pathway. J Hepatol 55:1400–1408

Lerat H, Honda M, Beard MR, Loesch K, Sun J, Yang Y et al (2002) Steatosis and liver cancer in transgenic mice expressing the structural and nonstructural proteins of hepatitis C virus. Gastroenterology 122:352–365

Machida K, Cheng KT, Lai CK, Jeng KS, Sung VM, Lai MM (2006) Hepatitis C virus triggers mitochondrial permeability transition with production of reactive oxygen species, leading to DNA damage and STAT3 activation. J Virol 80:7199–7207

Majumder M, Ghosh AK, Steele R, Zhou XY, Phillips NJ, Ray R, Ray RB (2002) Hepatitis C virus NS5A protein impairs TNF-mediated hepatic apoptosis, but not by an anti-FAS antibody, in transgenic mice. Virology 294:94–105

Mishra S, Murphy LC, Nyomba BL, Murphy LJ (2005) Prohibitin: a potential target for new therapeutics. Trends Mol Med 11:192–197

Miyamoto H, Moriishi K, Moriya K, Murata S, Tanaka K, Suzuki T et al (2007) Hepatitis C virus core protein induces insulin resistance through a PA28c-dependent pathway. J Virol 81:1727–1735

Miyoshi H, Fujie H, Shintani Y, Tsutsumi T, Shinzawa S, Makuuchi M, Kokudo N, Matsuura Y, Suzuki T, Miyamura T, Moriya K, Koike K (2005) Hepatitis C virus core protein exerts an inhibitory effect on suppressor of cytokine signaling (SOCS) -1 gene expression. J Hepatol 43:757–763

Moradpour D, Penin F, Rice CM (2007) Replication of hepatitis C virus. Nat Rev Microbiol 5:453–463

Moriishi K, Okabayashi T, Nakai K, Moriya K, Koike K, Murata S et al (2003) Proteasome activator

PA28 gamma-dependent nuclear retention and degradation of hepatitis C virus core protein. J Virol 77:10237–10249

Moriishi K, Mochizuki R, Moriya K, Miyamoto H, Mori Y, Abe T et al (2007) Critical role of PA28g in hepatitis C virus-associated steatogenesis and hepatocarcinogenesis. Proc Natl Acad Sci USA 104:1661–1666

Moriya K, Yotsuyanagi H, Shintani Y, Fujie H, Ishibashi K, Matsuura Y et al (1997) Hepatitis C virus core protein induces hepatic steatosis in transgenic mice. J Gen Virol 78:1527–1531

Moriya K, Fujie H, Shintani Y, Yotsuyanagi H, Tsutsumi T, Matsuura Y et al (1998) Hepatitis C virus core protein induces hepatocellular carcinoma in transgenic mice. Nat Med 4:1065–1068

Moriya K, Nakagawa K, Santa T, Shintani Y, Fujie H, Miyoshi H et al (2001a) Oxidative stress in the absence of inflammation in a mouse model for hepatitis C virus-associated hepatocarcinogenesis. Cancer Res 61:4365–4370

Moriya K, Todoroki T, Tsutsumi T, Fujie H, Shintani Y, Miyoshi H et al (2001b) Increase in the concentration of carbon 18 monounsaturated fatty acids in the liver with hepatitis C: analysis in transgenic mice and humans. Biophys Biochem Res Commun 281:1207–1212

Moriya K, Miyoshi H, Shinzawa S, Tsutsumi T, Fujie H, Goto K, Shintani Y, Yotsuyanagi H, Koike K (2010) Hepatitis C virus core protein compromises iron-induced activation of antioxidants in mice and HepG2 cells. J Med Virol 82:776–792

Naas T, Ghorbani M, Alvarez-Maya I, Lapner M, Kothary R, De Repentigny Y et al (2005) Characterization of liver histopathology in a transgenic mouse model expressing genotype 1a hepatitis C virus core and envelope proteins 1 and 2. J Gen Virol 86:2185–2196

Nijtmans LG, de Jong L, Artal Sanz M, Coates PJ, Berden JA, Back JW et al (2000) Prohibitins act as a membrane-bound chaperone for the stabilization of mitochondrial proteins. EMBO J 19:2444–2451

Nishina S, Hino K, Korenaga M, Vecchi C, Pietrangelo A, Mizukami Y, Furutani T, Sakai A, Okuda M, Hidaka I, Okita K, Sakaida I (2008) Hepatitis C virus-induced reactive oxygen species raise hepatic iron level in mice by reducing hepcidin transcription. Gastroenterology 134:226–238

Pasquinelli C, Shoenberger JM, Chung J et al (1997) Hepatitis C virus core and E2 protein expression in transgenic mice. Hepatology 25:719–727

Perlemuter G, Sabile A, Letteron P, Vona G, Topilco A, Koike K et al (2002) Hepatitis C virus core protein inhibits microsomal triglyceride transfer protein activity and very low density lipoprotein secretion: a model of viral-related steatosis. FASEB J 16:185–194

Perz JF, Armstrong GL, Farrington LA, Hutin YJ, Bell BP (2006) The contributions of hepatitis B virus and hepatitis C virus infections to cirrhosis and primary liver cancer worldwide. J Hepatol 45:529–538

Piccoli C, Scrima R, Quarato G, D'Aprile A, Ripoli M, Lecce L et al (2007) Hepatitis C virus protein expression causes calcium-mediated mitochondrial bioenergetic dysfunction and nitro-oxidative stress. Hepatology 46:58–65

Powell EE, Jonsson JR, Clouston AD (2005) Steatosis: co-factor in other liver diseases. Hepatology 42:5–13

Saito I, Miyamura T, Ohbayashi A, Harada H, Katayama T, Kikuchi S et al (1990) Hepatitis C virus infection is associated with the development of hepatocellular carcinoma. Proc Natl Acad Sci USA 87:6547–6549

Shintani Y, Fujie H, Miyoshi H, Tsutsumi T, Kimura S, Moriya K et al (2004) Hepatitis C virus and diabetes: direct involvement of the virus in the development of insulin resistance. Gastroenterology 126:840–848

Shirakura M, Murakami K, Ichimura T, Suzuki R, Shimoji T, Fukuda K et al (2007) E6AP ubiquitin ligase mediates ubiquitylation and degradation of hepatitis C virus core protein. J Virol 81:1174–1185

Suzuki R, Sakamoto S, Tsutsumi T, Rikimaru A, Tanaka K, Shimoike T et al (2005) Molecular determinants for subcellular localization of hepatitis C virus core protein. J Virol 79:1271–1281

Stocker R, Yamamoto Y, McDonagh AF, Glazer AN, Ames BN (1987) Bilirubin is an antioxidant of possible physiological importance. Science 235:1043–1046

Su AI, Pezacki JP, Wodicka L, Brideau AD, Supekova L, Thimme R et al (2002) Genomic analysis of the host response to hepatitis C virus infection. Proc Natl Acad Sci USA 99:15669–15674

Taguwa S, Kambara H, Fujita N, Noda T, Yoshimori T, Koike K, Moriishi K, Matsuura Y (2011) Dysfunction of autophagy participates in vacuole formation and cell death in cells replicating hepatitis C virus. J Virol 85:13185–13194

Theiss AL, Idell RD, Srinivasan S, Klapproth JM, Jones DP, Merlin D et al (2007) Prohibitin protects against oxidative stress in intestinal epithelial cells. FASEB J 21:197–206

Tsutsumi T, Suzuki T, Moriya K, Yotsuyanagi H, Shintani Y, Fujie H et al (2002) Intrahepatic cytokine expression and AP-1 activation in mice transgenic for hepatitis C virus core protein. Virology 304:415–424

Tsutsumi T, Suzuki T, Moriya K, Shintani Y, Fujie H, Miyoshi H et al (2003) Hepatitis C virus core protein activates ERK and p38 MAPK in cooperation with ethanol in transgenic mice. Hepatology 38:820–828

Tsutsumi T, Matsuda M, Aizaki H, Moriya K, Miyoshi H, Fujie H, Shintani Y, Yotsuyanagi H, Miyamura T, Suzuki T, Koike K (2009) Proteomics analysis of mitochondrial proteins reveals overexpression of a mitochondrial protein chaperone, prohibitin, in cells expressing hepatitis C virus core protein. Hepatology 50:378–386

Wakita T, Taya C, Katsume A et al (1998) Efficient conditional transgene expression in hepatitis C virus cDNA transgenic mice mediated by the Cre/loxP system. J Biol Chem 273:9001–9006

Waris G, Felmlee DJ, Negro F, Siddiqui A (2007) Hepatitis C virus induces proteolytic cleavage of sterol regulatory element binding proteins and stimulates their phosphorylation via oxidative stress. J Virol 81:8122–8130

Yotsuyanagi H, Shintani Y, Moriya K, Fujie H, Tsutsumi T, Kato T et al (2000) Virological analysis of non-B, non-C hepatocellular carcinoma in Japan: frequent involvement of hepatitis B virus. J Infect Dis 181:1920–1928

第 10 章　HCV 感染与肝癌的预防

E. J. Lim 和 J. Torresi

摘　要　肝细胞癌（HCC）是位列第五的、最为常见的癌症，是癌症死亡的第三大主要原因。目前，HCC 发病率仍在上升。大部分 HCC 与慢性病毒性肝炎有关。全球有超过 1.7 亿人慢性感染 HCV，诱发慢性肝病、肝硬化和肝癌，导致大量发病和死亡。因此，HCV 已经成为影响全球人口健康的重要病原。由于大部分 HCC 可发展成肝硬化，随着 HCV 感染人群的增加，与 HCV 相关的 HCC 问题也变得更加严重。为了减少诱发 HCC 的风险，在 HCV 感染者发生肝硬化之前，迫切需要给予抗病毒治疗。成功清除 HCV 感染的确与临床和组织学的改善紧密联系，并能够减少随后发生 HCC 的风险。即使在发生肝硬化后，清除病毒也可降低发生 HCC 的风险。目前，HCV 标准抗病毒治疗药物包括聚乙二醇化干扰素（IFN）-α 和利巴韦林，但是这种疗法的病毒清除率还不十分理想，特别是对于难治性 HCV 感染群体。最近，开发了一系列特异针对 HCV 的直接作用药物（DAA），这些药物能互相联合使用，或配合标准治疗方案使用，都可以提高 HCV 治愈率。针对 HCV 的预防和治疗性疫苗的研究正在进行中，并且已取得一些好的进展。

关键词　丙肝，肝细胞癌，肝硬化，抗病毒治疗，直接作用抗病毒药物，疫苗

1　引言

肝细胞癌（HCC）是世界第五大广泛发生的癌症，是癌症死亡的第三大因素（Parkin 2001）。HCC 发病率仍在增加（El-Serag and Rudolph 2007），世界上约 80% 的 HCC 与慢性病毒性肝炎有关（Thomas and Zhu 2005）。在美国，大概 1/3 的 HCC 患者是因为 HCV 感染，因此，HCV 已经成为 HCC 的主要风险因子（美

J. Torresi
Department of Infectious Diseases, Austin Hospital, Heidelberg, Victoria 3084, Australia
E. J. Lim (✉)
Department of Gastroenterology, Austin Hospital, Heidelberg, Victoria 3084, Australia
e-mail: josepht@unimelb.edu.au

国国立卫生研究院共同发展会议声明：丙型肝炎管理 2002）。虽然慢性 HCV 感染与 HCC 的发生存在密切相关性，但是 HCV 感染最终导致 HCC 的详细机制还不明确。然而，已有证据显示，无论 HCV 患者是否已经发生肝硬化，清除病毒都可以降低 HCC 发生的风险。

2　HCV 感染

全世界有超过 1.7 亿人慢性感染 HCV，造成每年约 47.6 万人死于与 HCV 感染相关的疾病（Dore et al. 2003）。HCV 通过血液传播。目前，在西方国家，HCV 感染主要是由于静脉注射毒品和纹身（Razali et al. 2007）；而在亚洲和非洲国家，HCV 感染主要是因为使用了被污染的血液制品和医疗器械。相对这些传播途径，性传播和母婴传播并不多见（Razali et al. 2007）。

HCV 感染后，高达 85%的患者因不能清除病毒而发展成慢性感染。约 20%的慢性感染患者最后发展为肝硬化（美国国立卫生研究院共同发展会议声明：丙型肝炎管理 2002）。图 10-1 表示 HCV 感染的自然史。大多数慢性感染的患者几十年不出现病症，因此，延迟了疾病的诊断和治疗。直到发展成肝硬化的并发症，如肝功能代偿不全和 HCC，这些患者才寻求医生进行治疗。HCV 感染导致肝功能衰竭，这已经成为美国、欧洲和澳大利亚肝移植的主要原因（Davis et al. 2003；Law et al. 2003），突显了慢性 HCV 感染对社会经济的影响。

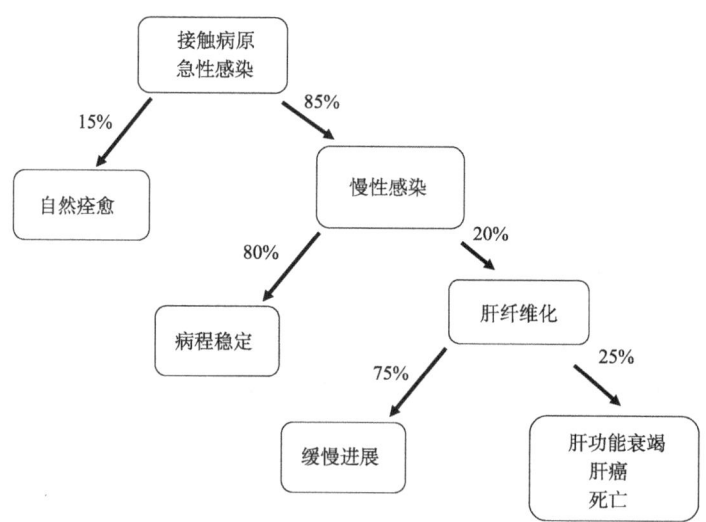

图 10-1　HCV 感染的自然史。参考 Alter 等（1995）。

HCV 属于黄病毒科（Flaviviridae）肝炎病毒属（*Hepacivirus*）（Forns and Bukh 1999）。HCV 基因组是单股正链 RNA，由约 9600 个核苷酸组成，编码一个约 3000 个氨基酸的多聚蛋白前体（Bartenschlager et al. 2011）。图 10-2 表示 HCV 基因组结构和各个病毒蛋白的主要功能。HCV 有 6 个主要基因型，其中基因 1 型在美国、欧洲和澳大利亚是主要流行的基因型（Simmonds et al. 2005）。基因 3 型在印度和东南亚较为流行，而 4 型多见于中东地区和非洲（Kamal and Nasser 2008）。根据序列差异，每个基因型可有多种亚型，用小写字母（a、b、c 等）表示。HCV 基因型影响药物治疗效果和肝病发生的严重程度，例如，1b 型 HCV 慢性感染更容易诱发肝纤维化、肝硬化和 HCC。对大量数据的综合分析表明，1b 型感染诱发 HCC 的概率是其他基因型的 2 倍（Raimondi et al. 2009）。

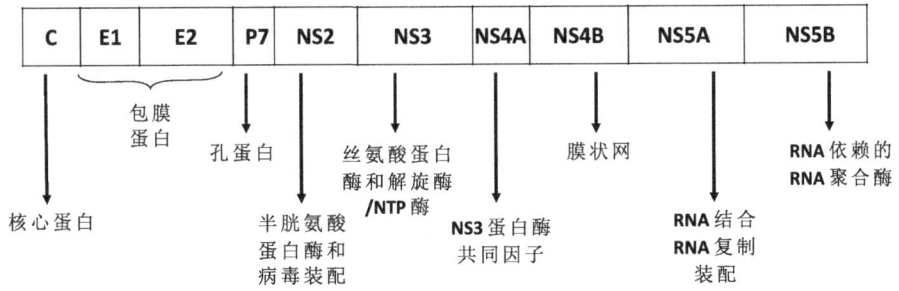

图 10-2　HCV 基因组结构和病毒蛋白功能。参考 Bartenschlager 等（2011）。

与其他 RNA 病毒类似，HCV 的 RNA 聚合酶缺少校正功能，因此，病毒基因组的复制容易出错，导致高突变率。结果产生大量遗传异质性的基因组，导致多样病毒准种的进化。病毒的这种多样性干扰宿主形成有效的抗病毒体液免疫，导致病毒持续存在于感染者体内（Forns and Bukh 1999）。

3　丙型肝炎和发生 HCC 的风险因子

HCV 是在全球范围发生 HCC 的主要原因。一个基于大量人群的前瞻性研究表明，感染 HCV 的个体中发生 HCC 的风险比无 HCV 感染的个体要高 20 倍（Sun et al. 2003）。早在 20 世纪 80 年代，人们还称 HCV 为"非甲非乙型肝炎"的时候，就已经认识到慢性 HCV 感染和 HCC 有密切联系（Kiyosawa et al. 1984）。几乎所有与 HCV 相关的 HCC 都是在肝硬化的情况下发生的，而肝硬化本身就是 HCC 重要的独立风险因子。在 HCV 肝硬化患者中，HCC 的年发生率为 2%~8%（Bruix et al. 2005）。在感染 HCV 很多年（通常 20~30 年）后，才发生 HCC。

然而，并不是所有 HCV 相关的 HCC 都发生于患有肝硬化的患者中。一个大的前瞻性研究表明，约17%的HCV阳性的HCC患者没有肝硬化。但是，在系列肝脏活检中，至少有一个伊沙克（Ishak）纤维化分数在3分或3分以上（Lok et al. 2009）。这表明，即使没有肝硬化，患有慢性肝炎和肝纤维化的HCV感染的个体也可能发生HCC。

与HCV相关的肝病发展成肝硬化和HCC的风险因子包括饮酒、在老年时感染、男性、与HIV或HBV共感染、免疫抵制、胰岛素抗性、非酒精性脂肪肝、肝活检时高度炎症和纤维化（Chen and Morgan 2006）。

感染HCV的女性每天摄入酒精>40g，男性每天摄入>60g，持续时间超过5年，发生肝硬化和失代偿性肝病的风险将增加2~3倍（Wiley et al. 1998）。此外，酒精摄入量>60g/d的HCV感染者比摄入量<60g/d的感染者发生HCC的风险高2倍（Donato et al. 2002）。而且，慢性HCV感染的酗酒者比慢性乙肝酗酒者更容易发生晚期肝病，而且死亡率升高（Mendenhall et al. 1991）。

患者感染HCV时的年龄，也是发展为更严重肝病的一个独立风险因子。那些>40岁的感染者比年轻感染者更容易发展成晚期肝纤维化（Poynard et al. 1997）。那些在感染时年龄超过39岁的患者的HCC发病率比那些感染时小于19岁的患者高29倍（Pradat et al. 2007）。

在HIV-HCV共感染的情况下，低CD4细胞数与高HCV病毒载量和肝硬化进程的加快有关（Di Martino et al. 2001）。其他来自免疫抵制的因素，如器官移植，也与肝纤维化进程加快有关（Berenguer et al. 2000）。最后，HCV-HBV共感染也可能是HCC发生的高风险因子（Cho et al. 2011）。

HCV感染导致发生HCC的机制还不清楚。有证据显示，HCV可能与细胞内各种信号转导通路相互作用或影响表观遗传的变化有关，从而改变肝细胞生理学特性，直接促进细胞恶性转化。例如，已经证明HCV核心蛋白与分裂素激活蛋白激酶（MARK）信号通路相互作用，从而促进细胞增殖（Hayashi et al. 2000）。在由HCV感染的HCC患者切除的肝脏肿瘤组织中，抑瘤基因p16INK4A高度甲基化，使p16INK4A失活；而在没有HCV感染的HCC患者中，没有发现p16INK4A失活（Li et al. 2004）。其次，免疫介导的肝脏炎症和HCV感染启动的细胞凋亡，导致补偿性刺激，使细胞增殖，以取代死亡的肝细胞。持续的细胞更新使肝细胞内的遗传突变积累，加上周围炎症环境，一起促进HCC发生（Hino et al. 2002）。

4 预防丙肝导致的肝硬化患者发生HCC

由于慢性HCV感染人数的增加、疾病并发症，以及因护理技术的提高使肝衰竭晚期患者存活更久等原因，与HCV感染相关的HCC在全球范围内的发病率还在持续上升。在HCV肝硬化的患者中，HCC的年发生率约为3%，四年的风险率为11.5%（Serfaty et al. 1998）。因此，在这些人群中进行HCC的筛查尤为重要。通过干扰素（IFN）治疗清除肝硬化患者中的HCV，可使HCC的发生率降低3倍（Bruno et al. 2007；Singal et al. 2010b），表明即使发生了肝硬化，成功进行抗病毒治疗仍然可以很大程度地降低HCC发生的风险。但是，即使清除了病毒，也并不能完全去除HCC发生的风险，因此，对肝硬化患者进行持续性的HCC筛查仍具有指导意义。相反，如果病毒清除不成功，IFN治疗不能降低HCC发生的风险。研究表明，对于那些经标准抗病毒治疗不能清除病毒的HCV肝硬化患者，维持半有效剂量聚乙二醇化IFN治疗可以降低患HCC的风险（Lok et al. 2011）。这个研究还发现，发生晚期肝纤维化但没有肝硬化的HCV感染者，HCC的发病率并没有降低。然而，来自包括1152名无应答者的四个研究数据表明，保持低剂量的IFN治疗或者不给予治疗，HCC发生的风险并没有统计学意义上的差异（Singal et al. 2010b）。

对HCV诱导肝硬化进而发展为HCC的患者进行Meta分析表明，通过原位组织消融或者外科手术切除对HCC进行治疗后，利用抗病毒治疗消除HCV可将HCC复发的风险从61%降低到35%（Singal et al. 2010a）。此外，用IFN和利巴韦林成功治疗HCV感染可以提高肝功能储备并延长存活率（3年内存活率：96% vs. 61%）（Ishikawa et al. 2012）。在因HCV感染导致HCC而进行肝移植的患者中，IFN治疗可将HCC复发的风险从27%降到4%（Kohli et al. 2012）。这些研究表明，在HCV诱发肝硬化的患者中，抗病毒治疗是预防HCC发生的重要补救措施。

5 预防慢性丙肝患者发生肝硬化和HCC

成功的抗病毒治疗使慢性丙肝患者得到的长期益处主要包括：血清转氨酶正常化，肝脏坏死性炎症和纤维化水平降低，健康生活质量改善和减少HCC发生的风险，所有这些都能提高患者的存活率（Patel et al. 2006）。我们知道，HCC主要发生于HCV肝硬化患者中，为了降低HCC发生的风险，在患者发展为肝硬化之前进行治疗，清除HCV感染，将成为首要目标。研究表明，大部分患者在进行抗病毒治疗成功后，临床和组织学都得到改善（Marcellin et al. 1997），同时降低发生肝硬化和HCC的风险（Pradat et al. 2007）。

在欧洲的一项多个中心机构参与的研究中，招募的HCV感染者中，无肝硬化的患者占89%。对这些患者进行抗病毒治疗研究发现，成功清除HCV后，肝硬化发生率仅为2.3%，没有患者发生HCC。无法清除病毒的患者发生肝硬化的比率为20%，其中4.2%的患者发展成HCC（Pradat et al. 2007）。在另一项研究中，无肝硬化的HCV感染者占90%，用IFN成功进行抗病毒治疗后，患HCC的年风险率从2.31%降低到0.24%（Maruoka et al. 2012）。这项研究还发现，那些用药物未能清除病毒的患者和不接受药物治疗的患者发生HCC的风险相同（Maruoka et al. 2012）。

对于那些IFN治疗失败但无肝硬化的HCV患者，进行单一IFN的长期治疗，可以降低HCC发生的风险。一个回顾性研究发现，在IFN治疗无效的感染HCV基因1型的患者中，93%的患者在治疗期间没有肝硬化，接受48周或更长时间IFN单一治疗可使HCC的10年发生率从16.4%降到11.5%（Takeyasu et al. 2012）。

6 丙型肝炎的抗病毒治疗

由于没有HCV疫苗，所以抗病毒治疗是防止肝硬化和HCC的唯一有效方法。治疗的目标是清除病毒，以阻止肝损伤和肝纤维化的发生。目前治疗慢性HCV感染的标准方法是聚乙二醇化IFN-α和利巴韦林联合治疗。最近，直接抗病毒药物（DAA）的应用明显改变了慢性丙肝抗病毒治疗的现状，可能提供了一种长期预防HCV相关的HCC更有效的方法。

6.1 标准治疗方法

目前治疗HCV感染的标准方法是，每周皮下注射IFN-α和每天口服利巴韦林（Fried et al. 2002）。现在，批准用于HCV治疗的聚乙二醇化IFN有两种，分别是聚乙二醇化IFN-α-2a（Pegasys，Hoffmann-La Roche，Nutley，NJ）和聚乙二醇化IFN-α-2b（Pegintron，Merck Sharp and Dohme，Whitehouse Station，NJ）；两者的疗效没有统计学意义的差异（McHutchison et al. 2009b）。IFN-α结合到IFN-α1和IFN-α2细胞表面受体，诱导JAK-STAT信号转导，发挥其免疫调节功能。一旦结合上配体，与受体关联的Janus激酶（JAK）酪氨酸激酶就被激活，导致转录因子的信号转导子和转录激活因子（STAT）家族成员磷酸化和激活（Kisseleva et al. 2002）。然后，这些转录因子转移到细胞核内，在肝细胞内转录参与细胞周期调控、凋亡和建立抗病毒状态的基因（Thomas et al. 2003）。除了直接作用于感染病毒的细胞外，IFN-α还通过增加$CD8^+$细胞毒性T细胞反应来对抗感染的肝细胞，以及通过加强B细胞分化增加对抗HCV的抗体产量，从而调节免疫系统（Thomas et al. 2003）。

利巴韦林（Copegus，Hoffmann-La Roche，Nutley，NJ；Rebetol，Merck Sharp and Dohme，Whitehouse Station，NJ）是合成的鸟嘌呤核苷类似物，可以在体外抵抗众多DNA和RNA病毒（Patterson and Fernandezlarsson 1990）。单独使用利巴韦林治疗慢性HCV患者时，它可以降低血清转氨酶水平，但没有抗病毒效果（Dibisceglie et al. 1995）。尽管有不少假说，但利巴韦林与聚乙二醇化IFN联合

使用时所表现出来的抗病毒作用的具体机制还不清楚。利巴韦林是口服的活性前体药物,在体内被代谢成类似嘌呤 RNA 核苷酸的形式。因此,利巴韦林可以在病毒 RNA 复制时加入到病毒 RNA 基因组中,使病毒的基因组高度变异,使病毒死亡(Crotty et al. 2002)。利巴韦林也可抑制 HCV 复制必需的、RNA 依赖的 RNA 聚合酶。利巴韦林还是一种肌苷一磷酸脱氢酶抑制剂,抑制这种细胞内酶可降低细胞内 GTP 水平,从而降低病毒蛋白合成和 RNA 复制水平(Streeter et al. 1973)。

6.2 聚乙二醇化 IFN/利巴韦林抗病毒应答的预测因子

有效而永久地清除病毒的成功治疗,被定义为在结束抗病毒治疗 24 周后,患者血清中检测不到 HCV RNA(Pradat et al. 2007),也称持续的病毒学应答(SVR)。经过治疗之后的第 4 周,血清中检测不到 HCV RNA,是快速病毒学应答(RVR)。RVR 预示将会有好的治疗效果,大于 86% 的 RVR 患者有 SVR(Yu et al. 2007)。如果在发展成肝硬化前清除病毒,在没有其他肝脏毒性因子存在的情况下,肝脏纤维化情况可以得到改善,患者发生 HCC 的风险也可以降到人群基线水平。

有很多宿主和病毒因子,可以在治疗前预测抗病毒治疗应答情况,其中最可靠的是 HCV 基因型。感染基因 2 型和 3 型 HCV 的患者清除病毒的比率明显高于感染基因 1 型的患者(Hadziyannis et al. 2004)。

位于 19 号染色体上的 *IL28B* 基因编码 IFN-λ3,这个基因内部不同位点的单核苷酸多态性被证明与 IFN 治疗应答有很强的关联性,特别是与基因 1 型 HCV 感染的治疗效果密切相关。在 IFN 和利巴韦林治疗中,*IL28B* 基因 rs12979860 位点多态性为 CC 的患者清除病毒的可能性比 CT 和 TT 型患者高 2 倍(Ge et al. 2009)。

除 HCV 基因型和 IL28B 核苷酸多态性外,治疗前 HCV 载量低(<600 000 IU/ml)通常也预示将有好的抗病毒治疗效果(Fried et al. 2002)。其他预示 IFN 和利巴韦林治疗效果不理想的因素包括:维生素 D 缺乏,胰岛素抗性或身体质量指数超过 30kg/m^2(Bressler et al. 2003;Romero-Gomez et al. 2005),存在肝硬化或失代偿性肝病(Fried et al. 2002;Manns et al. 2001)。

虽然聚乙二醇化 IFN 和利巴韦林联合治疗可以永久清除慢性丙型肝炎患者体内的病毒,但是这种治疗十分昂贵,而且有很多副作用。此外,这种标准疗法对 HCV 基因 1 型患者的 SVR 只有 40%~50%。与 HCV 2 型和 3 型患者 70%~80% 的 SVR,以及 4 型 70% 的 SVR 相比(Chevaliez and Pawlotsky 2007;Khuroo et al. 2004),基因 1 型患者的治疗效果难免令人失望。

6.3 直接作用抗病毒药物

最近,慢性 HCV 感染的治疗得到了很大发展。靶向 HCV 复制特定关键蛋白的直接作用抗病毒药物(DAA)的发展,显著提高了 SVR。DAA 对 *HCV 基因 1*

型患者、治疗前预后因素差的患者,以及对干扰素和利巴韦林治疗无应答的患者尤为有利。表 10-1 列出了一些正在使用或者正在研究的 DAA。

表 10-1 直接作用 HCV 抗病毒药物

DAA	抑制剂类型	研究阶段	作用基因型	抗药屏障	生产公司
Telaprevir	NS3/4A 蛋白酶抑制剂(第一代,第一期)	临床Ⅲ期	1	低	Vertex
Boceprevir	NS3/4A 蛋白酶抑制剂(第一代,第一期)	临床Ⅲ期	1	低	Merck Sharp and Dohme
Danoprevir	NS3/4A 蛋白酶抑制剂(第一代,第二期)	临床Ⅱb期	1	低	Roche/Genentech
Asunaprevir	NS3/4A 蛋白酶抑制剂(第一代,第二期)	临床Ⅲ期	1	低	Bristol-Myers Squibb
Vaniprevir	NS3/4A 蛋白酶抑制剂(第一代,第二期)	临床Ⅱb期	1	低	Merck Sharp and Dohme
MK-5172	NS3/4A 蛋白酶抑制剂(第二代)	临床Ⅱ期	1, 2, 3	中	Merck Sharp and Dohme
Mericitabine	NS5B 聚合酶(核苷)	临床Ⅱb期	1, 2, 3	高	Roche/Genentech
Sofosbuvir	NS5B 聚合酶(核苷)	临床Ⅲ期	1, 2, 3	高	Pharmasset/Gilead
BI207127	NS5B 聚合酶(非核苷)	临床Ⅱb期	1	低	Boehringer Ingelheim
VX-222	NS5B 聚合酶(非核苷)	临床Ⅱ期	1	低	Vertex
ABT-072	NS5B 聚合酶(非核苷)	临床Ⅱ期	1	低	Abbott Squibb
Daclatasvir	NS5A	临床Ⅱb期	1	低	Bristol-Myers Squibb

蛋白酶抑制剂:首先获得使用许可的 NS3/4A 抑制剂包括 telaprevir(Incivek,Vertex)和 boceprevir(Victrelis、Merck Sharp 和 Dohme),这两种药物仅对 HCV 基因 1 型感染有效。将蛋白酶抑制剂与标准疗法联合使用,对未经治疗的患者或者曾经治疗失败的患者,都可显著提高 SVR。

在一个采用随机、双盲、安慰剂对照的大型临床Ⅲ期试验中,对 *HCV* 基因 1 型初诊患者,用 telaprevir 和 IFN/利巴韦林联合治疗 12 周后,继续 IFN/利巴韦林治疗 12~36 周(Jacobson et al. 2011)。结果表明,加入 telaprevir 可使 SVR 从单纯应用标准疗法的 44%提高到 75%。即使对于治疗前有较高病毒载量的患者，加入 telaprevir 也可将 SVR 从 36%提高到 74%（Jacobson et al. 2011）。在另一个临床 III 期试验中，先用 IFN/利巴韦林进行导入期治疗 4 周，再加入 boceprevir，3 个药物联合治疗持续 28~44 周（boceprevir 在 24~44 周用药）（Poordad et al. 2011）。比起单纯使用 IFN/利巴韦林治疗，加入 boceprevir 将 SVR 从 38%提高到 66%。这两项研究结果显示，加入 telaprevir 可使未经治疗的肝硬化患者的 SVR 从 33%提高到 62%，加入 boceprevir 则由 38%提高到 52%（Poordad et al. 2011）。

对那些 IFN/利巴韦林治疗后 PCR 检测 HCV RNA 为阴性的复发患者，在 IFN/利巴韦林 48 周的疗程中，开始 12 周加入 telaprevir，可使 SVR 从 IFN/利巴韦林单独治疗 48 周的 24%提高到>80%（Zeuzem et al. 2011a）。在使用 IFN/利巴韦林进行 4 周导入期治疗后，加入 bocerevir 再治疗 44 周，可使 SVR 从 IFN/利巴韦林单独治疗 48 周的 29%提高到 75%（Bacon et al. 2011）。对经过治疗的有肝硬化的复发患者，telaprevir 可将 SVR 从 13%提高到 84%（Zeuzem et al. 2011a），boceprevir 可将 SVR 从 20%提高到 83%（Bacon et al. 2011）。

Telaprevir 治疗的常见副作用包括皮疹、贫血和胃肠道症状。Boceprevir 治疗的常见副作用包括贫血和味觉障碍（Jacobson et al. 2011；Poordad et al. 2011）。即使在治疗中应用了 boceprevir 和 telaprevir，利巴韦林的作用仍然很关键。证据显示，即使应用了高效 DAA，如果利巴韦林剂量不足，SVR 和病毒复发率仍然不理想（Kwo et al. 2010；McHutchison et al. 2009a）。虽然这些 DAA 药物可有效抑制 HCV 复制，但是很快就产生耐药 HCV 变异株，这些变异株还有可能与其他蛋白酶抑制剂有交叉抗性（Halfon and Locarnini 2011）。因此，这些抑制剂不能单独使用。

除了 telaprevir 和 boceprevir，不少 NS3/4A 的抑制剂，如 danoprevir（Roche/Genentech）、asunaprevir（Bristol-Myers Squibb）和 vanimprevir（Merck Sharp 和 Dohme）已经进入临床试验。这些第 II 期的第一代蛋白酶抑制剂拥有高效的抗病毒活性，与 telaprevir 和 boceprevir 相比，这些抑制剂还改善了药物代谢动力学和副作用。与 telaprevir 和 boceprevir 相似，这些药物对产生抗性的遗传障碍低，应该和 IFN/利巴韦林联合使用（Gane et al. 2011a）。第二代蛋白酶抑制剂 MK-5172（Merck Sharp 和 Dohme），在体外可抑制 *HCV* 基因 1、2 和 3 型的 NS3/4A 蛋白酶活性，可有效抑制已经对 telaprevir 和 boceprevir 产生抗性的 HCV。临床实验证明，MK-5172 对 *HCV* 基因 1 型和 3 型都有高效的抗病毒活性，有良好的机体耐受性，没有病毒反弹，因此，它难以产生抗药现象（Brainard et al. 2010）。

聚合酶抑制剂：抑制 HCV RNA 依赖的 RNA 聚合酶（NS5B）的活性位点的药物也在发展中。有两类聚合酶抑制剂，分别是核苷抑制剂和非核苷抑制剂。

核苷 NS5B 抑制剂：在 RNA 复制过程中，这些核苷抑制剂被 RNA 聚合酶加入到正在延伸的 HCV 基因组 RNA 中，导致未完成链提前终止。核苷抑制剂对产生药物抗性的遗传屏障高。HCV 聚合酶活性位点高度保守，因此，核苷酸抑制剂可对不同 HCV 基因型起作用（Buhler and Bartenschlager 2012）。Mericitabine（Roche/Genentech）被代谢为嘧啶（胞嘧呤）类似物，与干扰素/利巴韦林联合使用时，可以增加 SVR，而且不产生抗性变异毒株（Pockros et al. 2011）。另一个核苷抑制剂 sofosbuvir（Pharmasset/Gilead），是一种嘧啶（尿嘧啶）类似物，它可以高效抑制基因 1 型、2 型和 3 型 HCV（Lalezari et al. 2011；Nelson et al. 2011）。

非核苷 NS5B 抑制剂：这类 NS5B 抑制剂结合到病毒聚合酶催化中心外的 4 个变构位点中的 1 个，诱导酶构象改变，使酶活性丧失，阻止病毒复制。由于这些变构结合位点有基因型特异性，目前所有非核苷类 NS5B 抑制剂只能有效抑制基因 1 型 HCV。正在研发的这类药物包括 BI207127（Boehringer Ingelheim）、VX-222（Vertex）和 ABT-072（Abbott）。非核苷类 NS5B 药物的抗药遗传屏障低，单独使用会快速产生耐药变异株（Lagace et al. 2010）。

NS5A 抑制剂：NS5A 抑制剂结合到 NS5A 蛋白的结构域 I，但这些药物抑制 HCV 复制的机理还不清楚。临床 I 期实验显示，低浓度 daclatasvir（Bristol-Myers Squibb）即可高效地抑制 HCV 的复制，但单独使用这种药物会很快产生抗药性（Gao et al. 2010）。当 daclatasvir 与 IFN/利巴韦林联合使用时，对未经治疗的基因 1 型 HCV 感染的患者，可以达到 90%的病毒清除率（Pol et al. 2011）。

目前，几乎所有的 DAA 都是和 IFN/利巴韦林联合使用，以预防抗药 HCV 毒株的快速产生。因此，使用 DAA 比单独使用 IFN/利巴韦林治疗产生更多副作用。然而，随着开发出更多高效的 DAA，不含 IFN 的 DAA 联合使用策略，将实现既可以清除病毒，又不产生耐药性。最近，核苷类聚合酶抑制剂 RG7128 和蛋白酶抑制剂 danoprevir 的联合使用表明，在无 IFN/利巴韦林的条件下，可以快速降低 5 log10 IU/ml 的病毒载量，而且不产生耐药 HCV（Gane et al. 2010）。随后，另有研究表明，核苷类聚合酶抑制剂 sofosbuvir 和利巴韦林联合使用 12 周，不含 IFN，对感染基因 2 型和 3 型 HCV 的患者可达到 100%病毒清除率（Gane et al. 2011b）。对那些 IFN/利巴韦林治疗无应答的患者，DAA 联合使用可能是有效的治疗方法。研究发现，对 IFN/利巴韦林无应答的 HCV 基因 1 型患者（IFN/利巴韦林持续治疗 12 周后，HCV RNA 病毒载量减少小于 2 log IU/ml），NS5A 抑制剂 daclatasvir 和 NS3/4A 蛋白酶抑制剂 asunaprevir 联合治疗 24 周后，病毒清除率达到 90%（Chayama et al. 2012）。

6.4 靶向宿主的药物

6.4.1 干扰素 λ

干扰素 λ（IFN-λ）与 IFN-α 结合不同的细胞表面受体，但它们使用相同的胞内 JAK-STAT 信号通路来产生抗 HCV 作用。与广泛存在于大部分组织中的 IFN-α 受体不同，IFN-λ1 受体在肝细胞上丰富表达，在其他很多类型细胞中不表达，因此，它可以在肝内有更强的靶向作用（Sommereyns et al. 2008）。比较研究聚乙二醇化 IFN-α/利巴韦林和聚乙二醇化 IFN-λ/利巴韦林发现，IFN-λ 比 IFN-α 有更高的 RVR 和更完全的 EVR（高效病毒学应答率），副作用也更小（Zeuzem et al. 2011b）。这些结果提示，将来与 DAA 联合用药时，IFN-λ 可能是更有效和耐受性更好的干扰素。

6.4.2 亲环素类蛋白抑制剂

亲环素类蛋白是一个大的蛋白家族，在所有的细胞中含量丰富，承担多样化的功能，包括充当蛋白伴侣来保证蛋白质正确折叠，调节蛋白质功能和细胞内信号事件（Wang and Heitman 2005）。亲环素类蛋白对 HCV 复制起关键作用，其中 NS5A 与亲环素蛋白 A 相互作用（Hanoulle et al. 2009）。用环孢霉素抑制亲环素蛋白 A 可以抑制 HCV 复制，但是使用环孢霉素的治疗也抑制了钙调磷酸酶，会导致免疫抑制。后来，研发出不与钙调磷酸酶相互作用的环孢霉素，消除了免疫抑制作用。Alisporivir（Debiopharm/Novartis）可通过干扰 NS5A 与亲环素蛋白 A 相互作用，来抑制基因 1-4 型 HCV 感染患者的病毒载量（Flisiak et al. 2009）。然而，最近发现慢性 HCV 患者使用 alisporivir 可导致胰腺炎，故 alisporivir 的研发被迫停止。

6.5 治疗性疫苗

治疗性疫苗的作用是能刺激感染者的免疫系统产生 HCV 特异 T 细胞介导的应答，以提高抗病毒治疗的 SVR（Torresi et al. 2011）。虽然，目前的治疗性疫苗可以降低接种者的病毒载量，但单独使用时，只能有限度地清除病毒。正因如此，目前的治疗性疫苗主要作为标准抗病毒治疗的辅助方案。这种策略将有益于那些治疗前预后标志物差或者前期抗病毒治疗失败的患者。

旨在通过刺激 T 细胞抑制 HCV 的疫苗已经进入临床试验。这些疫苗包括基于合成的肽段抗原（IC41, Intercell AG）、tarmogens（GI-5005a, Globeimmune）、修饰的 HCV DNA（ChronVac-C, Tripep AB, Sweden）和改良痘苗 Ankara 病毒（TG4040, Transgene）。其他的策略，如利用重组的腺病毒和病毒样颗粒，正在临床前发展阶段（Torresi et al. 2011）。表 10-2 列出一些正在研发的 HCV 疫苗。

表 10-2　用于 HCV 预防和治疗的疫苗

疫苗	免疫原性	接种物质	结果	研究阶段	生产公司
IC41	诱导 HCV 特异 T 细胞反应	HCV 多肽疫苗与多聚精氨酸	完成	临床 II 期	Intercell AG
GI-5005a	降低 ALT 和体外病毒载量到 1.4 log	灭活重组酵母表达的 NS3 和 Core 融合蛋白	正在进行	临床 I 期	GlobeImmune
ChronVacC	安全、免疫原性和对病毒载量瞬时作用	DNA 疫苗结合电穿孔	正在招募患者	临床 IIa 期	Tripep AB
TG4040	T 细胞反应和降低病毒载量至 1.5 log	MVA 病毒表达非结构蛋白（NS3、NS4 和 NS5B）	正在招募患者	临床 I 期	Transgene
E1/E2 vaccine		重组的 E1 和 E2 蛋白	没有发表数据	临床 I 期	Chiron Corp

参考 Torresi 等（2011）

7　HCV 高发人群的预防

7.1　预防性疫苗

虽然 HCV 的发现已有 20 多年，但是还没有疫苗可以有效预防 HCV 感染，预防性疫苗的研发仍然是一个研究热点（Torresi et al. 2011）。我们知道，那些自主清除 HCV 感染的个体，产生针对 HCV 核心蛋白和非结构蛋白 NS3、NS4 和 NS5 的强烈而广谱的交叉反应的 $CD4^+$ 和 $CD8^+$ T 细胞（Lauer et al. 2004），并产生大量交叉反应中和抗体（Pestka et al. 2007）。因此，一个有应用前景的预防性疫苗需要对不同基因型 HCV 感染都能产生以上这些反应。除了致弱活病毒和病毒样颗粒，几乎没有疫苗能满足这些标准。

一个正在研发的整合重组 HCV E1 和 E2 包膜糖蛋白的疫苗，可以保护黑猩猩免受基因 1 型 HCV 感染（Vajdy et al. 2006）。另一个候选疫苗是利用重组 HCV 核心蛋白，但这个疫苗仍处于研发的早期阶段（Drane et al. 2009）。

7.2　公共卫生措施

由于缺乏安全有效的预防性疫苗，应该在高危人群中采用可减少 HCV 传播的措施。特别是减少静脉注射毒品者不安全注射行为的措施，如行为干预、提供无菌的针头和注射器、管理物品滥用，这些措施可以使 HCV 感染的风险降低约 75%（Hagan et al. 2011）。对血液捐献者进行全面的筛查，也是一个阻止由污染血液制品传播 HCV 的重要手段，如在卫生保健机构里坚持综合预防和严格的针刺抽血类操作。

8 小结

HCV 感染是当前一个严重的世界性健康问题，全球 3%的人口慢性感染。HCV 感染可引起肝硬化、肝纤维化、肝功能衰竭和肝癌，造成高发病率和死亡率。随着 HCV 感染人数的增加，HCV 相关的 HCC 发病情况也更加严重。多数 HCC 是在肝硬化的情况下发生的，因此，给还未发生肝硬化的 HCV 感染者提供抗病毒治疗来降低患 HCC 的风险是十分必要的。即使已经发展成为肝硬化，成功清除病毒仍然可以降低患 HCC 的风险。目前，正在快速发展的大量不同类别的 HCV 特异的 DAA，它们之间可以联合使用或者与标准疗法联合使用，来提高 HCV 的治愈率。预防和治疗性的 HCV 疫苗还在研发中，希望将来能得到一个有效的 HCV 疫苗来对抗 HCV 造成的感染。

（李义平，徐占雪，郑福祥 译）

参 考 文 献

Alter MJ (1995) Epidemiology of hepatitis c in the west. Semin Liver Dis 15 (1):5–14

Bacon BR, Gordon SC, Lawitz E, Marcellin P, Vierling JM, Zeuzem S, Poordad F, Goodman ZD, Sings HL, Boparai N, Burroughs M, Brass CA, Albrecht JK, Esteban R, Investigators HR (2011) Boceprevir for previously treated chronic HCV genotype 1 infection. N Engl J Med 364 (13):1207–1217

Bartenschlager R, Penin F, Lohmann V, Andre P (2011) Assembly of infectious hepatitis c virus particles. Trends Microbiol 19 (2):95–103

Berenguer M, Ferrell L, Watson J, Prieto M, Kim M, Rayon M, Cordoba J, Herola A, Ascher N, Mir J, Berenguer J, Wright TL (2000) HCV-related fibrosis progression following liver transplantation: Increase in recent years. J Hepatol 32 (4):673–684

Brainard DM, Petry A, Van Dyck K, Nachbar RB, De Lepeleire IM, Caro L, Stone JA, Sun P, Uhle M, Wagner FD, O'mara E, Wagner JA (2010) Safety and antiviral activity of MK-5172, a novel HCV N53/4a protease inhibitor with potent activity against known resistance mutants, in genotype 1 and 3 HCV-infected patients. Hepatology 52 (4):706A–707A

Bressler BL, Guindi M, Tomlinson G, Heathcote J (2003) High body mass index is an independent risk factor for nonresponse to antiviral treatment in chronic hepatitis c. Hepatology (Baltimore, Md.), vol 38 (3) pp 639–644

Bruix J, Sherman M, Practice Guidelines Committee A, A. F. T. S. O. L. D. (2005) Management of hepatocellular carcinoma. Hepatology (Baltimore, Md.) 42 (5): 1208–1236

Bruno S, Stroffolini T, Colombo M, Bollani S, Benvegno L, Mazzella G, Ascione A, Santantonio T, Piccinino F, Andreone P, Mangia A, Gaeta GB, Persico M, Fagiuoli S, Almasio PL, Italian Association of the Study of the Liver D (2007) Sustained virological response to interferonalpha is associated with improved outcome in HCV-related cirrhosis: A retrospective study. Hepatology (Baltimore, Md.), 45 (3): 579–587

Buhler S, Bartenschlager R (2012) New targets for antiviral therapy of chronic hepatitis c. Liver international: official J Int Assoc Liver, 32 Suppl 1, pp 9–16

Chayama K, Takahashi S, Toyota J, Karino Y, Ikeda K, Ishikawa H, Watanabe H, Mcphee F, Hughes E Kumada H (2012) Dual therapy with the nonstructural protein 5a inhibitor, daclatasvir, and the nonstructural protein 3 protease inhibitor, asunaprevir, in hepatitis c virus genotype 1b-infected null responders. Hepatology (Baltimore, Md.) 55 (3): 742–748

Chen SL, Morgan TR (2006) The natural history of hepatitis c virus (HCV) infection. Int J Med Sci 3 (2):47–52

Chevaliez S, Pawlotsky J-M (2007) Hepatitis c virus: virology, diagnosis and management of antiviral therapy. World J Gastroenterology:WJG 13 (17):2461–2466

Cho LY, Yang JJ, Ko K-P, Park B, Shin A, Lim MK, Oh J-K, Park S, Kim YJ, Shin H-R, Yoo KY, Park SK (2011) Coinfection of hepatitis b and c viruses and risk of hepatocellular carcinoma: systematic review and meta-analysis. Int J Cancer J Int du Cancer 128 (1):176–184

Crotty S, Cameron C, Andino R (2002) Ribavirin's antiviral mechanism of action: Lethal mutagenesis? J Molecular Med-Jmm 80 (2):86–95

Davis GL, Albright JE, Cook SF, Rosenberg DM (2003) Projecting future complications of chronic hepatitis c in the united states. Liver Transpl 9 (4):331–338

Di Martino V, Rufat P, Boyer N, Renard P, Degos F, Martinot-Peignoux M, Matheron S, Le Moing V, Vachon F, Degott C, Valla D, Marcellin P (2001) The influence of human immunodeficiency virus coinfection on chronic hepatitis c in injection drug users: A longterm retrospective cohort study. Hepatology (Baltimore, Md.) 34 (6), 1193–1199

Dibisceglie AM, Conjeevaram HS, Fried MW, Sallie R, Park Y, Yurdaydin C, Swain M, Kleiner DE, Mahaney K, Hoofnagle JH, Wright D (1995) Ribavirin as therapy for chronic hepatitisc—a randomized, double-blind, placebo-controlled trial. Ann Intern Med 123 (12), 897

Donato F, Tagger A, Gelatti U, Parrinello G, Boffetta P, Albertini A, Decarli A, Trevisi P, Ribero ML, Martelli C, Porru S, Nardi G (2002) Alcohol and hepatocellular carcinoma: the effect of lifetime intake and hepatitis virus infections in men and women. Am J Epidemiol 155 (4):323–331

Dore GJ, Law M, Macdonald M, Kaldor JM (2003) Epidemiology of hepatitis c virus infection in Australia. J Clin Virol 26 (2):171–184

Drane D, Maraskovsky E, Gibson R, Mitchell S, Barnden M, Moskwa A, Shaw D, Gervase B, Coates S, Houghton M, Basser R (2009) Priming of CD4 ? and CD8 ? t cell responses using a HCV core ISCOMATRIX vaccine: a phase I study in healthy volunteers. Human vaccines 5 (3):151–157

El-Serag HB, Rudolph KL (2007) Hepatocellular carcinoma: epidemiology and molecular carcinogenesis. Gastroenterology 132 (7):2557–2576

Flisiak R, Feinman SV, Jablkowski M, Horban A, Kryczka W, Pawlowska M, Heathcote JE, Mazzella G, Vandelli C, Nicolas-Metral V, Grosgurin P, Liz JS, Scalfaro P, Porchet H, Crabbe R (2009) The cyclophilin inhibitor Debio 025 combined with PEG IFnalpha2a significantly reduces viral load in treatment-naive hepatitis c patients. Hepatology (Baltimore, Md.) 49 (5), 1460–1468

Forns X, Bukh J (1999) The molecular biology of hepatitis c virus. Genotypes and quasispecies. Clinics in liver disease 3 (4), 693–716, vii

Fried MW, Shiffman ML, Reddy KR, Smith C, Marinos G, Goncales FL Jr, Haussinger D, DiagoM, Carosi G, Dhumeaux D, Craxi A, Lin A, Hoffman J, Yu J (2002) Peginterferon alfa-2a plus ribavirin for chronic hepatitis c virus infection. The New England J Med 347 (13):975–982

Gane EJ, Roberts SK, Stedman CAM, Angus PW, Ritchie B, Elston R, Ipe D, Morcos PN, Baher L, Najera I, Chu T, Lopatin U, Berrey MM, Bradford W, Laughlin M, Shulman NS, Smith PF (2010) Oral combination therapy with a nucleoside polymerase inhibitor (rg7128) and danoprevir for chronic hepatitis c genotype 1 infection (inform-1): a randomised, doubleblind, placebo-controlled, dose-escalation trial. Lancet 376 (9751):1467–1475

Gane EJ, Rouzier R, Stedman C, Wiercinska-Drapalo A, Horban A, Chang L, Zhang Y, Sampeur P, Najera I, Smith P, Shulman NS, Tran JQ (2011a) Antiviral activity, safety, and pharmacokinetics of danoprevir/ritonavir plus peg-IFN alpha-2a/RBV in hepatitis c patients. J Hepatol 55 (5): 972–979

Gane EJ, Stedman CA, Hyland RH, Sorensen RD, Symonds WT, Hindes R, Berrey MM (2011b) Once daily psi-7977 plus RBV: Pegylated interferon-alfa not required for complete rapid viral response in treatment-naive patients with HCV GT2 or GT3. Hepatology, 54 (377A–377A)

Gao M, Nettles RE, Belema M, Snyder LB, Nguyen VN, Fridell RA, Serrano-Wu MH, Langley DR, Sun J-H, O'boyle DR 2nd, Lemm JA, Wang C, Knipe JO, Chien C, Colonno RJ, Grasela DM, Meanwell NA, Hamann LG (2010) Chemical genetics strategy identifies an HCV NS5a inhibitor with a potent clinical effect. Nature 465 (7294):96–100

Ge D, Fellay J, Thompson AJ, Simon JS, Shianna KV, Urban TJ, Heinzen EL, Qiu P, Bertelsen AH,

Muir AJ, Sulkowski M, Mchutchison JG, Goldstein DB (2009) Genetic variation in IL28b predicts hepatitis c treatment-induced viral clearance. Nature 461 (7262):399–401

Hadziyannis SJ, Sette H, Jr, Morgan TR, Balan V, Diago M, Marcellin P, Ramadori G, Bodenheimer H, Jr, Bernstein D, Rizzetto M, Zeuzem S, Pockros PJ, Lin A, Ackrill AM & Group, P. I. S. (2004) Peginterferon-alpha2a and ribavirin combination therapy in chronic hepatitis c: A randomized study of treatment duration and ribavirin dose. Anna Intern Med 140 (5), 346–55

Hagan H, Pouget ER, Des Jarlais DC (2011) A systematic review and meta-analysis of interventions to prevent hepatitis c virus infection in people who inject drugs. J Infect Dis 204 (1):74–83

Halfon P, Locarnini S (2011) Hepatitis c virus resistance to protease inhibitors. J Hepatol 55 (1):192–206

Hanoulle X, Badillo A, Wieruszeski J-M, Verdegem D, Landrieu I, Bartenschlager R, Penin F, Lippens G (2009) Hepatitis c virus NS5a protein is a substrate for the peptidyl-prolyl cis/trans isomerase activity of cyclophilins a and b. J Biol Chem 284 (20):13589–13601

Hayashi J, Aoki H, Kajino K, Moriyama M, Arakawa Y, Hino O (2000) Hepatitis C virus core protein activates the MAPK/ERK cascade synergistically with tumor promoter TPA, but not with epidermal growth factor or transforming growth factor alpha. Hepatology (Baltimore, Md.) 32 (5), 958–961

Hino O, Kajino K, Umeda T, Arakawa Y (2002) Understanding the hypercarcinogenic state in chronic hepatitis: a clue to the prevention of human hepatocellular carcinoma. J Gastroenterol 37 (11):883–887

Ishikawa T, Higuchi K, Kubota T, Seki K-I, Honma T, Yoshida T, Kamimura T (2012) Combination peg-IFN a-2b/ribavirin therapy following treatment of hepatitis c virusassociated hepatocellular carcinoma is capable of improving hepatic functional reserve and survival. Hepatogastroenterology 59 (114):529–532

Jacobson IM, Mchutchison JG, Dusheiko G, Di Bisceglie AM, Reddy KR, Bzowej NH, Marcellin P, Muir AJ, Ferenci P, Flisiak R, George J, Rizzetto M, Shouval D, Sola R, Terg RA, Yoshida EM, Adda N, Bengtsson L, Sankoh AJ, Kieffer TL, George S, Kauffman RS, Zeuzem S, Team AS (2011) Telaprevir for previously untreated chronic hepatitis c virus infection. The New England J Med 364 (25):2405–2416

Kamal SM, Nasser IA (2008) Hepatitis c genotype 4: What we know and what we don't yet know. Hepatology (Baltimore, Md.), 47 (4), 1371–1383

Khuroo MS, Khuroo MS, Dahab ST (2004) Meta-analysis: a randomized trial of peginterferon plus ribavirin for the initial treatment of chronic hepatitis c genotype 4. Aliment Pharmacol Ther 20 (9):931–938

Kisseleva T, Bhattacharya S, Braunstein J, Schindler CW (2002) Signaling through the JAK/STAT pathway, recent advances and future challenges. Gene 285 (1–2):1–24

Kiyosawa K, Akahane Y, Nagata A, Furuta S (1984) Hepatocellular carcinoma after non-a, non-b posttransfusion hepatitis. Am J Gastroenterology 79 (10):777–781

Kohli V, Singhal A, Elliott L, Jalil S (2012) Antiviral therapy for recurrent hepatitis c reduces recurrence of hepatocellular carcinoma following liver transplantation. Transplant Int: official Journal of the European Society for Organ Transplantation 25 (2):192–200

Kwo PY, Lawitz EJ, Mccone J, Schiff ER, Vierling JM, Pound D, Davis MN, Galati JS, Gordon SC, Ravendhran N, Rossaro L, Anderson FH, Jacobson IM, Rubin R, Koury K, Pedicone LD, Brass CA, Chaudhri E, Albrecht JK (2010) Efficacy of boceprevir, an NS3 protease inhibitor, in combination with peginterferon alfa-2b and ribavirin in treatment-naive patients with genotype 1 hepatitis c infection (sprint-1): an open-label, randomised, multicentre phase 2 trial. Lancet 376 (9742):705–716

Lagace L, Cartier M, Laflamme G, Lawetz C, Marquis M, Triki I, Bernard M-J, Bethell R, Larrey DG, Lueth S, Trepo C, Stern JO, Boecher WO, Steffgen J, Kukolj G (2010) Genotypic and phenotypic analysis of the NS5b polymerase region from viral isolates of HCV chronically infected patients treated with bi 207127 for 5-days monotherapy. Hepatology 52 (4):1205A–1206A

Lalezari J, Lawitz E, Rodriguez-Torres M, Sheikh A, Freilich B, Nelson DR, Hassanein T, Mader M, Albanis E, Symonds W, Berrey MM (2011) Once daily psi-7977 plus pegIFN/RBV in a phase 2b trial: Rapid virologic suppression in treatment-naive patients with HCV GT2/GT3. J Hepatol 54 (S28–S28)

Lauer GM, Barnes E, Lucas M, Timm J, Ouchi K, Kim AY, Day CL, Robbins GK, Casson DR, Reiser M, Dusheiko G, Allen TM, Chung RT, Walker BD, Klenerman P (2004) High resolution analysis of cellular immune responses in resolved and persistent hepatitis c virus infection. Gastroenterology 127 (3):924–936

Law MG, Dore GJ, Bath N, Thompson S, Crofts N, Dolan K, Giles W, Gow P, Kaldor J, Loveday S, Powell E, Spencer J, Wodak A (2003) Modelling hepatitis c virus incidence, prevalence and long-term sequelae in Australia. Int J Epidemiol 32 (5):717–724

Li X, Hui A-M, Sun L, Hasegawa K, Torzilli G, Minagawa M, Takayama T, Makuuchi M (2004) P16INK4a hypermethylation is associated with hepatitis virus infection, age, and gender in hepatocellular carcinoma. Clinical Cancer Res: Official J Am Assoc Cancer Res 10 (22):7484–7489

Lok AS, Everhart JE, Wright EC, Di Bisceglie AM, Kim H.-Y, Sterling RK, Everson GT, Lindsay KL, Lee WM, Bonkovsky H. L, Dienstag JL, Ghany MG, Morishima C, Morgan TR & Group H.-C. T (2011) Maintenance peginterferon therapy and other factors associated with hepatocellular carcinoma in patients with advanced hepatitis c. Gastroenterology, 140 (3), 840–849

Lok AS, Seeff LB, Morgan TR, Di Bisceglie AM, Sterling RK, Curto TM, Everson GT, Lindsay KL, Lee WM, Bonkovsky HL, Dienstag JL, Ghany MG, Morishima C, Goodman Z D & Group, H.-C. T. (2009) Incidence of hepatocellular carcinoma and associated risk factors in hepatitis c-related advanced liver disease. Gastroenterology, 136 (1), 138–148

Manns MP, Mchutchison JG, Gordon SC, Rustgi VK, Shiffman M, Reindollar R, Goodman ZD, Koury K, Ling MH, Albrecht JK, & Int Hepatitis Interventional, T (2001) Peginterferon alfa-2b plus ribavirin compared with interferon alfa-2b plus ribavirin for initial treatment of chronic hepatitis c: A randomised trial. Lancet, 358 (9286), 958–965

Marcellin P, Boyer N, Gervais A, Martinot M, Pouteau M, Castelnau C, Kilani A, Areias J, Auperin A, Benhamou JP, Degott C, Erlinger S (1997) Long-term histologic improvement and loss of detectable intrahepatic HCV RNA in patients with chronic hepatitis c and sustained response to interferon-alpha therapy. Ann Intern Med 127 (10):875–881

Maruoka D, Imazeki F, Arai M, Kanda T, Fujiwara K, Yokosuka O (2012) Long-term cohort study of chronic hepatitis c according to interferon efficacy. J Gastroenterol Hepatol 27 (2):291–299

Mchutchison JG, Everson GT, Gordon SC, Jacobson IM, Sulkowski M, Kauffman R, Mcnair L, Alam J, Muir AJ (2009a) Telaprevir with peginterferon and ribavirin for chronic HCV genotype 1 infection (vol 360, pg 1827, 2009). New England J Med 361 (15), 1516–1516

Mchutchison JG, Lawitz EJ, Shiffman ML, Muir AJ, Galler GW, Mccone J, Nyberg LM, Lee WM, Ghalib RH, Schiff ER, Galati JS, Bacon BR, Davis MN, Mukhopadhyay P, Koury K, Noviello S, Pedicone LD, Brass CA, Albrecht JK, Sulkowski MS, Team IS (2009b) Peginterferon alfa-2b or alfa-2a with ribavirin for treatment of hepatitis c infection. The New England J Med 361 (6):580–593

Mendenhall CL, Seeff L, Diehl AM, Ghosn SJ, French S W, Gartside PS, Rouster SD, Buskell-Bales Z, Grossman CJ, Roselle GA (1991) Antibodies to hepatitis b virus and hepatitis c virus in alcoholic hepatitis and cirrhosis: Their prevalence and clinical relevance. The VA cooperative study group (no. 119). Hepatology (Baltimore, Md.) 14 (4 Pt 1), 581–589

National institutes of health consensus development conference statement: Management of hepatitis c (2002) (June 10–12, 2002). Gastroenterology, 123 (6):2082–2099

Nelson DR, Lalezari J, Lawitz E, Hassanein T, Kowdley K, Poordad F, Sheikh A, Afdhal N, Bernstein D, Dejesus E, Freilich B, Dieterich D, Jacobson I, Jensen D, Abrams GA, Darling J, Rodriguez-Torres M, Reddy R, Sulkowski M, Bzowej N, Demicco M, Strohecker J, Hyland R, Mader M, Albanis E, Symonds WT, Berrey MM (2011) Once daily psi-7977 plus peg-IFN/RBV in HCV GT1: 98% rapid virologic response, complete early virologic response: The proton study. J Hepatology, 54 (S544-S544)

Parkin DM (2001) Global cancer statistics in the year. Lancet Oncol 2 (9):533–543

Patel K, Muir AJ, Mchutchison JG (2006) Diagnosis and treatment of chronic hepatitis c infection.

BMJ (Clinical research ed.) 332 (7548):1013–1017

Patterson JL, Fernandezlarsson R (1990) Molecular mechanisms of action of ribavirin. Rev Infect Dis 12 (6):1139–1146

Pestka JM, Zeisel MB, Blaser E, Schurmann P, Bartosch B, Cosset F.-L, Patel AH, Meisel H, Baumert J, Viazov S, Rispeter K, Blum HE, Roggendorf M, Baumert TF (2007) Rapid induction of virus-neutralizing antibodies and viral clearance in a single-source outbreak of hepatitis C. Proc Nat Acad Sci United States Am 104 (14), 6025–6030

Pockros P, Jensen D, Tsai N, Taylor RM, Ramji A, Cooper C, Dickson R, Tice A, Stancic S, Ipe D, Thommes JA, Vierling JM (2011) First svr data with the nucleoside analogue polymerase inhibitor mericitabine (rg7128) combined with peginterferon/ribavirin in treatment-naive HCV G1/4 patients: Interim analysis from the jump-c trial. J Hepatology, 54 (S538–S538)

Pol S, Ghalib RH, Rustgi V, Martorell C, Everson G, Tatum H, Hezode C, Lim J, Bronowicki J.-P, Abrams G, Brau N, Morris D, Thuluvath P, Reindollar R, Yin P, Diva U, Hindes R, Mcphee F, Gao M, Thiry A, Schnittman S, Hughes E (2011) First report of SVR12 for a NS5a replication complex inhibitor, BMS-790052 in combination with peg-IFN-alfa-2a and RBV: Phase 2a trial in treatment-naive HCV-genotype 1 subjects. 46th annual meeting of the European association for the study of the liver (easl 2011) . J Hepatol 54, Suppl. 1 (S544–S545)

Poordad F, Mccone J Jr, Bacon BR, Bruno S, Manns MP, Sulkowski MS, Jacobson IM, Reddy KR, Goodman ZD, Boparai N, Dinubile MJ, Sniukiene V, Brass CA, Albrecht JK, Bronowicki J-P, Investigators S (2011) Boceprevir for untreated chronic HCV genotype 1 infection. N Engl J Med 364 (13):1195–1206

Poynard T, Bedossa P, Opolon P (1997) Natural history of liver fibrosis progression in patients with chronic hepatitis c. The obsvirc, metavir, clinivir, and dosvirc groups. Lancet 349 (9055):825–832

Pradat P, Tillmann HL, Sauleda S, Braconier JH, Saracco G, Thursz M, Goldin R, Winkler R, Alberti A, Esteban JI, Hadziyannis S, Rizzetto M, Thomas H, Manns MP, Trepo C, Grp H (2007) Long-term follow-up of the hepatitis C HENCORE cohort: Response to therapy and occurrence of liver-related complications. J Viral Hepatitis 14 (8):556–563

Raimondi S, Bruno S, Mondelli MU, Maisonneuve P (2009) Hepatitis c virus genotype 1b as a risk factor for hepatocellular carcinoma development: a meta-analysis. J Hepatol 50 (6):1142–1154

Razali K, Thein HH, Bell J, Cooper-Stanbury M, Dolan K, Dore G, George J, Kaldor J, Karvelas M, Li J, Maher L, Mcgregor S, Hellard M, Poeder F, Quaine J, Stewart K, Tyrrell H, Weltman M, Westcott O, Wodak A, Law M (2007) Modelling the hepatitis c virus epidemic in Australia. Drug Alcohol Depend 91 (2–3):228–235

Romero-Gomez M, Del Mar Viloria M, Andrade RJ, Salmeron J, Diago M, Fernandez-Rodriguez CM, Corpas R, Cruz M, Grande L, Vazquez L, Munoz-De-Rueda P, Lopez-Serrano P, Gila A,

Gutierrez ML, Perez C, Ruiz-Extremera A, Suarez E, Castillo J (2005) Insulin resistance impairs sustained response rate to peginterferon plus ribavirin in chronic hepatitis c patients. Gastroenterology 128 (3):636–641

Serfaty L, Aumaitre H, Chazouilleres O, Bonnand AM, Rosmorduc O, Poupon RE, Poupon R (1998) Determinants of outcome of compensated hepatitis c virus-related cirrhosis. Hepatology (Baltimore, Md.) 27 (5), 1435–1440

Simmonds P, Bukh J, Combet C, Deleage G, Enomoto N., Feinstone S, Halfon P, Inchauspe G, Kuiken C, Maertens G, Mizokami M, Murphy DG, Okamoto H, Pawlotsky J.-M, Penin F, Sablon E, Shin-I T, Stuyver LJ, Thiel H.-J, Viazov S, Weiner AJ, Widell A (2005) Consensus proposals for a unified system of nomenclature of hepatitis c virus genotypes. Hepatology (Baltimore, Md.) 42 (4), 962–973

Singal AK, Freeman DH Jr, Anand BS (2010a) Meta-analysis: Interferon improves outcomes following ablation or resection of hepatocellular carcinoma. Aliment Pharmacol Ther 32 (7):851–858

Singal AK, Singh A, Jaganmohan S, Guturu P, Mummadi R, Kuo Y-F, Sood GK (2010b) Antiviral therapy reduces risk of hepatocellular carcinoma in patients with hepatitis c virusrelated cirrhosis. Clinical Gastroenterology Hepatology: Official Clinical Prac J Am Gastroenterological Assoc 8 (2):192–199

Sommereyns C, Paul S, Staeheli P, Michiels T (2008) IFN-lambda (IFN-lambda) is expressed in a tissue-dependent fashion and primarily acts on epithelial cells in vivo. PLoS Pathog 4 (3):e1000017

Streeter DG, Witkowsk Jt, Khare GP, Sidwell RW, Bauer R J, Robins RK, Simon LN (1973) Mechanism of action of 1-beta-d-ribofuranosyl-1, 2, 4-triazole-3-carboxamide (virazole) —new broad-spectrum antiviral agent. Proc Nat Acad Sci United States Am 70 (4), 1174–1178

Sun C-A, Wu D-M, Lin C–C, Lu S-N, You S-L, Wang L-Y, Wu M-H, Chen C-J (2003) Incidence and cofactors of hepatitis c virus-related hepatocellular carcinoma: a prospective study of 12, 008 men in Taiwan. Am J Epidemiol 157 (8):674–682

Takeyasu M, Akuta N, Suzuki F, Seko Y, Kawamura Y, Sezaki H, Suzuki Y, Hosaka T, Kobayashi M, Kobayashi M, Arase Y, Ikeda K, Kumada H (2012) Long-term interferon monotherapy reduces the risk of HCV-associated hepatocellular carcinoma. J Med Virol 84 (8):1199–1207

Thomas H, Foster G, Platis D (2003) Mechanisms of action of interferon and nucleoside analogues. J Hepatology, 39 Suppl 1 (S93-8)

Thomas MB, Zhu AX (2005) Hepatocellular carcinoma: the need for progress. J Clinical Oncology: Official J Am Society Clinical Oncology 23 (13):2892–2899

Torresi J, Johnson D, Wedemeyer H (2011) Progress in the development of preventive and therapeutic vaccines for hepatitis c virus. J Hepatol 54 (6):1273–1285

Vajdy M, Selby M, Medina-Selby A, Coit D, Hall J, Tandeske L, Chien D, Hu C, Rosa D, Singh M, Kazzaz J, Nguyen S, Coates S, Ng P, Abrignani S, Lin Y-L, Houghton M, O'hagan DT (2006) Hepatitis c virus polyprotein vaccine formulations capable of inducing broad antibody and cellular immune responses. J Gen Virol 87 (Pt 8):2253–2262

Wang P, Heitman J (2005) The cyclophilins. Genome Biol 6 (7):226

Wiley TE, Mccarthy M, Breidi L, Layden TJ (1998) Impact of alcohol on the histological and clinical progression of hepatitis c infection. Hepatology (Baltimore, Md.) 28 (3), 805–9

Yu J-W, Wang G-Q, Sun L-J, Li X-G, Li S-C (2007) Predictive value of rapid virological response and early virological response on sustained virological response in HCV patients treated with pegylated interferon alpha-2a and ribavirin. J Gastroenterol Hepatol 22 (6):832–836

Zeuzem S, Andreone P, Pol S, Lawitz E, Diago M, Roberts S, Focaccia R, Younossi Z, Foster GR, Horban A, Ferenci P, Nevens F, Muellhaupt B, Pockros P, Terg R, Shouval D, Van Hoek B, Weiland O, Van Heeswijk R, De Meyer S, Luo D, Boogaerts G, Polo R, Picchio G, Beumont M, Team RS (2011a) Telaprevir for retreatment of HCV infection. N Engl J Med 364 (25):2417–2428

Zeuzem S, Arora S, Bacon B, Box T, Charlton M, Diago M, Dieterich D, Esteban Mur R, Everson GT, Fallón M, Ferenci P, Flisiak R, George J, Ghalib R, Gitlin N, Gladysz A, Gordon S, Greenbloom S, Hassanein T, Jacobson I, Jeffers L, Kowdley K, Lawitz E, Lee S, Leggett B, Lueth S, Nelson D, Pockros P, Rodriguez-Torres M, Rustgi V, Serfaty L, Sherman M, Shiffman M, Sola R, Sulkowski M, Vargas H, Vierling J, Yoffe B, Ishak L, Fontana D, Xu D, Lester J, Gray T, Horga A, Hillson J, Ramos E, Lopez-Talavera JC, Muir A (2011b) Pegylated interferon-lambda (pegIFN-l) shows superior viral response with improved safety and tolerability versus pegIFNa-2a in HCV patients (G1/2/3/4): Emerge phase IIb through week 12. J Hepatol, 54 Suppl. 1 (S538–S539)

第11章 人类乳头状瘤病毒在肿瘤发生中的作用

Kristen K. Mighty 和 Laimonis A. Laimins

摘 要 人类乳头状瘤病毒（HPV）是宫颈癌、生殖器癌及口腔癌的病原体。在美国，病毒诱导的肿瘤中约50%与HPV感染相关。HPV感染复层上皮，使病毒的生产复制与细胞分化相联系。病毒癌蛋白E6、E7和E5在病毒的生命周期中对于病毒功能的调控起着重要作用，也有助于肿瘤的发展。细胞的p53和Rb是HPV E6和E7癌蛋白的两个主要作用靶点，但其他细胞蛋白也参与重要的作用。E5则在促进肿瘤发生发展中起辅助作用。本章将讨论这些病毒蛋白的不同靶点以及它们在病毒致病机制中的作用。

1 引言

人类乳头状瘤病毒（HPV）是一种小的双链DNA病毒，包含长度约8 kb的环状基因组，编码约8个主要的开放阅读框（ORF）（Howley and Lowy 2007）。这种病毒易感染手、足，以及会阴处的鳞状上皮组织，它们利用宿主细胞的分化程序，通过不同寻常的生命周期进行增殖（zur Hausen and de Villiers 1994）。HPV具有生物多样性，迄今为止，已经发现了200种左右的HPV。尽管它们基因组各异，但都感染上皮组织，只是优先定位的靶组织有区别（zur Hausen and de Villiers 1994）。约40种HPV表现对生殖道上皮的嗜性，而其余的则特异性感染皮肤组织（Howley and Lowy 2007；Moody and Laimins 2010）。

生殖器感染的HPV可进一步分为两大类：高风险（HR）型和低风险（LR）型，这取决于病毒感染后引起恶性肿瘤进展的倾向性。HR型生殖器HPV包括16型、18型、31型、33型、45型和5型，常与宫颈癌的发生相关（zur Hausen and de Villiers 1994）。在超过99%的宫颈癌中发现HPV的DNA，而在癌前病变阶段HPV DNA则位于染色体外或以游离体形式存在。高达50%的HPV 16型阳性

K. K. Mighty _ L. A. Laimins (✉)
Department of Microbiology-Immunology, Feinberg School of Medicine,
Northwestern University, 303 E, Chicago Avenue, Morton 6-681, Chicago, IL 60611, USA
e-mail: l-laimins@northwestern.edu

和大部分 18 型阳性的肿瘤中 HPV DNA 以游离体存在（Parkin et al. 2000），而至少有 10 种 HPV 可以促进宫颈癌的发展，其中有三种是主要的贡献者：50%的宫颈癌中发现了 HPV 16，约 25%的宫颈癌中发现了 HPV 18，约 10%的病例中发现了 HPV 31（Fehrmann and Laimins 2003；Longworth and Laimins 2004a）。相反，LR 生殖器型 HPV 很少与恶性肿瘤有关，而主要是引起良性生殖器疣。这种 HPV 包括 6 型、11 型、42 型、43 型和 44 型，在 90%的生殖器疣中有 6 型和 11 型 HPV 感染（Lorincz et al. 1992）。

HR-HPV 是大多数宫颈癌的病原体（Stanley 2010）。宫颈癌占人类肿瘤的 5%，是全球第二大妇科常见肿瘤，每年有超过 50 万个新增病例。它也是第三大癌症杀手，每年造成近 30 万妇女死亡（Ferlay et al. 2008）。过去 50 年间，在美国因使用巴氏涂片检查减少了超过 80%的宫颈癌发病率（Moody and Laimins 2010）。此外，美国食品药品监督管理局（FDA）近日批准了两种预防性多克隆靶向疫苗（针对最常见的与宫颈癌和生殖器疣相关 HPV 类型）的使用。这些疫苗被批准用于 10~25 岁之间的男性和女性。加德西（Gardasil）是默克公司开发的针对 6 型、11 型、16 型和 18 型 HPV 的四价疫苗，卉妍康（Cervarix）是 GlaxoSmithKline 公司开发的针对 16 型、18 型 HPV 的二价疫苗。这两种疫苗都可有效地防止初始 HPV 感染（Markowitz et al. 2007）。由于这些疫苗仅能预防原发感染，不能用于治疗已发生的感染或肿瘤，因此被推荐只能用于从未有过滥交的个体。结合每年的定期巴氏涂片筛查，接种一种疫苗，这是最有效的预防策略。

HPV 感染通过性接触传播，并被列为最常见的性传播性病毒感染（Markowitz et al. 2007）。最近的分析表明，目前大约有 2000 万美国人感染 HPV。美国社会健康协会（American Social Health Association）进一步研究估计，15~49 岁间性生活活跃的人群中有 75%的人，在他们一生中的某个时刻已经感染 HPV。另据估计，超过一半的女性感染相关的肿瘤归因于 HPV（zur Hausen 2009）。总之，这些发现证实在美国和全球范围内重大的公共卫生影响着 HPV 感染和宫颈癌的发生。这也说明我们需要继续对 HPV 感染和 HPV 相关性肿瘤的预防与治疗进行研究。

因为病毒具有逃避先天免疫监视的能力，因而在大多数个体中生殖器型 HPV 感染可以持续 2 年之久，并且可以延缓宿主的适应性免疫应答。这种免疫逃避的部分原因是 HPV 感染的非细胞溶解性，以及病毒蛋白表达的水平极低（Bodily and Laimins 2011）。另外，HPV 诱导的先天免疫逃逸导致适应性免疫应答的延迟，从而促进病毒的持续性感染及生产性复制。最终，大多数人能产生有效的细胞免疫应答，从而清除病毒感染（Stanley 2008）。但是，仍然有高达 20%的妇女不能清除感染，而且具有发展为宫颈癌的高风险（Bodily and Laimins 2011）。虽然持续的高风险 HPV 感染是促进宫颈癌发展的一个重要因素，但其他风险因子如免疫抑制、吸烟、人类免疫缺陷病毒（HIV）感染也促进恶性肿瘤的进程（Markowitz et al. 2007；Bodily and Laimins 2011；zur Hausen 1996）。

宫颈癌的发展不是一个快速事件，通常需要几十年。初始感染如不被免疫监视清除，发展为典型的癌前病变需要十年，而宫颈癌的发生可能要经过数十年。要了解病毒感染是如何发展为宫颈癌的，首要的是检查病毒不同寻常的生命周期和基因组排列。

1.1 HPV 的生命周期

HPV 的生命周期与上皮细胞的分化程序密切相关（图 11-1）。要了解 HPV 不同寻常的生命周期，首先要了解正常上皮细胞的分化程序。对于正常上皮细胞，只有活跃的分裂细胞才位于复层上皮的基底层，复层上皮由短暂增殖（TA）细胞和干细胞组成。TA 细胞定义为增殖中的细胞，可以终极分化。与此相反，干细胞虽然具有无限增殖的潜能，但为了补充 TA 细胞池而不常分裂。一旦基底层细胞分裂，其中一个子细胞朝基底上部迁移并且发生分化，就失去了活跃的增殖能力。分化中的细胞将经历一系列事件，包括基因表达改变和剥离（Bodily and Laimins 2011）。

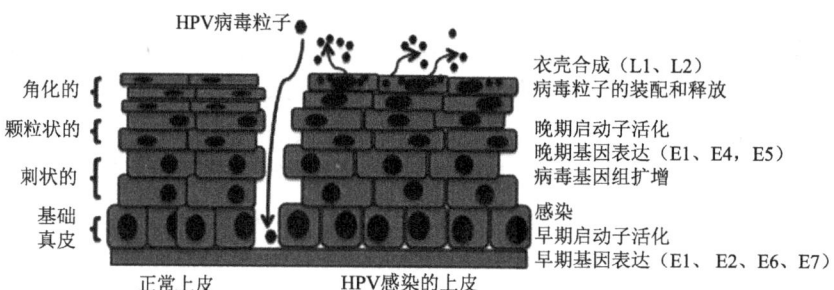

图 11-1 HPV 分化相关的生命周期。HPV 的生命周期与上皮细胞的分化程序紧密相关。HPV 感染经微磨损而活跃分裂的上皮中的基底层细胞进入细胞后，病毒基因的表达被激活，每个细胞中游离 HPV DNA 维持在约 50~100 个拷贝。然后 HPV 癌蛋白使感染细胞退出基底层以保持活跃的细胞周期。一旦感染细胞开始分化，晚期启动子即被激活，这导致病毒生命周期开始进入生产阶段。在这个阶段，病毒 DNA 复制，病毒蛋白表达升高。最后，在上皮最上面的分化层中进行病毒衣壳的合成与包装，其次是子代病毒粒子的释放。

病毒在感染过程中，能在被感染的宿主细胞的胞核内建立自己的双链 DNA 基因组（Howley and Lowy 2007）。上皮的基底层细胞因微损伤易暴露，HPV 则进入其中（Moody and Laimins 2010）。基底层感染后病毒持续感染，因为基底细胞是上皮中唯一能够活跃复制的细胞（Moody and Laimins 2010）。HPV 基因组只有 8kb，它们不编码病毒复制所需的聚合酶或其他酶。因此，必须依赖宿主细胞的复制机制来进行病毒 DNA 的合成（Moody and Laimins 2010）。进入细胞以后，病毒就以染色体外质粒或附加体的形式在细胞核内建立病毒基因组。在被感染的基底细胞，早期病毒基因表达活跃，每个细胞中基因组的拷贝数维持在 20~100（Moody and Laimins 2010）。如果 HPV 感染的基底细胞分裂，受感染的子细胞中其中一个保持在基底层，另一个子细胞则迁移远离基底层并开始分化，引起晚期病毒启动子的活化。这导致病毒生命周期进入生产阶段（包括病毒 DNA 扩增、每个细胞中 HPV DNA 的拷贝数上升至超过 100、衣壳基因表达开始）。最后，在顶端的上皮分化层中发生病毒衣壳的合成和病毒基因组的组装，最终导致释放子代病毒粒子。

在病毒生命周期中调控晚期事件的信号，其特征尚不十分清楚，但研究表明，HPV 癌蛋白能使基底上层中被感染细胞的细胞周期保持活跃状态、重新进入 S 期或停滞在 G_2/M 期，使病毒得以扩增。这种细胞周期调控的改变对于病毒生产性复制期的激活至关重要（Moody and Laimins 2010）。此外，研究表明病毒蛋白 E6、E7、E1^E4 和 E5 都需要这种活化过程。这种活化将简要总结如下。

1.2 HPV 基因组

所有 HPV 都具有小的双链 DNA 基因组，大小约 8kb。HPV 平均编码 8 个开放阅读框（ORF）（由单链 DNA 转录成的多顺反子 mRNA 表达而来）（Howley and Lowy 2007）（图 11-2）。早期蛋白 E1、E2、E6 和 E7 在未分化细胞中的病

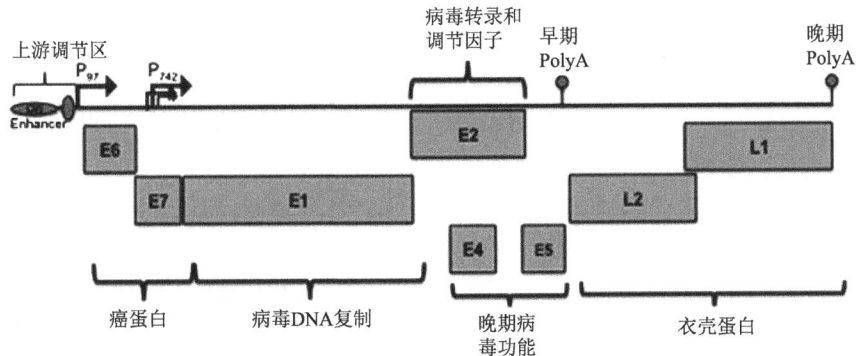

图 11-2 HPV 基因组的线性排列。HPV 基因组在这里是代表简单线性形式。其基因组为小的、环状、双链 DNA，大小为 8kb。由单链 DNA 转录成单一的多顺反子转录物，平均表达成 8 个开放阅读框（ORF）（E1、E2、E4、E5、E6、E7、L1 和 L2）。上游调节区（URR）位于非编码区，含有负责调节病毒转录和复制的序列。分化过程中被调节的 HPV 基因的三个一般基团分别是病毒早期启动子（P97）、分化依赖性晚期启动子（P742）和两个多腺苷酸信号（多聚 A）。P97 位于 E6 ORF 的上游，指导未分化细胞早期基因的表达。P742 位于 E7 的 ORF 中，宿主细胞分化时被激活，指导晚期基因产物的表达。E6 和 E7 是参与复制的癌基因。E1 和 E2 是参与病毒 DNA 复制及调控病毒转录的基因。E4 和 E5 是参与后期功能的基因。L1 和 L2 是衣壳蛋白。

毒感染早期表达，它们具有不同的功能。位于基因组中非编码区的上游调节区（URR）负责调控病毒的转录和复制。HPV 基因产物的表达由两个不同的启动子（早期启动子和晚期启动子）启动（Moody and Laimins 2010）。早期启动子在 HPV 31 中称为 P97，位于 E6 ORF 的上游，负责未分化细胞中早期基因产物的表达。早期基因产物包括 E1、E2、E6、E7、E1^E4 和 E5。HPV 信息的翻译通过一种叫渗漏扫描的机制（引起 E6 和 E7 高水平）来进行，而 E1^E4 和 E5 蛋白则处于低水平。E1 和 E2 蛋白在复制及转录调控中发挥作用，E1^E4 则调节晚期病毒的功能。HPV 31 中的晚期启动子——P742，位于 E7 ORF 内，控制晚期基因产物的表达。重要的是，P742 在上皮细胞分化时被激活。晚期蛋白（包括 L1、L2、E1^E4 和 E5）都是因 P742 活化而表达（Moody and Laimins 2010）。

1.3 癌蛋白：E5、E6 和 E7

E6 和 E7 蛋白在 HPV 初始感染宿主角化细胞时表达，而 E5 主要表达在病毒生命周期的晚期。尽管这些蛋白质都促进宿主细胞肿瘤的生长，但它们功能各异。如前面所讨论的，E1 和 E2 负责病毒复制和转录的调节，而 E6 和 E7 蛋白主要负责调节细胞周期进程。在 HR 型 HPV 中，E6 和 E7 扮演生殖器肿瘤发展所必需的癌蛋白的角色。相反，LR 型 HPV 蛋白则被证实无此功能。虽然 E6 和 E7 蛋白都定位于宿主细胞核，但在感染了 HPV 细胞的细胞质中也可检测到 E6 蛋白（Howley and Lowy 2007；Moody and Laimins 2010）。有研究表明，E6 蛋白的表达足够引起人类乳腺上皮细胞的无限增殖和 HIH3T3 纤维母细胞的转化。然而，人类角化细胞有效的无限增殖则需要 E6 和 E7 两种蛋白质的表达（Howley and Lowy 2007）。

E6 蛋白约含 150 个氨基酸（18kDa），有两个锌结合结构域，每个结构域由 4 个 Cys（半胱氨酸）-X-X-Cys 序列组成（Howley and Lowy 2007）。有研究已经证实，各种 E6 的活性是通过与十几个不同的蛋白质相互作用介导的。一个研究清楚的相互作用是 E6 蛋白与肿瘤抑制蛋白 p53 结合，影响 p53 依赖的细胞周期调控。p53 蛋白对于在 DNA 损伤后调节 G_1/S 和 G_2/M 细胞周期检测点非常重要（Slee et al. 2004；Oren 2003）。研究表明，E6 蛋白与 E3 细胞泛素连接酶、E6 相关蛋白（E6AP）和 p53 形成复合物，导致 p53 的 26S 蛋白酶体快速降解（Scheffner et al. 1990）。作为对 DNA 损伤或不定期复制诱导的正常反应，p53 通过各种修饰被激活。这种短暂的转录因子的活化导致细胞周期的调整，在某些情况下则导致凋亡过程的活化。活化的 p53 形成同源四聚体，转录激活细胞周期调节蛋白（如细胞周期蛋白激酶抑制剂 p21，负责诱导 G_1/S 期阻滞）的表达（Ko and Prives 1996）。p53 的活化也可诱导细胞程序性死亡（凋亡）。细胞周期阻滞允许细胞进入 S 期之前修复损伤的 DNA。如果损伤过于广泛，细胞则触发凋亡机制来防止细胞中损伤 DNA 的复制。此外，病毒感染后 p53 被活化。只要 HPV 依赖宿主细胞机制进入 S 期以复制其基因组，那么，它就在此前已经设计了一套机制来扰乱 p53 的正常功能。E6 介导的 p53 蛋白酶体降解引起细胞周期失调，这使得病毒可以持续存在并复制其基因组（Moody and Laimins 2010）。

高风险（HR）型 E6 的另一种活性是与 p300/CBP（p53 的共激活剂）相互作用（Patel et al. 1999；Zimmermann et al. 1999）。P300/CBP/ E6 的相互作用阻止 p53 基因乙酰化，从而阻断细胞周期停滞。P300/CBP 的结合不依赖于 E6 介导的 p53 降解（Patel et al. 1999；Zimmermann et al. 1999）。有趣的是，研究表明虽然 E6 突变体不引起 p53 的降解，但仍然可以使细胞永生化，而且永生化能力并不完全与 p53 依赖的机制有关；同样，具有正常降解活性的 E6 突变体也不能使细胞永生化（Kiyono et al. 1997）。

E6 的一个 p53 非依赖的功能是 HR 型 E6 蛋白可使端粒酶激活（Klingelhutz et al. 1996）。端粒酶是一种具有 4 个亚基的酶，这些亚基通过在染色体末端添加六聚体重复序列来复制端粒 DNA。其催化亚基的表达及人端粒酶逆转录酶（hTERT），在端粒酶活性调节中起重要作用（Liu 1999）。在连续的细胞分裂过程中，由于细胞衰老的诱导及不可逆的细胞生长阻滞，端粒变短并且失去功能，从而导致有限的细胞增殖。相反，在肿瘤中，hTERT 基因的再活化使端粒酶活性重建（Liu 1999）。研究表明，E6 通过 NFX1-123、Myc 和 SP-1 的作用来提高 hTERT 启动子的转录激活，从而进一步提高内源性 hTERT 的表达水平（Kyo et al. 2000；Howie et al. 2009；Gewin and Galloway 2001；Katzenellenbogen et al. 2009）。这种活性并不是宿主细胞有效永生化所需的唯一功能，而是 E6 的重要功能。

E6 蛋白对于细胞永生化的另一项重要功能是它与几个 PDZ 结构域蛋白相关。PDZ 结构域约含 90 个氨基酸，是许多蛋白质包括突触后密度蛋白（PSD-95）、果蝇圆盘大肿瘤抑制蛋白（Dlg1）和紧密连接蛋白-1（ZO-1）的结合域。在细胞-细胞接触区中负责细胞-细胞黏附和细胞信号的蛋白质中经常可以发现这些结合域。研究表明，PDZ 蛋白 MUPP-1、hDLG、hScribble，以及 MAGI-1、2、3 与 HR 型 E6 蛋白的 C 端结合，导致 PDZ 蛋白的降解（Lee et al. 1997，2000）。虽然 PDZ 蛋白与 E6 蛋白的相互作用可能促进细胞恶性进程，但其中的机制目前尚不得而知。

在其他各种与细胞因子（包括桩蛋白 paxillin、假定钙结合蛋白 E6-BP 和干扰素调节因子 IRF-3）相互作用的分子中也可以见到 HR 型 E6 蛋白的身影（Patel et al. 1999；Ronco et al. 1998）。有几项研究已经鉴定了许多与 LR 型 E6 结合的细胞内分子伴侣如 MCM7、Bak、zyxin 和 GPS2（Kuhne and Banks 1998；Kukimoto et al. 1998；Thomas and Banks 1999）。由于将 E6 从基因组中敲除可以导致游离体不能维持，那么，从大量的 E6 结合伙伴及其活性特征可以明显看出，在病毒生命周期中这种病毒蛋白是至关重要的（Thomas et al. 1999）。

第二个癌蛋白 E7，约由 100 个氨基酸组成，并能通过其 C 端形成二聚体。HR 型 E7 蛋白由三个保守区组成：位于 N 端的 CR1、含有一个 LXCXE 模式并能与视网膜母细胞瘤蛋白（Rb）结合的 CR2、含有两个锌指样模式的 CR3（Dyson et al. 1992）。CR1 和 CR2 结构域与腺病毒 E1A 中的 CR1 和 CR2 保守区域具有序列同源性。E7 本身能转化成纤维细胞 NIH3T3，或者与 E6 共表达能提高转化 NIH3T3 的有效性。与 E6 对比，E7 癌蛋白单独表达时，能够使人类角化细胞永生化。不过，永生化发生的频率很低（Howley and Lowy 2007；Munger et al. 1989；Riley et al. 2003）。

E7 蛋白的主要活性体现在与 Rb 蛋白家族的相关性（Dyson et al. 1989）。Rb、p107 和 p130 都是这个家族的成员，它们在整个细胞周期表达，调节细胞周期进程。要了解 E7 如何避开 Rb 调节的细胞周期进程，首要的是要了解正常情况下 Rb 是如何调节细胞周期的。未磷酸化的 Rb 蛋白和 E2F/ DP1 转录因子形成复合物，以抑制 S 期进程（DNA 合成）或细胞凋亡的基因转录。E2F 转录因子调节正常细胞 DNA 合成所需的蛋白质的转录。Rb 蛋白被细胞周期蛋白激酶复合物磷酸化后，引起 E2F 复合物释放 Rb 蛋白，减轻了参与 DNA 合成基因的转录抑制，这时从 G_1 到 S 期的转换被触发。

E7 通过与 Rb 结合而使其无法与 E2F/ DP1 复合物结合，来促进 E2F 调控基因群的表达，从而改变对 G_1 / S 期的调节。这样既减轻了转录抑制，又允许 DNA 合成所需的基因得到转录（Edmonds and Vousden 1989；Weintraub et al. 1995）。此外，E7 能够使靶向 Rb 的、泛素介导的蛋白酶体降解，而这又允许 E2F 调节的基因群转录，从而促进 DNA 的合成（Howley and Lowy 2007；Moody and Laimins 2010）。上皮细胞分化过程中，Rb 基因还负责调控从细胞周期退出，因此，E7 介导的对 Rb 功能的阻断有利于维持细胞周期活动。这种活性对于分化的上皮细胞中的病毒复制是必要的（Thomas et al. 1999）。Rb-E7 对于未分化细胞中病毒维持其游离体基因组也是必需的（Longworth and Laimins 2004b）。

E7 蛋白影响细胞周期进程的另一种方式是通过与细胞周期蛋白（cyclin）和周期蛋白依赖性激酶（cdk）抑制剂结合。例如，多项研究已经阐明了 E7 与细胞周期蛋白 A、E，以及 cdk 抑制剂 p21、p27 结合（Davies et al. 1993；Funk et al. 1997；Jones et al. 1997；Ruesch and Laimins 1998；Tommasino et al. 1993；Zerfass-Thome et al. 1996）。这些细胞蛋白通过这种相关性不但影响 Rb 蛋白的磷酸化状态，而且促进细胞周期进程。具体来说，E7 蛋白可以与细胞周期蛋白 A、E、p21、p27 结合，引起细胞周期蛋白 A 和 E 水平增加，同时导致 p21 和 p27 蛋白水平下降（Jones et al. 1997；Ruesch and Laimins 1998；Tommasino et al. 1993）。这种相互作用的效应是驱动细胞周期进程，而这种驱动效应对于促进分化上皮中 HPV 的生命周期是必要的。

Rb 磷酸化状态的改变不仅是影响 E2F 反应性启动子的唯一手段，它们还可以因组蛋白脱乙酰酶（HDAC）的作用而被抑制。E7 影响细胞周期调控的另一种机制是以 I 类 HDAC 为靶点（Longworth and Laimins 2004a，b；Brehm et al. 1998）。HDAC 是泛表达的转录共阻遏因子，可以将核小体中组蛋白富含赖氨酸的 N 端尾巴的乙酰基团移去。此外，HDAC 还可以直接将 E2F 响应因子脱去乙酰化而导致其功能丧失。HDAC 根据序列同源性和在细胞中的定位可以分为三类。I 类 HDAC 位于细胞核，包括 HDAC 1、2、3 和 8。这类 HDAC 需要与共作用因子蛋白结合，要么改变自身的活性，要么定位在作用位点。HRE7 蛋白通过其 C 端锌指区域的序列与辅助蛋白 Mi2b 直接结合来间接同 HDAC 相联系（Brehm et al. 1998）。这种 HDAC/E7 的相互作用特异性地引起分化细胞中 E2F 反应性转录水平的升高，这种升高使细胞维持细胞周期活动（Longworth and Laimins 2004b）。E7 与 HDAC 的结合对促进病毒生命周期也很重要。研究显示，因为突变的 HPV31 病毒因 E7/HDAC 相互作用的丧失而变得生长缓慢，游离体的维持功能出现缺陷，寿命也变得有限（Longworth and Laimins 2004b）。

许多肿瘤表现出基因组不稳定性的增强，HPV 诱发的肿瘤中也可以见到类似的效应。HR 型 E7 的表达是引起肿瘤细胞基因组不稳定的因素。在 HPV 阳性肿瘤的活检组织中，可以观察到较高的非整倍体水平，这表明染色体数目的改变可以促进从低级别损伤发展为恶性肿瘤。在正常细胞分裂过程中，中心体将染色体平均分配到子细胞中。人类角化细胞中 E7 的表达引起含异常中心体数目的细胞增多，这表明 E7 是引起染色体错误分离的主要诱导者（Duensing et al. 2000）。此外，在 P130、Rb 和 p107 缺失的细胞中，还发现 E7 诱导其染色体异常，这说明这种作用不依赖于 E7 结合 Rb 和/或降解 Rb 的功能（Duensing and Munger 2003）。

第三个癌蛋白 E5 是一个小的疏水性膜蛋白，主要定位于内质网，但在高尔基体和胞膜也有发现（Conrad et al. 1993；Disbrow et al. 2005）。HPV E5 蛋白约含 84 个氨基酸，主要表达在病毒生命周期的晚期。相对于其他病毒蛋白而言，人们对 E5 在病毒生命周期中的功能知之甚少，不过，已经开始有 E5 促进肿瘤发生发展的研究。单独表达牛乳头状瘤病毒（BPV）的 E5 蛋白，可使啮齿动物的成纤维细胞具有高效转化能力（Petti et al. 1991）。相比之下，HR-HPV E5 蛋白单独表达时表现的转化能力则非常微弱。然而，当 HR-HPV E5 蛋白与 E6 和 E7 蛋白同时表达时，则可以增强细胞转化能力（Stoppler et al. 1996；Valle and Banks 1995；Bouvard et al. 1994）。E5 蛋白的潜在致癌性在雌激素治疗的转基因小鼠（只表达 E5，迅速发展为宫颈癌）试验中得到了清楚的证实（Maufort et al. 2007）。尽管这不是 HPV 促进肿瘤发生的唯一途径，但这些研究显示 E5 蛋白对于病毒的存活是至关重要的，很可能作为宫颈癌治疗的潜在靶点（Valle and Banks 1995；Bouvard et al. 1994；DiMaio and Mattoon 2001）。

大量的研究已经确定了与 E5 有关的蛋白质。一种是表皮生长因子受体（EGFR），E5 与之结合，随后改变 EGFR 的活性（Straight et al. 1995）。此外，E5 还能够与液泡质子-ATP 酶 16 kDa 的亚基相互作用，这会改变其内部 pH 和内吞作用的发生，并可能有助于改变 EGFR 的生成（Conrad et al. 1993；Disbrow et al. 2005；Straight et al. 1993）。研究也已经阐明 E5 在病毒生命周期的生产阶段对于激活其后期功能的重要性。这是通过用含有 HPV 31 基因组（携带野生型或翻译终止突变的 E5 序列）的稳定转染角化细胞系来证实的（Fehrmann et al. 2003）。最近，一个分裂-泛素酵母双杂交系统新鉴定到与 E5 结合的伴侣蛋白，包括参与膜蛋白转运调节的 B 细胞受体蛋白（BAP31）。已经证明这种相互作用对于 HPV 感染的细胞分化后增殖能力的保持非常重要（Regan and Laimins 2008）。

2　小结

人类乳头状瘤病毒是诱导多种肿瘤的重要病原体。尽管引进了针对 HPV 的疫苗，它们只是防止 HPV 初始感染。除了外科手术，目前没有其他可用于 HPV 感染损伤的治疗。E6 和 E7 蛋白在病毒的生命周期中具有重要功能，并且在促进恶性肿瘤进程中起主要作用。E6 和 E7 的细胞靶点是 p53、Rb、p300、端粒酶，以及其他各种因子。膜相关的 E5 蛋白也可以促进向恶性化发展，虽然其作用机理尚不清楚。了解 HPV 癌蛋白的作用模式可以为治疗 HPV 相关性肿瘤提供重要靶标。

（杨静，卢建红 译）

参 考 文 献

Bodily J, Laimins LA (2011) Persistence of human papillomavirus infection: keys to malignant progression. Trends Microbiol 19(1):33–39. doi:10.1016/j.tim.2010.10.002

Bouvard V, Storey A, Pim D, Banks L (1994a) Characterization of the human papillomavirus E2 protein: evidence of trans-activation and trans-repression in cervical keratinocytes. EMBO J 13(22):5451–5459

Bouvard V, Matlashewski G, Gu ZM, Storey A, Banks L (1994b) The human papillomavirus type 16 E5 gene cooperates with the E7 gene to stimulate proliferation of primary cells and increases viral gene expression. Virology 203(1):73–80

Brehm A, Miska EA, McCance DJ, Reid JL, Bannister AJ, Kouzarides T (1998) Retinoblastoma protein recruits histone deacetylase to repress transcription. Nature 391(6667):597–601. doi:10.1038/35404

Conrad M, Bubb VJ, Schlegel R (1993) The human papillomavirus type 6 and 16 E5 proteins are membrane-associated proteins which associate with the 16-kilodalton pore-forming protein. J Virol 67(10):6170–6178

Davies R, Hicks R, Crook T, Morris J, Vousden K (1993) Human papillomavirus type 16 E7 associates with a histone H1 kinase and with p107 through sequences necessary for transformation. J Virol 67(5):2521–2528

DiMaio D, Mattoon D (2001) Mechanisms of cell transformation by papillomavirus E5 proteins. Oncogene 20(54):7866–7873. doi:10.1038/sj.onc.1204915

Disbrow GL, Hanover JA, Schlegel R (2005) Endoplasmic reticulum-localized human papillomavirus type 16 E5 protein alters endosomal pH but not trans-Golgi pH. J Virol 79(9):5839–5846. doi:10.1128/JVI.79.9.5839-5846.2005

Duensing S, Munger K (2003) Human papillomavirus type 16 E7 oncoprotein can induce abnormal centrosome duplication through a mechanism independent of inactivation of retinoblastoma protein family members. J Virol 77(22):12331–12335

Duensing S, Lee LY, Duensing A, Basile J, Piboonniyom S, Gonzalez S, Crum CP, Munger K (2000) The human papillomavirus type 16 E6 and E7 oncoproteins cooperate to induce mitotic defects and genomic instability by uncoupling centrosome duplication from the cell division cycle. Proce Natl Acad Sci USA 97(18):10002–10007. doi:10.1073/pnas.170093297 Dyson N, Howley PM, Munger K, Harlow E (1989) The human papilloma virus-16 E7 oncoprotein is able to bind to the retinoblastoma gene product. Science 243(4893):934–937 (New York)

Dyson N, Guida P, Munger K, Harlow E (1992) Homologous sequences in adenovirus E1A and human papillomavirus E7 proteins mediate interaction with the same set of cellular proteins. J Virol 66(12):6893–6902

Edmonds C, Vousden KH (1989) A point mutational analysis of human papillomavirus type 16 E7 protein. J Virol 63(6):2650–2656

Fehrmann F, Laimins LA (2003) Human papillomaviruses: targeting differentiating epithelial cells for malignant transformation. Oncogene 22(33):5201–5207. doi:10.1038/sj.onc.1206554

Fehrmann F, Klumpp DJ, Laimins LA (2003) Human papillomavirus type 31 E5 protein supports cell cycle progression and activates late viral functions upon epithelial differentiation. J Virol 77(5):2819–2831

Ferlay J, Shin HR, Bray F, Forman D, Mathers C, Parkin DM (2010) Estimates of worldwide burden of cancer in 2008: GLOBOCAN 2008. Int J Cancer 127(12):2893–2917. doi:10.1002/ijc.25516

Funk JO, Waga S, Harry JB, Espling E, Stillman B, Galloway DA (1997) Inhibition of CDK activity and PCNA-dependent DNA replication by p21 is blocked by interaction with the HPV-16 E7 oncoprotein. Genes Dev 11(16):2090–2100

Gewin L, Galloway DA (2001) E box-dependent activation of telomerase by human papillomavirus type 16 E6 does not require induction of c-myc. J Virol 75(15):7198–7201. doi:10.1128/JVI.75.15.7198-7201.2001

Howie HL, Katzenellenbogen RA, Galloway DA (2009) Papillomavirus E6 proteins. Virology 384(2):324–334. doi:10.1016/j.virol.2008.11.017

Howley PM, Lowy DR (2007) Papillomaviruses. Wolters Kluwer Health/Lippincott Williams & Wilkins, Philadelphia

Jones DL, Alani RM, Munger K (1997) The human papillomavirus E7 oncoprotein can uncouple cellular differentiation and proliferation in human keratinocytes by abrogating p21Cip1-mediated inhibition of cdk2. Genes Dev 11(16):2101–2111

Katzenellenbogen RA, Vliet-Gregg P, Xu M, Galloway DA (2009) NFX1-123 increases hTERT expression and telomerase activity posttranscriptionally in human papillomavirus type 16 E6 keratinocytes. J Virol 83(13):6446–6456. doi:10.1128/JVI.02556-08

Kiyono T, Hiraiwa A, Fujita M, Hayashi Y, Akiyama T, Ishibashi M (1997) Binding of high-risk human papillomavirus E6 oncoproteins to the human homologue of the Drosophila discs large tumor suppressor protein. Proc Natl Acad Sci USA 94(21):11612–11616

Klingelhutz AJ, Foster SA, McDougall JK (1996) Telomerase activation by the E6 gene product of human papillomavirus type 16. Nature 380(6569):79–82. doi:10.1038/380079a0

Ko LJ, Prives C (1996) p53: puzzle and paradigm. Genes Dev 10(9):1054–1072

Kuhne C, Banks L (1998) E3-ubiquitin ligase/E6-AP links multicopy maintenance protein 7 to the ubiquitination pathway by a novel motif, the L2G box. J Biol Chem 273(51):34302–34309

Kukimoto I, Aihara S, Yoshiike K, Kanda T (1998) Human papillomavirus oncoprotein E6 binds to the C-terminal region of human minichromosome maintenance 7 protein. Biochem Biophys Res Commun 249(1):258–262. doi:10.1006/bbrc.1998.9066

Kyo S, Takakura M, Taira T, Kanaya T, Itoh H, Yutsudo M, Ariga H, Inoue M (2000) Sp1 cooperates with c-Myc to activate transcription of the human telomerase reverse transcriptase gene (hTERT). Nucleic Acid Res 28(3):669–677

Lee SS, Weiss RS, Javier RT (1997) Binding of human virus oncoproteins to hDlg/SAP97, a mammalian homolog of the Drosophila discs large tumor suppressor protein. Proc Natl Acad Sci USA 94(13):6670–6675

Lee SS, Glaunsinger B, Mantovani F, Banks L, Javier RT (2000) Multi-PDZ domain protein MUPP1 is a cellular target for both adenovirus E4-ORF1 and high-risk papillomavirus type 18 E6 oncoproteins. J Virol 74(20):9680–9693

Liu JP (1999) Studies of the molecular mechanisms in the regulation of telomerase activity. FASEB J 13(15):2091–2104

Longworth MS, Laimins LA (2004a) Pathogenesis of human papillomaviruses in differentiating epithelia. Microbiol Mol Biol Rev 68(2):362–372. doi:10.1128/MMBR.68.2.362-372.2004

Longworth MS, Laimins LA (2004b) The binding of histone deacetylases and the integrity of zinc finger-like motifs of the E7 protein are essential for the life cycle of human papillomavirus type 31. J Virol 78(7):3533–3541

Lorincz AT, Reid R, Jenson AB, Greenberg MD, Lancaster W, Kurman RJ (1992) Human papillomavirus infection of the cervix: relative risk associations of 15 common anogenital types. Obstet Gynecol 79(3):328–337

Markowitz LE, Dunne EF, Saraiya M, Lawson HW, Chesson H, Unger ER (2007) Quadrivalent human papillomavirus vaccine: recommendations of the advisory committee on immunization practices (ACIP). MMWR Recomm Rep 56(RR-2):1–24 (Morbidity and mortality weekly report Recommendations and reports/Centers for Disease Control)

Maufort JP, Williams SM, Pitot HC, Lambert PF (2007) Human papillomavirus 16 E5 oncogene contributes to two stages of skin carcinogenesis. Cancer Res 67(13):6106–6112. doi:10.1158/0008-5472.CAN-07-0921

Moody CA, Laimins LA (2010) Human papillomavirus oncoproteins: pathways to transforma- tion. Nat Rev 10(8):550–560. doi:10.1038/nrc2886

Munger K, Phelps WC, Bubb V, Howley PM, Schlegel R (1989) The E6 and E7 genes of the human papillomavirus type 16 together are necessary and sufficient for transformation of primary human keratinocytes. J Virol 63(10):4417–4421

Oren M (2003) Decision making by p53: life, death and cancer. Cell Death Differ 10(4):431–442. doi:10.1038/sj.cdd.4401183

Parkin DM, Bray F, Ferlay J, Pisani P (2000) Estimating the world cancer burden: Globocan. Int J Cancer 94(2):153–156

Patel D, Huang SM, Baglia LA, McCance DJ (1999) The E6 protein of human papillomavirus type 16 binds to and inhibits co-activation by CBP and p300. EMBO J 18(18):5061–5072. doi:10.1093/emboj/18.18.5061

Petti L, Nilson LA, DiMaio D (1991) Activation of the platelet-derived growth factor receptor by the bovine papillomavirus E5 transforming protein. EMBO J 10(4):845–855

Regan JA, Laimins LA (2008) Bap31 is a novel target of the human papillomavirus E5 protein. J Virol 82(20):10042–10051. doi:10.1128/JVI.01240-08

Riley RR, Duensing S, Brake T, Munger K, Lambert PF, Arbeit JM (2003) Dissection of human papillomavirus E6 and E7 function in transgenic mouse models of cervical carcinogenesis. Cancer Res 63(16):4862–4871

Ronco LV, Karpova AY, Vidal M, Howley PM (1998) Human papillomavirus 16 E6 oncoprotein binds to interferon regulatory factor-3 and inhibits its transcriptional activity. Genes Dev 12(13):2061–2072

Ruesch MN, Laimins LA (1998) Human papillomavirus oncoproteins alter differentiation- dependent cell cycle exit on suspension in semisolid medium. Virology 250(1):19–29. doi: 10.1006/viro.1998.9359

Scheffner M, Werness BA, Huibregtse JM, Levine AJ, Howley PM (1990) The E6 oncoprotein encoded by human papillomavirus types 16 and 18 promotes the degradation of p53. Cell 63(6):1129–1136. doi:0092-8674(90)90409-8

Slee EA, O'Connor DJ, Lu X (2004) To die or not to die: how does p53 decide? Oncogene 23(16):2809–2818. doi:10.1038/sj.onc.1207516

Stanley M (2008) Immunobiology of HPV and HPV vaccines. Gynecol Oncol 109(2):S15–S21. doi:10.1016/j.ygyno.2008.02.003

Stanley M (2010) HPV: immune response to infection and vaccination. Infect Agent Cancer 5:19. doi:10.1186/1750-9378-5-19

Stoppler MC, Straight SW, Tsao G, Schlegel R, McCance DJ (1996) The E5 gene of HPV-16 enhances keratinocyte immortalization by full-length DNA. Virology 223(1):251–254. doi: 10.1006/viro.1996.0475

Straight SW, Hinkle PM, Jewers RJ, McCance DJ (1993) The E5 oncoprotein of human papillomavirus type 16 transforms fibroblasts and effects the downregulation of the epidermal growth factor receptor in keratinocytes. J Virol 67(8):4521–4532

Straight SW, Herman B, McCance DJ (1995) The E5 oncoprotein of human papillomavirus type 16 inhibits the acidification of endosomes in human keratinocytes. J Virol 69(5):3185–3192

Thomas M, Banks L (1999) Human papillomavirus (HPV) E6 interactions with Bak are conserved amongst E6 proteins from high and low risk HPV types. J Gen Virol 80(Pt 6):1513–1517

Thomas JT, Hubert WG, Ruesch MN, Laimins LA (1999) Human papillomavirus type 31 oncoproteins E6 and E7 are required for the maintenance of episomes during the viral life cycle in normal human keratinocytes. Proc Natl Acad Sci USA 96(15):8449–8454

Tommasino M, Adamczewski JP, Carlotti F, Barth CF, Manetti R, Contorni M, Cavalieri F, Hunt T, Crawford L (1993) HPV16 E7 protein associates with the protein kinase p33CDK2 and cyclin A. Oncogene 8(1):195–202

Valle GF, Banks L (1995) The human papillomavirus (HPV)-6 and HPV-16 E5 proteins cooperate with HPV-16 E7 in the transformation of primary rodent cells. J Gen Virol 76(Pt 5):1239–1245

Weintraub SJ, Chow KN, Luo RX, Zhang SH, He S, Dean DC (1995) Mechanism of active transcriptional repression by the retinoblastoma protein. Nature 375(6534):812–815. doi: 10.1038/375812a0

Zerfass-Thome K, Zwerschke W, Mannhardt B, Tindle R, Botz JW, Jansen-Durr P (1996) Inactivation of the cdk inhibitor p27KIP1 by the human papillomavirus type 16 E7 oncoprotein. Oncogene 13(11):2323–2330

Zimmermann H, Degenkolbe R, Bernard HU, O'Connor MJ (1999) The human papillomavirus type 16 E6 oncoprotein can down-regulate p53 activity by targeting the transcriptional coactivator CBP/p300. J Virol 73(8):6209–6219

zur Hausen H (1996) Papillomavirus infections–a major cause of human cancers. Biochim Biophys Acta 1288(2):F55–F78

zur Hausen H (2009) Papillomaviruses in the causation of human cancers: a brief historical account. Virology 384(2):260–265. doi:10.1016/j.virol.2008.11.046

zur Hausen H, de Villiers EM (1994) Human papillomaviruses. Annu Rev Microbiol 48:427–447. doi:10.1146/annurev.mi.48.100194.002235

第12章　通过疫苗接种控制HPV感染及其相关性肿瘤

Nam Phuong Tran, Chien-Fu Hung, Richard Roden 和 T.-C. Wu

摘　要　人乳头瘤病毒（HPV）是最常见的性传播病毒，与多种疾病相关，在超过6亿感染的个体中持续引起显著的发病率和死亡率。预防性疫苗已经取得了重大进展，美国FDA批准的两个基于L1病毒样颗粒（VLP）疫苗的功效和交叉反应已经有了临床数据。然而，已批准疫苗的成本限制了它们在发展中国家的广泛使用，而发展中国家的HPV相关性疾病的发生却最严重。此外，已批准的HPV预防性疫苗仅包含两个高风险型HPV（HPV-16和HPV-18），最多只可以保护75%的子宫颈癌。因此，希望第二代预防性候选疫苗能够解决成本的问题，并通过使用更多有意义的L1-VLP、疫苗制剂或替代性抗原（如L1衣壳蛋白、L2衣壳蛋白和嵌合VLP）来拓宽保护范围。预防性疫苗对于控制HPV的传播是至关重要的，但已有数以亿计具有HPV相关性病变的感染个体正在悄然向恶性肿瘤发展。这就增加了HPV治疗性疫苗的需求，此种疫苗可触发针对HPV病变、包括HPV转化的肿瘤细胞的T细胞杀伤。为了刺激这种抗肿瘤免疫反应，治疗性候选疫苗通过采用各种细菌、病毒、蛋白质、多肽、树突状细胞，以及基于DNA的载体，在体内释放HPV抗原。本章将评论市售预防性疫苗——目前第二代候选疫苗，并讨论开发治疗性HPV疫苗的进展。

N. P. Tran _ C.-F. Hung _ R. Roden _ T.-C. Wu
Department of Pathology, The Johns Hopkins School of Medicine, Cancer Research Building II, Room 310, 1550 Orleans Street, Baltimore, MD 21231, USA

C.-F. Hung _ R. Roden _ T.-C. Wu
Departments of Oncology, The Johns Hopkins School of Medicine, Cancer Research Building II, Room 307, 1550 Orleans Street, Baltimore, MD 21231, USA

R. Roden _ T.-C. Wu
Departments of Obstetrics and Gynecology, The Johns Hopkins School of Medicine, Cancer Research Building II, Room 308, 1550 Orleans Street, Baltimore, MD MD 21231, USA

T.-C. Wu (✉)
Department Molecular Microbiology and Immunology, The Johns Hopkins Medical Insitutions, Cancer Research Building II, Room 309, 1550 Orleans Street, Baltimore, MD 21231, USA
e-mail: wutc@jhmi.edu

关键词 人乳头瘤病毒（HPV），疫苗，肿瘤，免疫治疗，病毒样颗粒（VLP）

1 引言

为什么拥有控制人类乳头瘤病毒（HPV）感染的有效方法在全球范围都非常重要？据估计，目前全球有 6.6 亿人感染 HPV，HPV 感染是人类最常见的生殖道病毒感染（Brooks 2010）。黏膜感染特异性的 HPV 可以在人体引起从良性尖锐湿疣到转移性宫颈癌的各种疾病。良性菌株，特别是 HPV-6 和 HPV-11 可导致肛门生殖器湿疣及喉乳头状瘤。这些病变在自然界并不具有内在的致瘤性。然而，高风险型 HPV 毒株（HPV-16、18、31、33、35、45 等）是 99.7%宫颈癌、90%肛门生殖器癌、40%阴茎癌和 42%~60%口咽癌的必要病因（Brooks 2010；Kwak et al. 2010；Simard et al. 2012）。

上述 HPV 相关的疾病中，宫颈癌每年引起了最大数量的死亡（Lowy and Schiller 2012）。宫颈癌在全世界妇女最常见的肿瘤中处于第三位，每年导致超过 40 万妇女死亡（Brooks 2010；Jemal et al. 2011）。85%的宫颈癌发生在发展中国家的妇女中，但她们也是最不可能获得疫苗接种、筛查或治疗方案的人群（Lowy and Schiller 2012）。在发达国家，由于早期监测和治疗，自 20 世纪 50 年代至今，宫颈癌发病率已降低了 27%~77%（不同区域有差异）；然而，在发达国家妇女一生中感染 HPV 致癌毒株的风险仍然大于 80%，且治疗与发病率相关（Echelman and Feldman 2012；Trimble and Frazer 2009）。另外，头颈部肿瘤发病率的上升归因于 HPV 感染是令人担忧的（Chaturvedi et al. 2011），特别是口腔癌没有像宫颈癌筛查那样进行巴氏涂片检测（Trimble and Frazer 2009）。必须采取行动来控制这种致瘤病毒。对 HPV 相关性恶性肿瘤中 HPV 作为病因学因素的认识已经引出了通过接种 HPV 疫苗来控制这些肿瘤的概念。

我们对 HPV 分子生物学认识的不断增长，带动了针对 HPV 疫苗的开发。HPV 是双链 DNA 病毒，属于乳头瘤病毒家族，在人类宿主中特异复制。HPV DNA 是环形的，约包含 8000 个碱基对，含有早期（E）和晚期（L）基因的遗传密码。早期基因（E1、E2、E4 和 E6）对病毒 DNA 复制和转录具有调控功能，而两个晚期基因（L1 和 L2）则编码病毒衣壳蛋白。非编码区（或 URR）调节表达，并包含病毒的复制原点。一旦进入宿主细胞，早期基因就执行病毒复制和转录必不可少的过程，但一些早期基因直接参与对宿主细胞的致瘤性转化。早期蛋白 E1 和 E2 都参与病毒 DNA 复制和 RNA 转录，而 E4 则参与细胞骨架重塑。E5 是一个癌蛋白，已经发现其能增强 EGFR 的活化，限制宿主细胞内的再循环，引起细胞-细胞融合，导致人角化细胞永生化（DiMaio and Mattoon 2001）。E6 下调 p53

蛋白（细胞周期检查点蛋白）的表达，而 E7 与 Rb 蛋白螯合，这两个过程有助于引起感染细胞的增殖失调并转化为宫颈癌。在大多数宫颈癌中，HPV 基因组整合到宿主染色体 DNA 中，并导致病毒 E2 基因受到破坏。E2 是 E6 和 E7 基因的转录调节因子。因此，E2 功能的丧失引起 E6 和 E7 蛋白的失控表达，又通过分别与 p53 和 Rb 的交互作用导致正常细胞周期调控的破坏。进一步，细胞周期不受控制、基因组不稳定及细胞凋亡被抑制，共同促进发展为 HPV 相关的宫颈癌（zur Hausen 2002）。在晚期基因中，L1 作为病毒衣壳的主要结构蛋白，用于市售预防性疫苗的研发。L2 是次要的病毒衣壳蛋白，将在后面的章节（下一代预防性疫苗）中讨论（Roden and Wu 2006）。

HPV 具有组织嗜性，因为它们在特定黏膜上皮优先复制。早期和晚期基因表达与角化细胞分化相关：从基底层中表达早期蛋白的新感染基底细胞和中间层中的角化细胞，到表达 L1 和 L2 病毒衣壳蛋白并最终分化为角质形成细胞的角化细胞（利于病毒从表层细胞释放）（Roden and Wu 2006）。HPV 感染仅限于上皮，这使得人免疫系统难以启动潜在的 HPV 特异性免疫应答来根除感染，因为 HPV 损伤停留在基底膜之上，循环系统或淋巴系统中没有 HPV 抗原。此外，HPV 不会激发强有力的炎症反应，而是似乎逃脱了"雷达"监测范围之外。预防性疫苗的目标是提供 HPV L1 和/或 L2 衣壳抗原以刺激中和抗体的免疫，阻止 HPV 感染上皮细胞。HPV 抗体尽管可以有效地防止感染，但无法杀死 HPV 已经感染的和/或转化的细胞。需要特异性细胞毒性 T 细胞（CTL）和辅助 T 细胞的作用才能消除感染的和/或转化的细胞（Hung and Wu 2003）。治疗性 HPV 疫苗依赖于 T 细胞介导的免疫活化，这个过程通过 MHC I 类和 II 类分子的作用，经抗原提呈细胞（如树突状细胞），将 HPV 抗原提呈给 HPV 抗原特异性 T 细胞。这些 HPV 生命周期的特征，对于制定预防性和治疗性疫苗的战略非常重要。

靶抗原的选择也是需要考虑的一个重要因素。L1 和 L2 都是预防性疫苗开发的合适目标，而不是治疗性 HPV 疫苗开发的理想目标，因为它们在感染 HPV 的基底细胞中不表达。另一方面，早期病毒蛋白，特别是 E6 和 E7，在病毒感染早期表达并帮助推动恶性进程。因此，治疗性疫苗的目标应该是针对早期蛋白 E6 和 E7，使产生 T 细胞介导的免疫反应（Lin et al. 2010）。此外，E6 和 E7 共表达是转化的关键所在，而且它们在正常细胞中不表达。因此，E6 和 E7 代表治疗性 HPV 疫苗开发的理想目标。

2 目前市售的预防性疫苗

在过去十年中，两种预防性 HPV 疫苗（葛兰素史克公司的 Cervarix™ 和默克公司的 Gardasil）的成功开发，提供了预防 HPV 传播的机会。两种疫苗都已经商品化，每一种疫苗在 6 个多月内使用 3 个剂量的给药方案。此外，这两种疫苗都使用 L1 病毒样颗粒（VLP）——无病毒基因组的非感染性乳头瘤病毒粒子（Campo and Roden 2010；Roden and Wu 2006）。Cervarix™ 是二价疫苗，在昆虫细胞（粉纹夜蛾）中采用杆状病毒表达载体系统和佐剂系统 04（单磷酸脂 A 和氢氧化铝盐），可以产生 HPV-16 和 HPV-18 的 VLP。Gardasil 是四价疫苗，在酵母细胞（酿酒酵母）中采用非晶体羟基磷酸铝盐佐剂可以产生 HPV-6、11、16 和 18 的 VLP（Einstein et al. 2009）。因此，这种四价疫苗可以保护患者免受致瘤性 HPV-16 和 HPV-18，以及引起常见的尖锐湿疣的 HPV-6 和 HPV-11 的感染。在两个疫苗的比较研究中，将 1106 名妇女按年龄层次分组，使用二价疫苗 Cervarix™ 或者四价疫苗 Gardasil 治疗，结果在所有年龄层次中，二价疫苗诱导的 HPV-16 和 HPV-18 中和性抗体的几何平均滴度（GMT 水平）比四价疫苗高 2.3~9.1 倍，而且产生的循环记忆 B 细胞的数目也比四价疫苗的多（Einstein et al. 2009）。在这些患者接种疫苗后 12~24 个月的后续研究中，Einstein 等在 2011 年再次发现，和四价疫苗相比，二价疫苗的 HPV-16 GMT 升高了 2.4~5.8 倍，HPV-18 GMT 升高了 7.7~9.4 倍（表 12-1）。

表 12-1　治疗性疫苗的比较

类型	优点	缺点	发展阶段	参考文献
基于活载体	高免疫原性定制	载体特异性中和抗体或先前存在的载体特异性免疫力，安全问题，类似流感的不利影响	ADXS11-001 在 Ⅱ 期试验阶段	Maci et al.（2009），NCI（2012b），Radulovic et al.（2009）
			MVA 在 Ⅱ 期试验阶段	Corona Gutierrez et al.（2004）
			TA-HPV 完成了 Ⅰ/Ⅱ 试验	Kaufmann et al.（2002）
			TG4001-R3484 完成了 Ⅰ/Ⅱ 期试验	Brun et al.（2011）
基于肽段	安全，易于生产，稳定	HLA 的限制，弱免疫原性	HPV-16 E7 为 HLA-A*0201 完成 Ⅰ 期试验	Kente et al.（2008），Muderspach et al.（2000）
			重叠肽临床试验	Kente et al.（2008），Kente et al.（2009），Welte et al.（2010），Welter et al.（2008）
基于蛋白	安全，易于生产，稳定	弱免疫原性	HspE7 完成 Ⅰ 期和 Ⅱ 期临床试验	Derka et al.（2005），Einste et al.（2007），Goldstone et al.（2002），Van Doorslaer et al.（2009）
			TA-CIN 完成 Ⅱ 期临床试验	Daayana et al.（2010）

续表

类型	优点	缺点	发展阶段	参考文献
基于 DC	高免疫原性	个性化和劳动力密集,潜在的致癌性	HPV-16 和-18 E7 致敏 DC 疫苗完成 I 期临床试验	Wang et al.（2009）
基于 DNA	易生产,稳定,长期表达抗原,能重复给药	弱免疫原性,潜在致癌	ZYC101a 完成 II 期临床试验	Garcia et al.（2004）,Matijevic et al.（2011）,Sheets et al.（2003）
			VGX-300 在 II 期临床试验	Inovio（2012）
			pNGVL4a-SIG/ E7/ HSP70 完成 I 期临床试验	Trimble et al.（2009）

来自每种疫苗的 III 期临床试验的 4 年随访研究中,关于两种疫苗的功效数据最近已经发表。在 4 年的试验中,女性 17 622 人,年龄为 16~26 岁,发现四价疫苗可有效地防止由 HPV-6、11、16 和 18 引起的病变发展：96%为 CIN1（宫颈上皮内瘤 1）,100%为 VIN1 和 VAIN1（外阴和阴道上皮内瘤 1）,99%为尖锐湿疣（Dillner et al. 2010）。然而,针对不包含在内的 HPV 毒株,四价疫苗的保护能力不强；不管针对何种 HPV 类型,其保护 HPV 损伤的宫颈癌、外阴癌、阴道上皮内瘤变和湿疣的有效率分别为 30%、75%、48%和 3%,这表明四价疫苗对其他 HPV 毒株具有较低的交叉反应性。对二价疫苗进行的 4 年随访研究中,女性 18 644 人,年龄 15~25 岁,发现二价疫苗对预防 HPV 16 和 HPV18 引起的 CIN3 及 AIS 的有效性为 100%,对预防任何型 HPV 引起的 CIN3 病变的保护效应可达 93.2%。然而,在一个分析相同数据的同一研究中,二价疫苗预防 CIN2+病变（由非 HPV 16 和 18 株引起的）的交叉保护性功效在 HPV 初始感染患者（接受了 3 倍剂量的疫苗）中是不同的：对 HPV-31,84.3%有效；对 HPV-33,59.4%有效,对 HPV-39、45、52、58、59 和 68 具有统计学意义（Wheeler et al. 2012）。因此,该二价疫苗的交叉反应性,如同四价疫苗一样,也受到了限制。二价疫苗能更加有效地预防 HPV 感染引起的 AIS 和 CIN3+病变,但不能有效预防非 HPV-16 和 HPV-18 毒株引起的 CIN2+病变,这提示,大部分高级别的病变是由 HPV-16 和 HPV-18 毒株引起的（Wheeler et al. 2012）。在两项研究中,发现二价疫苗预防 CIN2+和 CIN3+病变的有效性在 15~17 岁年龄组是最高的,且随着年龄的增加而下降,这支持目前疫苗使用要年轻化的建议（Lehtinen et al. 2012；Wheeler et al. 2012）。

两种商业化疫苗目前按 3 剂量方案销售。然而,最近一项涉及 960 个学科的随机试验比较了二价疫苗 2 剂量和标准的 3 剂量方案。如果几何平均抗体滴度（GMT）的比值大于 2 倍差异,则认为 3 剂量方案更优越。结果表明,接种 2 剂量的二价疫苗（并不低于标准的 3 剂量方案中的疫苗浓度）1 个月和 24 个月后都可引发抗体反应。这表明，接种 2 剂量的当前二价疫苗 24 个月后会与标准的 3 剂量方案产生同等的预防作用（Romanowski et al. 2011）。

尽管开发商业化 HPV 疫苗的主要目的是为了在妇女中预防宫颈癌的发生，四价疫苗可用于防止男性 HPV-6 和 HPV-11 引起的尖锐湿疣及肛门生殖器病变。因此，男性也可能从预防 HPV-16 和 HPV-18 的感染（易引发阴茎癌、肛门癌和口咽癌）中受益（Giuliano et al. 2011）。在一项随机的双盲试验中，有 4065 名 16~26 岁的男性参与，以安慰剂作对照，对四价疫苗预防外生殖器病变的效率进行了测试。在意向接受治疗组，受试者试验前可能是 HPV 血清反应阳性，也可能是 HPV 血清反应阴性，至少接受一剂量疫苗或安慰剂治疗。相比安慰剂组的 89 例病变，HPV 接种疫苗组可见 36 例外生殖器病变，总效率达 60.2%（95% CI, 40.8~73.8）。在符合方案的男性群体中，接种疫苗前血清阴性并完成了所有 3 个剂量四价疫苗治疗的，预防 HPV-6、11、16 和 18 病变的有效率为 90.4%（95% CI, 69.2~98.1），这表明四价疫苗可以有效预防男性 HPV 相关的生殖器病变（Giuliano et al. 2011）。

3 第二代预防性疫苗的开发

有效的 HPV 疫苗提供的临床结果是令人鼓舞的，但问题仍然存在。85%的宫颈癌发生在发展中国家（Jemal et al. 2011）。在这些发展中国家，不仅多数居民无法负担目前的商业疫苗，许多人甚至没有居住在存储并分发这些疫苗（通过冷藏物流链）的地区中。预防性疫苗的另一个限制性因素是它们限制许多致瘤性 HPV 毒株的交叉反应。接种疫苗的患者将免受 HPV-16 和 HPV-18 的感染，70%以上的宫颈癌由这两种病毒引发，但也有十几个其他致癌毒株可以感染那些防护能力有限或没有防护能力的患者。未来针对致癌性 HPV 毒株的 HPV 疫苗将会覆盖更广阔的国家或地区。因此，努力改进现有 HPV 疫苗有更多优势。

已有几种方法用于下一代的预防性 HPV 疫苗，具体包括：①更多的基于 VLP 的多价疫苗；②基于 L1 的衣壳蛋白；③基于 L2 的疫苗；④L1-L2 嵌合疫苗。图 12-1 总结了当前的各种策略，以及下一代预防性 HPV 疫苗。多价 VLP 疫苗建立在最初的将二价和四价疫苗（Cervarix™ 和 Gardasil®）商业化的想法上。如果高风险型 HPV-16 和 HPV-18 的病毒株 VLP 具有保护性，那么为什么不增加更多的 VLP 来拓宽覆盖面？目前，比较 VLP 疫苗（没有价的区分）和四价疫苗的试验正在进行（Merck 2011）。增加更多的 VLP 可能会增加生产成本；然而，有好几项工作已在细菌体内高效生产 HPV VLP。

另一个新的预防性疫苗其开发的潜在途径涉及创建 L1 衣壳蛋白疫苗——潜在的成本效益替代型 VLP 疫苗。衣壳蛋白是病毒衣壳的基本结构部件，而 HPV 的 L1 VLP 由 360 拷贝的 L1 蛋白组成，装配一个五价衣壳体只需要 5 个单体。此

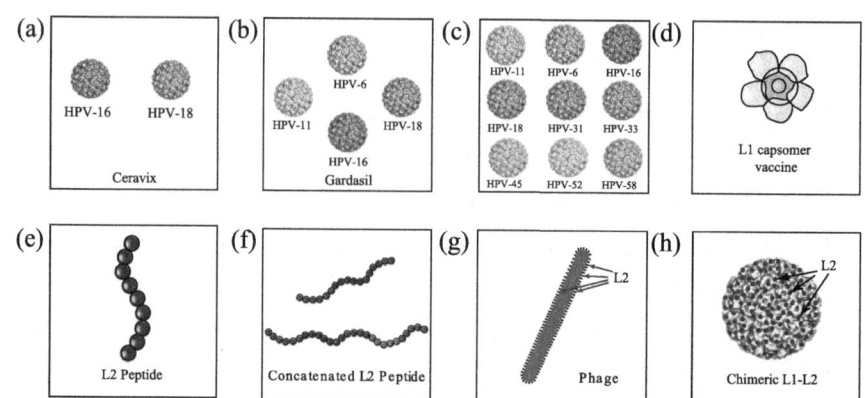

图 12-1　下一代预防性 HPV 疫苗的示意图。（a）由 HPV-16 和 HPV-18 VLP 组成的疫苗。（b）由 HPV-6、HPV-11、HPV-16 和 HPV-18 VLP 组成的加德西（Gardasil）。（c）由 HPV-6、HPV-11、HPV-16、HPV-18、HPV-31、HPV-33、HPV-45、HPV-52 和 HPV-58 VLP 组成的多价 VLP 疫苗。（d）L1 衣壳疫苗。（e）L2 肽疫苗。（f）多个 L2 肽连接的疫苗。（g）L2 的噬菌体表面展示疫苗。（h）表面表达 L2 的嵌合 L1-L2 VLP 疫苗。

外，这些衣壳蛋白可在细菌体内产生，因此比在昆虫或酵母细胞中产生 VLP 成本更低。在临床前模型中，大肠杆菌、重组麻疹病毒或重组沙门氏菌中制成的 L1 衣壳蛋白已成功诱导保护性抗体，这些遗传修饰的活疫苗可能是降低成本的另一种方法，并可能降低免疫接种的次数（Chen et al. 2000；Fraillery et al. 2007；Li et al. 1997；Rose et al. 1998）。

开发第二代预防性疫苗的另一种方法涉及用 L2 的 VLP 代替 L1 的 VLP。在不同类型的 HPV 中 L2 是高度保守的，一个 HPV 毒株上的 L2 很可能通过交叉中和抗体甚至交叉物种诱导更广泛的预防效应。已经表明，在动物免疫中，大肠杆菌中产生 L2 的氨基末端肽产生中和抗体，保护动物对体内同源乳头瘤病毒的攻击（Embers et al. 2002；Gaukroger et al. 1996）、对体外具有交叉中和的异源类型病毒（Kawana et al. 1999；Pastrana et al. 2005；Roden et al. 2000）的攻击，并赋予体内交叉保护作用（Gambhira et al. 2007）。

L2 也被用于其他形式。在临床前期试验中，串联的、多类型的 L2 融合蛋白在不同的组合中使用[3 种 HPV 型（6、16 和 18）的 L2 11~200 残基，5 种 HPV 型（1、5、6、16 和 18）的 L2 11~88 残基，或 5 个皮肤型、2 个黏膜低风险型及 15 种致癌性 HPV 的 L2 17~36 残基]（Jagu et al. 2009）。在小鼠和兔体内用级联多类型的 L2 与不同佐剂进行接种，比仅用 HPV-16 的氨基末端的 L2 多肽、HPV-16 的 L1 VLP、疫苗株 Gardasil，或阴性对照接种能引起更高的中和抗体滴度（Jagu et al. 2009）。接种这些级联多类型 L2 融合蛋白的小鼠 4 个月后也具有挑战 HPV-16

假病毒的免疫力。此外，HPV-16 的 L2 肽能够产生抵消 HPV-18、31、45 和 58 的抗血清，从而证实了 L2 的交叉反应（Jagu et al. 2009）。通常，L2 的免疫原性低于 L1，这种限制促使 Tumban 等于 2011 年创建了含有 PP7 噬菌体的 VLP 疫苗，此疫苗表现出 8 个不同 HPV 类型的 L2 蛋白质的中和表位（Tumban et al. 2011）。接种展示 PP7 的 HPV-16 L2 肽疫苗两次和接种展示 PP7 的 HPV-18 L2 肽疫苗能激活产生广谱抗 L2 IgG 的几何平均滴度为 $10^4 \sim 10^5$。此外，这些抗 L2 的抗体可以防护阴道对 HPV-16 或 HPV-18 假病毒的攻击，以及与合成工程化的 HPV L2 肽的交叉反应（Tumban et al. 2011）。尽管它们可能有更大的交叉反应性，但 L2 蛋白的免疫原性低，因此目前正在探讨更有效的佐剂和抗原展示技术。

L1 疫苗的高度免疫原性和 L2 介导的广泛的交叉保护作用的优势使二者可以嵌合型 L1-L2 VLP 的形式组合。L2 是一个主要在病毒颗粒内部发现的不太丰富的蛋白质，通常用 L1 免疫表位可替换 VLP 表面的一些区域，能产生更多的免疫原性，以及对多种基因型 HPV 的交叉保护免疫反应。嵌合体模型中，L2 中和表位在 L1 VLP 表面的表达很关键，因为在其 VLP 内正常位置表达的 L1 和 L2 不会引起 L2 抗体的产生。嵌合了 L2 肽的 L1-L2 VLP 的兔，不仅可以诱导中和 HPV-16 抗体，还可以产生 HPV-18、31、52、58 假病毒的交叉中和抗体（Kondo et al. 2008）。此外，接种了嵌合型 HPV-16 L1-L2 VLP 疫苗的兔和鼠也表现出对 HPV-16 进化来的高风险和低风险型的交叉中和反应（Schellenbacher et al. 2009）。将 L2 的免疫中和表位嵌入 L1 VLP，将使下一代预防性 HPV 疫苗诱导抗 HPV 的广谱中和抗体具有广阔的应用前景。

4 治疗性疫苗的临床开发策略

4.1 治疗性疫苗的概念和目标

HPV 预防性疫苗尽管可以有效阻断 HPV 感染，但不能消除已有的 HPV 感染或 HPV 相关性损伤，因此没有治疗作用（Lin et al. 2010）。鉴于几乎所有的宫颈癌都是由高危型 HPV 引起的事实，靶向 HPV 的治疗性疫苗极有可能通过免疫治疗来高度特异性地消除 HPV 感染的细胞和 HPV 相关性肿瘤。如前面章节所讨论的，潜伏的 HPV 感染进展到浸润癌需要很多年，幸运的是，大多数女性清除了感染。但是，如果患有高级别 CIN 病变的妇女因症状不明显而且没经过筛查，她们可能不知道肿瘤正在她们的子宫颈内发展。在持续的慢性感染中，有一个相当大的窗口是对细胞学筛查/HPV DNA 检测之后发现的感染进行的二次预防性治疗。在肿瘤进展的长时间内，非常需要能主动攻击 HPV 感染细胞的有效治疗性 HPV 疫苗，以预防恶性肿瘤的发展并进行治疗。如果治疗性疫苗可消除早期转化的细胞，HPV 相关的恶性肿瘤经过侵入性治疗引起的发病率和死亡率可能会大幅减少。

许多不同的平台已用于治疗性 HPV 疫苗的研发，每个都在测试和临床试验的不同阶段。为比较各种候选疫苗的应用可能性，研究者必须牢记理想的治疗性疫苗的特性。具体包括：①安全性；②触发有效的 HPV 抗原特异性细胞毒性 T 细胞介导的靶向病变组织的能力；③针对肿瘤细胞的特异性；④反应功效的持续时间长；⑤批量生产和存储成本更低；⑥所需剂量较少。治疗性疫苗触发特异性 T 细胞介导的杀伤能力对于疫苗靶向转化细胞而非健康细胞的功效是非常重要的。生产和储存成本的降低是一个非常吸引人的特点，这将在全球范围内让更多的肿瘤患者得到治疗。目前，能按市售二价或四价疫苗的要求开始并且完成所有三次注射的患者只有约 25%[综述见 Trimble and Frazer（2009）]。因此，传送过程的简单化将大大增加治疗性疫苗的坚持使用率。

正如前面所提到的，E6 和 E7 是治疗性疫苗的理想靶点。已经研究和开发了很多治疗性 HPV 疫苗，包括基于活载体、多肽、蛋白质、树突状细胞、DNA，以及靶向 E6 和/或 E7 抗原的联合疫苗。

4.2 基于活载体的治疗性 HPV 疫苗

活载体疫苗的概念包括细菌和病毒载体的使用，从而有效地感染宿主细胞，并为抗原提呈细胞提供 E6 和/或 E7 抗原。已经探索了好几个细菌载体用于治疗性 HPV 疫苗，其中革兰氏阳性的产单核细胞李氏菌，人们已经对其产生了浓厚的兴趣，因为它能够利用孔形成毒素李斯特菌融胞素 O（LLO）侵入巨噬细胞并藏在吞噬体内部，从而逃避吞噬作用。来自产单核细胞李氏菌感染的抗原在两个 MHC（Ⅰ类和Ⅱ类）途径都可以加工。基于产单核细胞李氏菌的 HPV E7 疫苗已经显示出可以刺激更多的 E7 特异性的 $CD8^+$ T 细胞，可治疗转基因小鼠和野生型小鼠的实体瘤（Gunn et al. 2001；Hussain and Paterson 2004；Sewell et al. 2004；Souders et al. 2007）。这一研究已经向临床试验转化。ADXS11-001，以前称为 Lovaxin C 或 Lm-LLO-E7，是一种活的、可分泌 HPV-16 E7 并融合至 LLO 的致弱产单核细胞李氏菌载体。在Ⅰ期试验中，ADXS11-001 使用的剂量限制在只出现流感样症状的毒性，被认为是安全的，而且可接受性良好（Maciag et al. 2009；Radulovic et al. 2009）。目前，ADXS11-001 两项注册的临床试验正在进行。一项随机的、单盲、以安慰剂为对照的Ⅱ期研究的首要目标是确定 3 剂量的 ADXS11-001 是否可以安全地逆转外科手术确定的 CIN2/3 病变（NCI 2012d）。另一项正在进行的Ⅱ期临床试验涉及测试 ADXS11-001 在治疗持续或复发宫颈癌患者并提高其一年生存率的安全性和有效性（NCI 2012b）方面的作用。

除了细菌，活病毒载体因具有高免疫原性也一直在被研究。已有几个病毒载体用于提呈 HPV E7 抗原，但牛痘病毒（一种有包膜的双链 DNA 病毒，属痘病毒科家族），因其基因组大、感染性高而表现为特别有希望的病毒载体。一项 I/II 期临床试验评估了表达 HPV-16 和 HPV-18 E6/E7 抗原（TA-HPV）的重组痘病毒疫苗，试验的肿瘤包括早期宫颈癌（Kaufmann et al. 2002）、晚期宫颈癌（Borysiewicz et al. 1996）、外阴上皮内瘤样病变（Davidson et al. 2003）及阴道上皮内肿瘤（Baldwin et al. 2003）。TA-HPV 被认为可以安全而有效地刺激牛痘病毒特异性抗体和 HPV 抗原特异性 CTL 反应（Adams et al. 2001；Borysiewicz et al. 1996；Kaufmann et al. 2002）。

另一个基于牛痘病毒的治疗性 HPV 疫苗是 MVA-E2——一个细长的、编码牛乳头瘤病毒型 1（BPV-1）E2 的重组痘病毒（Corona Gutierrez et al. 2004）。在一项 I/II 期临床试验中，4 倍宫内剂量的 MVA E2 对 CIN 病变的患者有显著作用。据报道，36 个受试者中有 34 个表现 CIN 病变完全消退，而其他 2 个受试者的病变级别从 CIN3 降低到 CIN1（Corona Gutierrez et al. 2004）。几种可能的解释也许可以说明观察到的治疗效果。第一，在感染的早期阶段，例如，CIN 病变时受感染细胞中 HPV 的基因组还没有被整合到宿主基因组中，感染的细胞仍然可以在其表面表达 E2 抗原肽，进一步使通过治疗处理产生的 E2 特异性 CTL，得到磨炼和获得攻击能力。但是，目前尚不清楚 CIN 病变受感染的细胞通过 MVA-E2 治疗产生的 BPV-1 E2 特异性 CTL 是否能够识别 HPV E2 靶点。第二，来自 MVA-E2 的 E2 可能充当转录抑制子来抑制 E6 和 E7 的表达。第三，高免疫原性的活载体如 MVA-E2 通过局部给药，可能激发 HPV 相关病变中的微环境产生更强的免疫应答。虽然最初的观察结果令人鼓舞，但还需要进一步的验证来建立这种控制 CIN 病变的方法。

另一种基于牛痘病毒的疫苗经过修饰改造，使用安卡拉载体以及佐剂 IL-2（TG4001/R3484）来表达 HPV-16 E6 和 E7 抗原。一项 II 期临床试验的结果认为，TG4001/R3484 在 HPV-16 阳性 CIN2/3 的妇女中的临床反应是既安全又有希望的。在试验中，10/21 女性接种半年后再也检测不到 CIN2/3。在 12 个月的随访中，观察到无复发或 HPV-16 抗原的持续存在（Brun et al. 2011）。虽然活载体疫苗已显示出可喜的结果，但它们本质上造成了潜在的安全风险，特别是对于免疫力低下的个体。活载体也可能因为重复给药而诱导载体特异性中和抗体和/或预先存在的载体特异性免疫而只能有限使用。

4.3 基于多肽的治疗性 HPV 疫苗

HPV 短肽抗原连同佐剂可以被提呈到树突状细胞，然后将这些抗原提呈到 MHC I 类分子，从而激活抗原特异性 T 细胞免疫。这些短肽疫苗的产生涉及对现有的特异性 CTL 和 HPV 抗原 CD4[+] T 辅助表位的鉴定。基于多肽疫苗稳定、易于生产，并具有较高的安全性，目前的研究重点集中在解决这些疫苗的主要缺陷，即低免疫原性和MHC限制。

基于多肽的HPV疫苗，其免疫原性可随佐剂的使用而增强，佐剂包括免疫球蛋白G片段（Qin et al. 2005）、链霉融合至鼠4-1BBL的胞外域（Sharma et al. 2009）、树突状细胞因子刺激苔藓抑素（Yan et al. 2010）和Toll样受体（TLR）激动剂（Daftarian et al. 2006；Wu et al. 2010；Zhang et al. 2010；Zwaveling et al. 2002）。例如，HPV-16的E7（氨基酸43-77），同时包含CTL和辅助T表位，佐剂为TLR9激动剂CpG寡聚脱氧核苷酸，结果显示在接种的小鼠中可激发E7特异性$CD4^+$和$CD8^+$ T细胞功能，以及产生有效的抗肿瘤效应（Zwaveling et al. 2002）。MHC限制是要克服的另一问题。由于HLA-A 0201是最常见的人类MHC I类分子，基于多肽的HPV治疗性疫苗的研究集中在HPV-16的E7 HLA-A 0201 CTL表位。一项I期临床试验发现，对HLA-A 0201特异性的HPV-16 E7多肽疫苗配以佐剂能够刺激10/16 HLA-A2阳性宫颈或外阴上皮瘤（CIN/VIN）2/3期患者的免疫应答，以及3/18 CIN病变患者症状完全消退（Muderspach et al. 2000）。然而，这些多肽疫苗仅仅对HLA-A 0201的患者有效。

长的重叠多肽包含CTL的一些HPV E6和E7蛋白的抗原表位，还提供了CD4的Th表位，因此规避了MHC限制问题。由13个代表HPV-16 E6和E7抗原组成的重叠肽的疫苗辅以佐剂能够引起终末期宫颈癌患者的广泛T细胞应答（Kenter et al. 2008）。相对于未接种疫苗的患者，具有多个抗原表位的疫苗可增加早期宫颈癌患者HPV-16特异的$CD4^+$和$CD8^+$ T细胞应答（Welters et al. 2008）。一项以非安慰剂为对照的II期临床试验证实，相同疫苗对HPV-16阳性的高级别外阴上皮瘤（VIN）具有显著的功效，一半经病理证实为HPV-16阳性的VIN3患者显示其病灶完全消退（Kenter et al. 2008）。其解释可能归因于HPV-16特异性的效应T细胞的数量与HPV-16特异性$CD4^+CD25^+Foxp3^+$调节性T细胞数量所占的比例。科学家们已经发现$Foxp3^+$ T细胞与恶性肿瘤免疫功能受损相关（Welters et al. 2010）。

4.4 基于蛋白质的疫苗

基于蛋白质的疫苗也已经被开发为宫颈癌潜在的治疗性疫苗。它们比基于活载体的疫苗更安全且优于多肽疫苗，因为它们包含结合到所有单倍型MHC I类和II类分子的表位。然而，基于蛋白质的疫苗其缺点是：免疫原性差，以产生抗体为主而不是CTL应答。科学家们对许多增加蛋白质疫苗效力的策略进行了研究，其中包括使用多样化的佐剂和融合蛋白。佐剂包括脂质体-聚阳离子-DNA（LPD）佐剂（Cui and Huang 2005）、基于皂苷的ISCOMATRIX（Frazer et al. 2004），以及Toll样受体激动剂（Kang et al. 2010）。

在临床试验中探索的几种基于蛋白质的候选治疗性HPV疫苗之一的HspE7，

是由 HPV-16 E7 与卡介苗热激蛋白（Hsp65）连接的嵌合蛋白，引起了人们极大的兴趣。在针对各型 HPV 病变的 I 和 II 期临床试验中，都发现 HspE7 具有良好的可接纳性。在一项 II 期临床试验中，有 27 例高级别肛门鳞状上皮瘤患者接种 HspE7，结果 21%的受试者病灶完全消退，71%的几乎完全消退（Goldstone et al. 2002）。在一项研究 CIN3 病变消退的 II 期临床试验中，13/58 受试者经病理检查完全消退，而 32/58 皮下注射 HspE7 疫苗的受试者病变部分消退（Einstein et al. 2007；Roman et al. 2007；Van Doorslaer et al. 2009）。然而，感染 HPV-16 与未感染 HPV-16 受试者的病变消退无显著差异，因此病变消退的确切原因不清楚（Einstein et al. 2007）。在另外的一项 II 期试验中，研究了 27 例复发性呼吸道乳头状瘤病（其中大部分由 HPV-6 和 HPV-11 引起），HspE7 使手术的间隔时间增长 93%，从而减少手术所需的频率（Derkay et al. 2005）。引起这些结果的原因可能是因为热激蛋白的非特异性免疫原性，或来自 HPV-16 的 E7 蛋白提供的针对 HPV-6 和 HPV-11 的交叉保护。

另一种基于蛋白质的疫苗 TA-CIN 也显示出对 HPV 感染有效，这是一种含 HPV-16 的 L2-E6-E7 组成的融合蛋白。最近的一项 II 期临床试验评估了给高级别 VIN 患者肌肉注射 TA-CIN 结合咪喹莫特的疗效。这种组合治疗的可接受性良好，无不良影响，并且"应答"到 HPV 相关的病变部位内部，局部出现高水平的 $CD4^+$ 和 $CD8^+$ T 细胞。结果还显示咪喹莫特增加 T 细胞浸润，导致 63%的患者在治疗一年后 VIN 病灶完全消退。此外，36%VIN 病变的患者表现出 HPV 完全清除，79%的妇女保持无症状（Daayana et al. 2010）。还需要 III 期临床试验来评估本组合方法的效果。

4.5 基于树突状细胞的疫苗

树突状细胞（DC）是专职的抗原提呈细胞，通过加工抗原并装载到抗原特异性 T 细胞而诱导适应性免疫应答。DC 可随来自体外的多肽、蛋白质或 DNA 编码抗原的变化而波动。体外制备好的 DC 被回输到体内，可激发细胞介导的免疫应答。已经证明，了解 DC 的成熟和抗原提呈对于探索 DC 作为免疫治疗手段是卓有成效的[参阅综述（Santin et al. 2005）]。

近几年出现了一些增强 DC 疫苗免疫原性和功效的策略，包括一系列佐剂如霍乱毒素（Nurkkala et al. 2010）和 Toll 样受体激动剂（Chen et al. 2010）。在一个基于 DC 的 HPV 疫苗的 I 期临床试验中，使用 HPV-16 E7 和/或 HPV-18 的 E7 蛋白评估了治疗性疫苗在确诊为早期宫颈癌患者中应用的安全性和免疫原性。将体外分离的树突状细胞装填 HPV 蛋白 E6 和 E7，重新输入患者体内后激发了特异性 T 细胞应答。受试者对三个免疫 HPV-16 E7 特定区域（氨基酸序列 46~70、47~70 及 76~98）均产生了特异性 $CD4^+$T 细胞免疫。但是，一个患者产生的 T 细胞应答是针对 E7 氨基酸 58~68 的新抗原的（Wang et al. 2009）。这个新发现的 $CD4^+$ Th 细胞表位可以在未来基于 DC 的 HPV 治疗性疫苗策略，以及在基于多肽的 HPV 疫苗中应用。

4.6 基于 DNA 的疫苗

在不同形式的治疗性 HPV 疫苗中，DNA 疫苗因其安全、稳定和简单等特性已引起人们的注意。DNA 疫苗接种需要将编码兴趣抗原的质粒 DNA 导入宿主细胞。所编码抗原的表达可引起针对编码抗原的细胞和/或体液免疫应答。DNA 疫苗相比活载体如细菌或病毒，具有较小的急性安全风险，但其整合仍然是一个潜在问题。裸 DNA 相对容易生产，并且在靶细胞内维持抗原表达的时间较长。此外，DNA 疫苗不会像活载体疫苗那样产生中和抗体，因此能够重复操作给药。然而，DNA 疫苗的免疫原性有限，需要改善提呈到目标树突状细胞（DC）的策略，即使用抗原特异性免疫应答的强效激活剂。一般情况下，这些策略可以分为：①增加抗原表达/负载抗原的 DC 的数目；②改善 HPV 抗原的表达、加工和在 DC 中的呈现；③提高 DC 和 T 细胞的相互作用[参阅综述（Lin et al. 2010）]。

增加抗原表达或负载抗原的 DC 数目的策略包括通过基因枪、微胶囊和电穿孔等方法增强 DNA 疫苗的配送方式。特别令人感兴趣的是 ZYC101，它是一种编码 HPV-16 的 E7 HLA-A2 限制性多肽的质粒，包被在聚乳酸共乙交酯（PLG）构成的微粒中。一项 I 期临床试验表明，ZYC101 使 5/15 患者产生完全的组织学回归，在 11/15 患者中有显著的 HPV 特异性 T 细胞反应且无严重不良反应（Sheets et al. 2003）。一个最近的研究显示，ZYC101a（编码 HPV-16 和 HPV-18 E6 及 E7 的抗原多肽的一种质粒）在一项涉及 127 例高级别 CIN 的 II 期临床试验中得到应用。该疫苗的可接受性良好，相比安慰剂组（70% vs. 23%），可以促进 2/3 的 CIN 患者（年龄低于 25 岁）的分辨力（Garcia et al. 2004）。最近，一项 ZYC101a 的 II 期临床试验涉及 21 例 CIN2/3，结果表明有 11 例 $CD8^+$ T 细胞对 HPV-16 和 HPV-18 的反应升高了；然而在 CIN 损伤清除方面，安慰剂组和免疫组之间并无显著差异（Matijevic et al. 2011）。

除了 DNA 疫苗微胶囊，肌内注射加之随后的电穿孔也被证实为一种配送方式（Inovio 2012）。VGX-3100 是一种用包含针对 HPV-16/18 E6 和 E7 蛋白的质粒制备的 DNA 疫苗，通过肌内注射提呈，然后在接种区域使用装置进行电穿孔。在一项高级别 CIN 病变的 I 期临床试验中，VGX-3100 能在 13/18 患者中引起 T 细胞应答。目前，一个双盲、随机、以安慰剂为对照的 II 期临床试验正在招募经组织学确定为 HPV-16/18 相关的高级别 CIN 患者（Inovio 2012）。

在提高抗原提呈到 DC 方面，DNA 疫苗提呈的不同方式正在各种临床试验中进行测试。目前，一项头对头的、使用三种不同给药途径的 DNA 疫苗的免疫原性比较试验正在招募 HPV-16⁺的 CIN2/3 女性患者。在该疫苗中，钙网蛋白编码 DNA 与非致瘤形式的 HPV-16 E7 连接在一起[称为 pNGVL4a-CRT/ E7（detox）]。受试者将被分组，通过基因枪在皮内、肌内或子宫颈病灶内注射不同剂量的相同疫苗，比较它们产生 HPV-16 E7 抗原特异性免疫应答的能力和治疗效果（NCI 2012c）。

另一种提高 DNA 疫苗功效的策略是将 HPV 抗原与能够靶向专职抗原提呈细胞的分子连接起来，改善这种连接抗原的相互激活作用。热激蛋白 70 就是一种这样的分子。一项 I 期临床试验在 15 例高级别 CIN 受试者中研究了肌肉注射 pNGVL4a-Sig/E7（detox）/HSP70 的效果。这个 DNA 疫苗含有定位于内质网的信号编码序列，含有致弱形式的 HPV-16 E7 及 HSP70（Trimble et al. 2009）。结果表明，4/15 受试者和 5/9 接受最高剂量疫苗接种的受试者（6 个月之后）都有 HPV-16 的 E7 特异性 T 细胞应答。尽管免疫反应较弱，但 33%接种高剂量 pNGVL4a-SIG/E7（detox）/HSP70（3mg）的患者出现了组织学完全消退（Trimble et al. 2009）。同样的疫苗还在 HPV-16 阳性的头颈部肿瘤患者（20%与 HPV 感染相关）中进行了探讨（Gilison and Wu，个人交流）。这些早期临床试验证实 pNGVL4a-SIG/E7（detox）对于 HPV 引起的 CIN2/3 和头颈部肿瘤具有高安全性和低副作用。

还可以将 HPV 治疗性 DNA 疫苗与佐剂结合用于提高 DNA 疫苗的效力（Chuang et al. 2010）。已证明一个这样的佐剂，即 TLR7 激动剂咪喹莫特，能促进抗原提呈细胞的活化，诱导细胞因子的产生（干扰素 α、IL-6 和 TNF-α），并促进适应性免疫细胞的分化（Bilu and Sauder 2003）。目前，一项正在进行的 I 期临床试验在 HPV-16 阳性 CIN3 病变患者中，使用 pNGVL4a-Sig/E7（detox）/HSP70 DNA 疫苗，结合局部使用咪喹莫特和 TA-HPV 用来提升疫苗效果（NCI 2012a）。使用多个疫苗和佐剂一起进行测试，是为了产生更强的 HPV 抗原特异性免疫应答和更好的治疗效果。

4.7 联合策略

治疗性 HPV 疫苗可与其他疗法结合以提高疫苗效力。治疗性 HPV 疫苗与化疗、放疗和/或手术等方法联合可有效提高肿瘤细胞特别是微小残留病灶的治疗。例如，对钙网蛋白（CRT）编码 DNA 与 HPV-16 E7 融合的（CRT/E7）DNA、结合放疗对小鼠的治疗中，与单用 HPV DNA 疫苗或放疗相比，E7 特异性 CD8⁺ T 细胞应答，以及针对 E7 表达肿瘤的抗肿瘤效应显著增加（Tseng et al. 2009）。另一种联合疗法使用表达重组 HPV E6 和 E7 的腺病毒疫苗（Ad-p14）、联合以下系统性免疫调节试剂之一使用：咪喹莫特、CD4 抗体、α-干扰素或 GITR 抗体。在 E6/E7 表达的 TC-1 小鼠模型，将 Ad-p14 与 GITR 抗体结合使用可观察到显著的抗肿瘤效果，所有的 TC-1 肿瘤得以完全、永久性的根除（Hoffmann et al. 2010）。

化疗与治疗性 HPV DNA 疫苗结合是另一种有前途的方法。在临床前期研究中，对荷瘤小鼠使用常见化疗药物顺铂，与治疗性 HPV DNA 疫苗（CRT/E7）联合治疗。顺铂使 E7 表达的肿瘤细胞发生细胞介导的裂解，从而增加了为 T 细胞准备的 E7 抗原。结果还表明，E7 特异性 $CD8^+$ T 细胞前体（能够增殖并迁移到肿瘤位置）的数量有所增加（Tseng et al. 2008）。最近，一种抗氧化的黄酮类化合物、具抗炎和抗环氧合酶活性的化疗剂芹黄素，被用来与编码 HPV-16 E7 和热激蛋白 70（E7/ HSP70）的 DNA 疫苗联合使用（Chuang et al. 2009）。将 E7/HSP70 的 DNA 联合芹黄素注射 TC-1 荷瘤小鼠，结果证明，相比对照组，可以大大提高 E7 特异的效应性和记忆性 $CD8^+$ T 细胞的数目。用芹黄素治疗还可以剂量依赖性的方式增强肿瘤细胞的凋亡。疫苗接种和化疗最可能导致肿瘤对 E7 特异性细胞毒性免疫产生易感性，从而导致肿瘤体积减小并增加存活率（Chuang et al. 2009）。在临床前模型，化疗和/或放射疗法与治疗性 HPV 疫苗的联合应用产生了令人鼓舞的抗肿瘤效果，因此值得 HPV 相关性恶性肿瘤患者进行未来的测试。

5　小结

HPV 感染令人难以置信地在世界各地普遍存在，因此，开发有效、特异、可用的控制 HPV 感染及其恶性转化的方法具有挑战性。目前市售的预防性疫苗代表 HPV 研究领域的重大成功。然而，在以下宫颈癌的控制方面仍然有很大的改进空间：①制造更广谱、成本低、单剂量、热稳定，以及可广泛获得的预防性疫苗；②应用关于 HPV 感染的免疫学知识来构建有效的 HPV 治疗性疫苗。各种创新策略已经用于开发治疗性 HPV 疫苗，这促成了多个 I/II 期临床试验的开展。要确定合适的治疗性 HPV 候选疫苗来控制已确定的 HPV 感染和 HPV 相关性损伤，进一步推进这些试验是非常重要的。对高级别 HPV 相关性恶性肿瘤的控制将最有可能使用治疗性 HPV 疫苗与常规的如外科手术、化疗和放射治疗相结合的联合治疗法。毫无疑问，预防性和治疗性 HPV 疫苗的进展每年可救助数以亿计暴露于 HPV 的个体。

（杨静，卢建红　译）

参 考 文 献

Adams M, Borysiewicz L, Fiander A, Man S, Jasani B, Navabi H, Lipetz C, Evans AS, Mason M (2001) Clinical studies of human papilloma vaccines in pre-invasive and invasive cancer. Vaccine 19:2549–2556

Baldwin PJ, van der Burg SH, Boswell CM, Offringa R, Hickling JK, Dobson J, Roberts JS,

Latimer JA, Moseley RP, Coleman N et al (2003) Vaccinia-expressed human papillomavirus 16 and 18 e6 and e7 as a therapeutic vaccination for vulval and vaginal intraepithelial neoplasia. Clin Cancer Res 9:5205–5213

Bilu D, Sauder DN (2003) Imiquimod: modes of action. Br J Dermatol 149(Suppl 66):5–8

Borysiewicz LK, Fiander A, Nimako M, Man S, Wilkinson GW, Westmoreland D, Evans AS, Adams M, Stacey SN, Boursnell ME et al (1996) A recombinant vaccinia virus encoding human papillomavirus types 16 and 18, E6 and E7 proteins as immunotherapy for cervical cancer. Lancet 347:1523–1527

Brooks G, Carroll KC, Butel JS, Morse SA, Mietzneron TA (eds) (2010) Jawetz, Melnick, & Adelberg's Medical Microbiology, 25th edn. McGraw-Hill Medical, New York

Brun JL, Dalstein V, Leveque J, Mathevet P, Raulic P, Baldauf JJ, Scholl S, Huynh B, Douvier S, Riethmuller D et al (2011) Regression of high-grade cervical intraepithelial neoplasia with TG4001 targeted immunotherapy. Am J Obstet Gynecol 204:161–168

Campo MS, Roden RB (2010) Papillomavirus prophylactic vaccines: established successes, new approaches. J Virol 84:1214–1220

Chaturvedi AK, Engels EA, Pfeiffer RM, Hernandez BY, Xiao W, Kim E, Jiang B, Goodman MT, Sibug-Saber M, Cozen W et al (2011) Human papillomavirus and rising oropharyngeal cancer incidence in the United States. J Clin Oncol 29:4294–4301

Chen XS, Garcea RL, Goldberg I, Casini G, Harrison SC (2000) Structure of small virus-like particles assembled from the L1 protein of human papillomavirus 16. Mol Cell 5:557–567

Chen XZ, Mao XH, Zhu KJ, Jin N, Ye J, Cen JP, Zhou Q, Cheng H (2010) Toll like receptor agonists augment HPV 11 E7-specific T cell responses by modulating monocyte-derived dendritic cells. Arch Dermatol Res 302:57–65

Chuang CM, Monie A, Wu A, Hung CF (2009) Combination of apigenin treatment with therapeutic HPV DNA vaccination generates enhanced therapeutic antitumor effects. J Biomed Sci 16:49

Chuang CM, Monie A, Hung CF, Wu TC (2010) Treatment with imiquimod enhances antitumor immunity induced by therapeutic HPV DNA vaccination. J Biomed Sci 17:32

Corona Gutierrez CM, Tinoco A, Navarro T, Contreras ML, Cortes RR, Calzado P, Reyes L, Posternak R, Morosoli G, Verde ML et al (2004) Therapeutic vaccination with MVA E2 can eliminate precancerous lesions (CIN 1, CIN 2, and CIN 3) associated with infection by oncogenic human papillomavirus. Hum Gene Ther 15:421–431

Cui Z, Huang L (2005) Liposome-polycation-DNA (LPD) particle as a carrier and adjuvant for protein-based vaccines: therapeutic effect against cervical cancer. Cancer Immunol Immunother 54:1180–1190

Daayana S, Elkord E, Winters U, Pawlita M, Roden R, Stern PL, Kitchener HC (2010) Phase II trial of imiquimod and HPV therapeutic vaccination in patients with vulval intraepithelial neoplasia. Br J Cancer 102:1129–1136

Daftarian P, Mansour M, Benoit AC, Pohajdak B, Hoskin DW, Brown RG, Kast WM (2006) Eradication of established HPV 16-expressing tumors by a single administration of a vaccine composed of a liposome-encapsulated CTL-T helper fusion peptide in a water-in-oil emulsion. Vaccine 24:5235–5244

Davidson EJ, Boswell CM, Sehr P, Pawlita M, Tomlinson AE, McVey RJ, Dobson J, Roberts JS, Hickling J, Kitchener HC et al (2003) Immunological and clinical responses in women with vulval intraepithelial neoplasia vaccinated with a vaccinia virus encoding human papillomavirus 16/18 oncoproteins. Cancer Res 63:6032–6041

Derkay CS, Smith RJ, McClay J, van Burik JA, Wiatrak BJ, Arnold J, Berger B, Neefe JR (2005) HspE7 treatment of pediatric recurrent respiratory papillomatosis: final results of an open-label trial. Ann Otol Rhinol Laryngol 114:730–737

Dillner J, Kjaer SK, Wheeler CM, Sigurdsson K, Iversen OE, Hernandez-Avila M, Perez G, Brown DR, Koutsky LA, Tay EH et al (2010) Four year efficacy of prophylactic human papillomavirus quadrivalent vaccine against low grade cervical, vulvar, and vaginal intraepithelial neoplasia and anogenital warts: randomised controlled trial. BMJ 341:c3493

DiMaio D, Mattoon D (2001) Mechanisms of cell transformation by papillomavirus E5 proteins. Oncogene 20:7866–7873

Echelman D, Feldman S (2012) Management of cervical precancers: a global perspective. Hematol Oncol Clin North Am 26:31–44

Einstein MH, Kadish AS, Burk RD, Kim MY, Wadler S, Streicher H, Goldberg GL, Runowicz CD (2007) Heat shock fusion protein-based immunotherapy for treatment of cervical intraepithelial neoplasia III. Gynecol Oncol 106:453–460

Einstein MH, Baron M, Levin MJ, Chatterjee A, Edwards RP, Zepp F, Carletti I, Dessy FJ, Trofa AF, Schuind A et al (2009) Comparison of the immunogenicity and safety of Cervarix and Gardasil human papillomavirus (HPV) cervical cancer vaccines in healthy women aged 18–45 years. Hum Vaccin 5:705–719

Einstein MH, Baron M, Levin MJ, Chatterjee A, Fox B, Scholar S, Rosen J, Chakhtoura N, Meric D, Dessy FJ et al (2011) Comparative immunogenicity and safety of human papillomavirus (HPV)-16/18 vaccine and HPV-6/11/16/18 vaccine: Follow-up from Months 12–24 in a Phase III randomized study of healthy women aged 18–45 years. Hum Vaccin 7:1343–1358

Embers ME, Budgeon LR, Pickel M, Christensen ND (2002) Protective immunity to rabbit oral and cutaneous papillomaviruses by immunization with short peptides of L2, the minor capsid protein. J Virol 76:9798–9805

Fraillery D, Baud D, Pang SY, Schiller J, Bobst M, Zosso N, Ponci F, Nardelli-Haefliger D (2007) Salmonella enterica serovar Typhi Ty21a expressing human papillomavirus type 16 L1 as a potential live vaccine against cervical cancer and typhoid fever. Clin Vaccine Immunol 14:1285–1295

Frazer IH, Quinn M, Nicklin JL, Tan J, Perrin LC, Ng P, O'Connor VM, White O, Wendt N, Martin J et al (2004) Phase 1 study of HPV16-specific immunotherapy with E6E7 fusion protein and ISCOMATRIX adjuvant in women with cervical intraepithelial neoplasia. Vaccine 23:172–181

Gambhira R, Karanam B, Jagu S, Roberts JN, Buck CB, Bossis I, Alphs H, Culp T, Christensen ND, Roden RB (2007) A protective and broadly cross-neutralizing epitope of human papillomavirus L2. J Virol 81:13927–13931

Garcia F, Petry KU, Muderspach L, Gold MA, Braly P, Crum CP, Magill M, Silverman M, Urban RG, Hedley ML et al (2004) ZYC101a for treatment of high-grade cervical intraepithelial neoplasia: a randomized controlled trial. Obstet Gynecol 103:317–326

Gaukroger JM, Chandrachud LM, O'Neil BW, Grindlay GJ, Knowles G, Campo MS (1996) Vaccination of cattle with bovine papillomavirus type 4 L2 elicits the production of virus-neutralizing antibodies. J Gen Virol 77:1577–1583

Giuliano AR, Palefsky JM, Goldstone S, Moreira ED Jr, Penny ME, Aranda C, Vardas E, Moi H, Jessen H, Hillman R et al (2011) Efficacy of quadrivalent HPV vaccine against HPV Infection and disease in males. N Engl J Med 364:401–411

Goldstone SE, Palefsky JM, Winnett MT, Neefe JR (2002) Activity of HspE7, a novel immunotherapy, in patients with anogenital warts. Dis Colon Rectum 45:502–507

Gunn GR, Zubair A, Peters C, Pan ZK, Wu TC, Paterson Y (2001) Two Listeria monocytogenes vaccine vectors that express different molecular forms of human papilloma virus-16 (HPV-16) E7 induce qualitatively different T cell immunity that correlates with their ability to induce regression of established tumors immortalized by HPV-16. J Immunol 167:6471–6479

Hoffmann C, Stanke J, Kaufmann AM, Loddenkemper C, Schneider A, Cichon G (2010) Combining T-cell vaccination and application of agonistic anti-GITR mAb (DTA-1) induces complete eradication of HPV oncogene expressing tumors in mice. J Immunother 33:136–145 Hung CF, Wu TC (2003) Improving DNA vaccine potency via modification of professional antigen presenting cells. Curr Opin Mol Ther 5:20–24

Hussain SF, Paterson Y (2004) CD4+CD25+ regulatory T cells that secrete TGFbeta and IL-10 are preferentially induced by a vaccine vector. J Immunother 27:339–346

Inovio (2012) A study of VGX-3100 DNA vaccine with electroporation in patients with cervical intraepithelial neoplasia grade 2/3 or 3 (HPV-003). http://clinicaltrials.gov/ct2/show/NCT01304524?term=NCT01304524&rank=1

Jagu S, Karanam B, Gambhira R, Chivukula SV, Chaganti RJ, Lowy DR, Schiller JT, Roden RB (2009) Concatenated multitype L2 fusion proteins as candidate prophylactic pan-human papillomavirus vaccines. J Natl Cancer Inst 101:782–792

Jemal A, Bray F, Center MM, Ferlay J, Ward E, Forman D (2011) Global cancer statistics. CA Cancer J Clin 61:69–90

Kang TH, Monie A, Wu LS, Pang X, Hung CF, Wu TC (2010) Enhancement of protein vaccine potency by in vivo electroporation mediated intramuscular injection. Vaccine 29:1082–1089

Kaufmann AM, Stern PL, Rankin EM, Sommer H, Nuessler V, Schneider A, Adams M, Onon TS, Bauknecht T, Wagner U et al (2002) Safety and immunogenicity of TA-HPV, a recombinant vaccinia virus expressing modified human papillomavirus (HPV)-16 and HPV-18 E6 and E7 genes, in women with progressive cervical cancer. Clin Cancer Res 8:3676–3685

Kawana K, Yoshikawa H, Taketani Y, Yoshiike K, Kanda T (1999) Common neutralization epitope in minor capsid protein L2 of human papillomavirus types 16 and 6. J Virol 73:6188–6190

Kenter GG, Welters MJ, Valentijn AR, Lowik MJ, Berends-van der Meer DM, Vloon AP, Drijfhout JW, Wafelman AR, Oostendorp J, Fleuren GJ et al (2008) Phase I immunotherapeutic trial with long peptides spanning the E6 and E7 sequences of high-risk human papillomavirus 16 in end-stage cervical cancer patients shows low toxicity and robust immunogenicity. Clin Cancer Res 14:169–177

Kenter GG, Welters MJ, Valentijn AR, Lowik MJ, Berends-van der Meer DM, Vloon AP, Essahsah F, Fathers LM, Offringa R, Drijfhout JW et al (2009) Vaccination against HPV-16 oncoproteins for vulvar intraepithelial neoplasia. N Engl J Med 361:1838–1847

Kondo K, Ochi H, Matsumoto T, Yoshikawa H, Kanda T (2008) Modification of human papillomavirus-like particle vaccine by insertion of the cross-reactive L2-epitopes. J Med Virol 80:841–846

Kwak K, Yemelyanova A, Roden RB (2010) Prevention of cancer by prophylactic human papillomavirus vaccines. Curr Opin Immunol 23:244–251

Lehtinen M, Paavonen J, Wheeler CM, Jaisamrarn U, Garland SM, Castellsague X, Skinner SR, Apter D, Naud P, Salmeron J et al (2012) Overall efficacy of HPV-16/18 AS04-adjuvanted vaccine against grade 3 or greater cervical intraepithelial neoplasia: 4-year end-of-study analysis of the randomised, double-blind PATRICIA trial. Lancet Oncol 13:89–99

Li M, Cripe TP, Estes PA, Lyon MK, Rose RC, Garcea RL (1997) Expression of the human papillomavirus type 11 L1 capsid protein in Escherichia coli: characterization of protein domains involved in DNA binding and capsid assembly. J Virol 71:2988–2995

Lin K, Roosinovich E, Ma B, Hung CF, Wu TC (2010) Therapeutic HPV DNA vaccines. Immunol Res 47:86–112

Lowy DR, Schiller JT (2012) Reducing HPV-associated cancer globally. Cancer Prev Res (Phila) 5:18–23

Maciag PC, Radulovic S, Rothman J (2009) The first clinical use of a live-attenuated Listeria monocytogenes vaccine: a Phase I safety study of Lm-LLO-E7 in patients with advanced carcinoma of the cervix. Vaccine 27:3975–3983

Matijevic M, Hedley ML, Urban RG, Chicz RM, Lajoie C, Luby TM (2011) Immunization with a poly (lactide co-glycolide) encapsulated plasmid DNA expressing antigenic regions of HPV 16 and 18 results in an increase in the precursor frequency of T cells that respond to epitopes from HPV 16, 18, 6 and 11. Cell Immunol 270:62–69

Merck (2011) Phase III clinical trial: broad spectrum HPV (Human Papillomavirus) vaccine study in 16-to 26-year-old women (V503-001 AM2)

Muderspach L, Wilczynski S, Roman L, Bade L, Felix J, Small LA, Kast WM, Fascio G, Marty V, Weber J (2000) A phase I trial of a human papillomavirus (HPV) peptide vaccine for women with high-grade cervical and vulvar intraepithelial neoplasia who are HPV 16 positive. Clin Cancer Res 6:3406–3416

NCI (2012a) A Phase I efficacy and safety study of HPV16-specific therapeutic DNA-vaccinia vaccination in combination with topical imiquimod, in patients with HPV16+ high grade cervical dysplasia (CIN3). http://www.cancer.gov/clinicaltrials/search/view?cdrid= 617261&version=HealthProfessional&protocolsearchid=10105493

NCI (2012b) Phase II study of live-attenuated listeria monocytogenes cancer vaccine ADXS11- 001 in patients with persistent or recurrent squamous cell or non-squamous cell carcinoma of the cervix. http://cancer.gov/clinicaltrials/search/view?cdrid=691288&version= healthprofessional

NCI (2012c) A pilot study of pnGVL4a-CRT/E7 (Detox) for the treatment of patients with HPV16+ cervical intraepithelial neoplasia 2/3 (CIN2/3). http://clinicaltrials. gov/ct2/show/NCT00988559?term=trimble&rank=1

NCI (2012d) A randomized, single blind, placebo controlled phase 2 study to assess the safety of ADXS11-001 for the treatment of cervical intraepithelial neoplasia grade 2/3. http://clinicaltrials.gov/ct2/show/NCT01116245

Nurkkala M, Wassen L, Nordstrom I, Gustavsson I, Slavica L, Josefsson A, Eriksson K (2010) Conjugation of HPV16 E7 to cholera toxin enhances the HPV-specific T-cell recall responses to pulsed dendritic cells in vitro in women with cervical dysplasia. Vaccine 28:5828–5836

Pastrana DV, Gambhira R, Buck CB, Pang YY, Thompson CD, Culp TD, Christensen ND, Lowy DR, Schiller JT, Roden RB (2005) Cross-neutralization of cutaneous and mucosal Papillomavirus types with anti-sera to the amino terminus of L2. Virology 337:365–372

Qin Y, Wang XH, Cui HL, Cheung YK, Hu MH, Zhu SG, Xie Y (2005) Human papillomavirus type 16 E7 peptide(38–61) linked with an immunoglobulin G fragment provides protective immunity in mice. Gynecol Oncol 96:475–483

Radulovic S, Brankovic-Magic M, Malisic E, Jankovic R, Dobricic J, Plesinac-Karapandzic V,

Maciag PC, Rothman J (2009) Therapeutic cancer vaccines in cervical cancer: phase I study of Lovaxin-C. J Buon 14(Suppl 1):S165–S168

Roden R, Wu TC (2006) How will HPV vaccines affect cervical cancer? Nat Rev Cancer 6:753–763

Roden RB, Yutzy WHt, Fallon R, Inglis S, Lowy DR, Schiller JT (2000) Minor capsid protein of human genital papillomaviruses contains subdominant, cross-neutralizing epitopes. Virology 270:254–257

Roman LD, Wilczynski S, Muderspach LI, Burnett AF, O'Meara A, Brinkman JA, Kast WM, Facio G, Felix JC, Aldana M et al (2007) A phase II study of Hsp-7 (SGN-00101) in women with high-grade cervical intraepithelial neoplasia. Gynecol Oncol 106:558–566

Romanowski B, Schwarz TF, Ferguson LM, Peters K, Dionne M, Schulze K, Ramjattan B, Hillemanns P, Catteau G, Dobbelaere K et al (2011) Immunogenicity and safety of the HPV-16/18 AS04-adjuvanted vaccine administered as a 2-dose schedule compared to the licensed 3-dose schedule: Results from a randomized study. Hum Vaccin 7:1374–1386

Rose RC, White WI, Li M, Suzich JA, Lane C, Garcea RL (1998) Human papillomavirus type 11 recombinant L1 capsomeres induce virus-neutralizing antibodies. J Virol 72:6151–6154

Santin AD, Bellone S, Roman JJ, Burnett A, Cannon MJ, Pecorelli S (2005) Therapeutic vaccines for cervical cancer: dendritic cell-based immunotherapy. Curr Pharm Des 11:3485–3500 Schellenbacher C, Roden R, Kirnbauer R (2009) Chimeric L1–L2 virus-like particles as potential broad-spectrum human papillomavirus vaccines. J Virol 83:10085–10095

Sewell DA, Shahabi V, Gunn GR 3rd, Pan ZK, Dominiecki ME, Paterson Y (2004) Recombinant Listeria vaccines containing PEST sequences are potent immune adjuvants for the tumor-associated antigen human papillomavirus-16 E7. Cancer Res 64:8821–8825

Sharma RK, Elpek KG, Yolcu ES, Schabowsky RH, Zhao H, Bandura-Morgan L, Shirwan H (2009) Costimulation as a platform for the development of vaccines: a peptide-based vaccine containing a novel form of 4–1BB ligand eradicates established tumors. Cancer Res 69:4319–4326

Sheets EE, Urban RG, Crum CP, Hedley ML, Politch JA, Gold MA, Muderspach LI, Cole GA, Crowley-Nowick PA (2003) Immunotherapy of human cervical high-grade cervical intraepithelial neoplasia with microparticle-delivered human papillomavirus 16 E7 plasmid DNA. Am J Obstet Gynecol 188:916–926

Simard EP, Ward EM, Siegel R, Jemal A (2012) Cancers with increasing incidence trends in the United States: 1999 through 2008. CA Cancer J Clin. doi:10.3322/caac.20141

Souders NC, Sewell DA, Pan ZK, Hussain SF, Rodriguez A, Wallecha A, Paterson Y (2007) Listeria-based vaccines can overcome tolerance by expanding low avidity CD8+ T cells capable of eradicating a solid tumor in a transgenic mouse model of cancer. Cancer Immun

7:2–14

Trimble CL, Frazer IH (2009) Development of therapeutic HPV vaccines. Lancet Oncol 10:975–980

Trimble CL, Peng S, Kos F, Gravitt P, Viscidi R, Sugar E, Pardoll D, Wu TC (2009) A phase I trial of a human papillomavirus DNA vaccine for HPV16？cervical intraepithelial neoplasia 2/3. Clin Cancer Res 15:361–367

Tseng CW, Hung CF, Alvarez RD, Trimble C, Huh WK, Kim D, Chuang CM, Lin CT, Tsai YC, He L et al (2008) Pretreatment with cisplatin enhances E7-specific CD8？T-Cell-mediated antitumor immunity induced by DNA vaccination. Clin Cancer Res 14:3185–3192

Tseng CW, Trimble C, Zeng Q, Monie A, Alvarez RD, Huh WK, Hoory T, Wang MC, Hung CF, Wu TC (2009) Low-dose radiation enhances therapeutic HPV DNA vaccination in tumor-bearing hosts. Cancer Immunol Immunother 58:737–748

Tumban E, Peabody J, Peabody DS, Chackerian B (2011) A pan-HPV vaccine based on bacteriophage PP7 VLPs displaying broadly cross-neutralizing epitopes from the HPV minor capsid protein, L2. PLoS One 6:e23310

Van Doorslaer K, Reimers LL, Studentsov YY, Einstein MH, Burk RD (2009) Serological response to an HPV16 E7 based therapeutic vaccine in women with high-grade cervical dysplasia. Gynecol Oncol 116(2):208–212

Wang X, Santin AD, Bellone S, Gupta S, Nakagawa M (2009) A novel CD4 T-cell epitope described from one of the cervical cancer patients vaccinated with HPV 16 or 18 E7-pulsed dendritic cells. Cancer Immunol Immunother 58:301–308

Welters MJ, Kenter GG, Piersma SJ, Vloon AP, Lowik MJ, Berends-van der Meer DM, Drijfhout JW, Valentijn AR, Wafelman AR, Oostendorp J et al (2008) Induction of tumor-specific CD4+ and CD8+ T-cell immunity in cervical cancer patients by a human papillomavirus type 16 E6 and E7 long peptides vaccine. Clin Cancer Res 14:178–187

Welters MJ, Kenter GG, de Vos van Steenwijk PJ, Lowik MJ, Berends-van der Meer DM, Essahsah F, Stynenbosch LF, Vloon AP, Ramwadhdoebe TH, Piersma SJ et al (2010) Success or failure of vaccination for HPV16-positive vulvar lesions correlates with kinetics and phenotype of induced T-cell responses. Proc Natl Acad Sci U S A 107:11895–11899

Wheeler CM, Castellsague X, Garland SM, Szarewski A, Paavonen J, Naud P, Salmeron J, Chow SN, Apter D, Kitchener H et al (2012) Cross-protective efficacy of HPV-16/18 AS04-adjuvanted vaccine against cervical infection and precancer caused by non-vaccine oncogenic HPV types: 4-year end-of-study analysis of the randomised, double-blind PATRICIA trial. Lancet Oncol 13:100–110

Wu CY, Monie A, Pang X, Hung CF, Wu TC (2010) Improving therapeutic HPV peptide-based vaccine potency by enhancing CD4+ T help and dendritic cell activation. J Biomed Sci 17:88

Yan W, Chen WC, Liu Z, Huang L (2010) Bryostatin-I: A dendritic cell stimulator for chemokines induction and a promising adjuvant for a peptide based cancer vaccine. Cytokine 52:238–244

Zhang YQ, Tsai YC, Monie A, Hung CF, Wu TC (2010) Carrageenan as an adjuvant to enhance peptide-based vaccine potency. Vaccine 28:5212–5219

zur Hausen H (2002) Papillomaviruses and cancer: from basic studies to clinical application. Nat Rev Cancer 2:342–350

Zwaveling S, Ferreira Mota SC, Nouta J, Johnson M, Lipford GB, Offringa R, van der Burg SH, Melief CJ (2002) Established human papillomavirus type 16-expressing tumors are effectively eradicated following vaccination with long peptides. J Immunol 169:350–358

第13章 HTLV-1 与白血病：成人 T 细胞白血病发生中的病毒-细胞相互作用

Linda Zane 和 Kuan-The Jeang

摘 要 人类嗜 T 淋巴细胞白血病病毒 I 型（HTLV-1）最初是在 20 世纪 80 年代早期被发现的。该病毒是第一个被确定的与人类肿瘤有因果关系的逆转录病毒。HTLV-1 目前在全世界感染约 2000 万人。在本章中，我们将对近 30 年来有关 HTLV-1 的感染、复制、基因表达和细胞转化等方面的进展进行综述。

1 引言

HTLV-1 是第一个被鉴定的人类逆转录病毒。HTLV-1 属于逆转录病毒科慢病毒亚科的 δ 逆转录病毒属。慢病毒亚科的成员还有 HTLV-2、HTLV-3、HTLV-4（Mahieux and Gessain 2005；Mahieux and Gessain 2009）、牛白血病病毒（BLV）和类人猿 T 细胞白血病病毒（STLV）。HTLV-1 是 1980~1981 年间在对患有 T 细胞白血病（ATL）的患者进行 T 细胞分析时发现的（Poiesz et al. 1980；Hinuma et al. 1981；Miyoshi et al. 1981；Yoshida 1982；Watanabe et al. 1983；Gallo 2005）。ATL 首先在日本被报道，是一种快速致死性疾病（Takatsuki 2005）。从那时起，就已确定了 HTLV-1 与 ATL 之间的因果关系（Gallo 2005）。目前，HTLV-1 是已知的唯一与人类肿瘤直接相关的逆转录病毒。除了与肿瘤有关，该病毒也能引起炎症性疾病，如 HTLV-1 相关性骨髓病（HAM）/热带痉挛性截瘫（TSP）、眼色素层炎、传染性皮炎和肌炎（Gessain 2011；Goncalves et al. 2010）。

L. Zane _ K.-T. Jeang (✉)
Molecular Virology Section, Laboratory of Molecular Microbiology, The National Institutes of Allergy and Infectious Diseases, The National Institutes of Health, Bethesda, MD 20892-0460, USA
e-mail: KJEANG@nih.gov

2 HTLV-1 的感染

2.1 流行病学

全世界大约有 2000 万人感染 HTLV-1（Proietti et al. 2005），但该病毒在世界范围内并不是均匀分布，流行率最高的地区主要在日本南部、加勒比地区、南美和中非部分地区、中东少数聚集区和澳大利亚（Goncalves et al. 2010）。目前仍然不清楚为什么呈现这种分布（Proietti et al. 2005）。在 HTLV-1 感染的人群中，病毒经过长达 30~60 年的潜伏感染，有 2%~5% 的人会患 ATL，而大约 0.25%~5% 的人会患 HAM/TSP。感染者患 ATL 或 TSP/HAM 不受 HTLV-1 亚型的影响（Watanabe 2011；Ono et al. 1994）。实际上，尽管 HTLV-1 有 6 个亚型（A~F 亚型）的报道，但绝大多数的感染是由全球分布的 A 亚型病毒引起的。

HTLV-1 有三种传播途径：①母-婴传播，主要是通过长期的哺乳进行传播（大于 6 个月）；②性传播，主要由男性传播给女性，但并不绝对；③通过被病毒感染的淋巴细胞的血液制品传播（Goncalves et al. 2010；Matsuura et al. 2010）。男性和在儿童早期受到感染的儿童患 ATL 的风险最高（Goncalves et al. 2010；Matsuura et al. 2010）。

2.2 嗜性和受体

在体外，HTLV-1 能感染多种细胞，包括几种非淋巴肿瘤细胞系，如人成骨肉瘤细胞、肺癌细胞、宫颈癌细胞（HeLa 细胞）、人胃癌 HGC-27 细胞、人早幼粒细胞白血病 HL60 细胞，以及原代内皮细胞、单核细胞、小神经胶质细胞和乳腺上皮细胞（Clapham et al. 1983；Hayami et al. 1984；Ho et al. 1984；Hiramatsu et al. 1986；Akagi et al. 1988；LeVasseur et al. 1998）。然而在体内，HTLV-1 主要在 $CD4^+$ 和 $CD8^+$ T 淋巴细胞中被发现（Nagai et al. 2001），很少在其他类型细胞中被发现，如单核细胞、内皮细胞、髓系细胞和浆细胞样树突状细胞（Macatonia et al. 1992；Koyanagi et al. 1993；Jones et al. 2008），以及 $CD34^+$ 造血干细胞（Banerjee et al. 2008，2010；Feuer et al. 1996；Grant et al. 2002；Tripp et al. 2003，2005）。在 2003 年发现转运蛋白 GLUT1 是 HTLV-1 的受体以前，人们对 HTLV-1 进入细胞的受体知之甚少（Manel et al. 2003）。目前，从多个不同实验室发表的论文来看，实验数据支持 HTLV-1 进入细胞的模式是多受体模式的观点（图 13-1）。有三个细胞表面蛋白参与 HTLV-1 进入感染细胞：葡萄糖转运蛋白 1（GLUT1）、神经纤毛蛋白-1（NRP-1）和硫酸乙酰肝素蛋白多糖（HSPG）（Jones et al. 2011）。下面的程序可以解释 HTLV-1 如何进入细胞。首先，病毒编码的黏膜糖蛋白的表面亚单位（SU）与硫酸乙酰肝素蛋白多糖/神经纤毛蛋白-1 复合物相互作用；随后，这种分子之间的相互作用触发 SU 的空间构象发生改变，导致 SU 结合到 GLUT1 上；最后发生膜融合，使病毒进入到靶细胞中（Jones et al. 2005，2011；Pinon et al. 2003；Ghez et al. 2006；Lambert et al. 2009）。

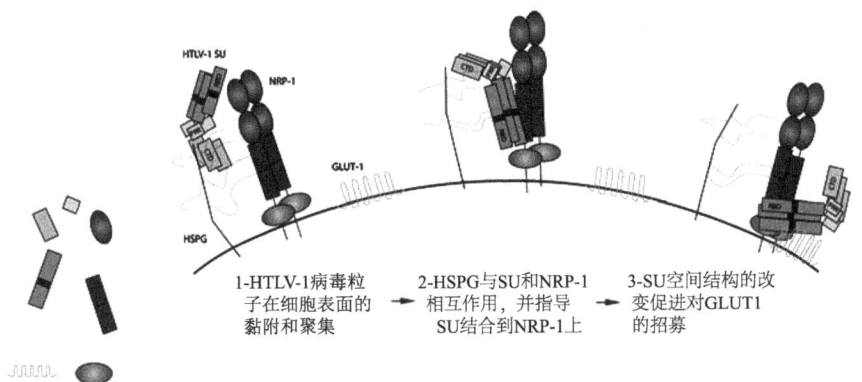

图 13-1　HTLV-1 进入细胞的多受体模式。HSPG，硫酸乙酰肝素蛋白多糖；SU，HTLV-1 黏膜糖蛋白亚单位；NRP-1，神经纤毛蛋白-1；GLUT-1，葡萄糖转运蛋白 1；CTD，C 端区；RBD，受体结合区；PRR，富脯氨酸区。此模式图引自 Jones 等（2012），并进行了修改。

2.3　病毒增殖

在细胞水平，HTLV-1 主要通过两条途径进行传播：一是通过细胞之间相互接触（水平传播）；二是通过 HTLV-1 感染的细胞克隆化扩增（垂直传播）。

2.3.1　细胞-细胞间的传播

在自然条件下，被感染的 T 淋巴细胞几乎不产生游离的病毒颗粒，并且这些无细胞的游离病毒颗粒的感染性很低。在体内，HTLV-1 在细胞之间的传播，如水平的、以逆转录为基础的复制，需要细胞之间紧密接触。至今已报道有三种传播机制（图 13-2）。第一种是 Igakura 等在 2003 年证明的"病毒学突触"的形成，包括在 HTLV-1 感染和传播的靶细胞之间的接触点，需要多种病毒的和细胞的分子参与（Igakura et al. 2003；Nejmeddine et al. 2005）。第二种是 Pais-Correia 等报道的，具体过程如下：病毒出芽后，在细胞外进行包括胶原蛋白、集聚蛋白和连接蛋白（如 tetherin 和 galectin-3）在内的病毒组装期间，HTLV-1 病毒粒子仍然停留在感染细胞的表面（Pais-Correia et al. 2010）。当 HTLV-1 病毒感染的细胞与未感染的细胞接触时，存在于感染细胞外的类似生物膜结构中的病毒颗粒会快速转移到靶细胞的表面，并导致靶细胞感染（Pais-Correia et al. 2010）。第三种模式最近由 Franchini 和他的同事证明。HTLV-1 在其 pX 区编码一种蛋白质,即 $p12^I$。在加工处理 $p12^I$ 时产生 $p8^I$,这个蛋白质通过聚集淋巴细胞功能相关抗原-1(LFA-1)增加了 T 细胞间的接触,通过 LFA-1 与细胞间的黏附分子 1(ICAM-1)相互作用,促进 T 细胞聚集,从而通过诱导形成细胞导管而增强 HTLV-1 在细胞间的传播(Van Prooyen et al. 2010;Fukumoto et al. 2009)。

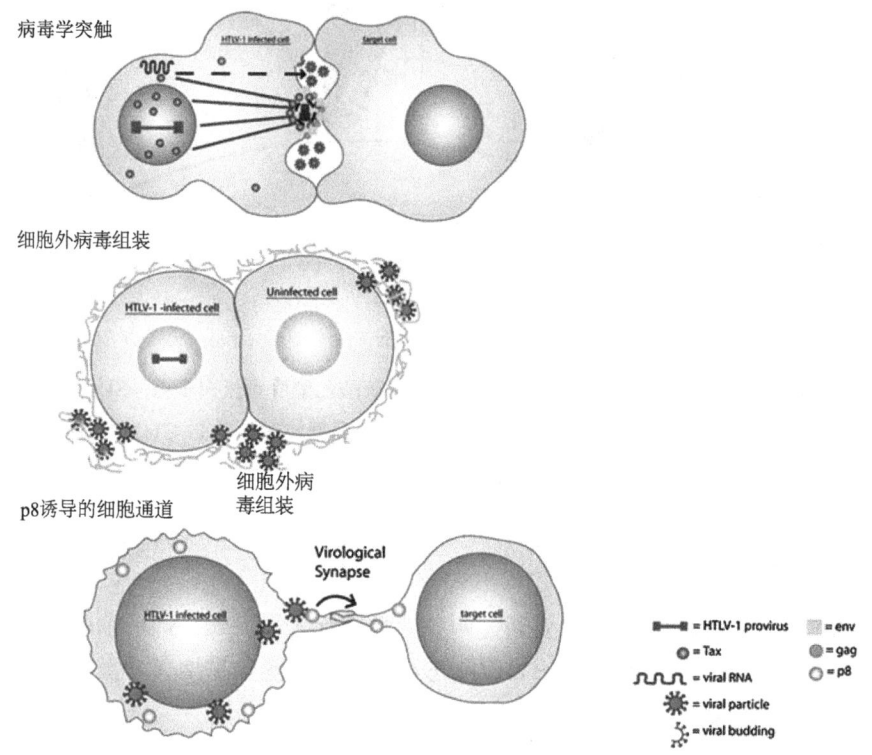

图 13-2　HTLV-1 在细胞间传播机制。此模式图引自 Yasunaga 和 Matsuoka(2011)并做了修改。

2.3.2　克隆扩增

HTLV-1 的感染与不断提高的原病毒数量、在细胞间传播率极低和病毒遗传物质稳定有关。HTLV-1 和其他 δ 逆转录病毒一样,其遗传物质的高稳定性是由于病毒的增殖通过在体内感染细胞的克隆扩增而实现(Wattel et al. 1995;Cavrois et al. 1996;Cavrois et al. 1996;Wattel et al. 1996;Zane et al. 2009)。实际上,与采用可引起错配的病毒逆转录机制不同,HTLV-1 原病毒基因组的复制是随细胞 DNA 的合成而复制。由于 HTLV-1 基因组在多数情况下随机整合到宿主基因组中,对整合位点的序列分析证明 HTLV-1 感染的细胞的增殖是克隆化的,并具有持续性（Etoh et al. 1997；Cavrois et al. 1998）。在一些动物模型中，例如，在实验中分别用 HTLV-1 和 BLV（牛白血病病毒）感染松鼠猴（*Saimiri sciureus*）和羊，结果表明，δ 逆转录病毒的感染分两步：第一步包括免疫反应建立之前的逆转录早期（早期感染）和瞬时期；第二步是感染的细胞通过克隆扩增而持续增殖（Mortreux et al. 2001；Pomier et al. 2008）。克隆化细胞存活时间长，已经发现 ATL 起源于这些出现在早期感染中的细胞克隆（Moules et al. 2005）。

2.4 病毒的基因表达

如图 13-3 所示，HTLV-1 原病毒基因组含有逆转录病毒的结构基因和非结构基因。病毒的 gag、pro、pol 和 env 基因的两端含有长的末端重复序列（LTR），有一个区域命名为 pX，位于 env 基因和 3′端 LTR 之间。5′ LTR 是病毒基因转录的启动子。Pol 基因开放阅读框编码逆转录酶、蛋白酶和整合酶。Gag 基因编码病毒粒子核心蛋白，Env 基因参与病毒的感染。pX 区含有 4 个部分重叠的开放阅读框（ORF）；利用选择性剪接和内部起始密码子，该区域编码几种调节蛋白。Orf-I 编码 $p12^I$ 蛋白，在酶解作用下，在蛋白质的氨基端进行剪切，生成 $p8^I$ 蛋白；同时，对 Orf-II 的 mRNA 进行差异化剪切，生成 $p13^{II}$ 和 $p30^{II}$ 蛋白。Orf-III 和 Orf-IV

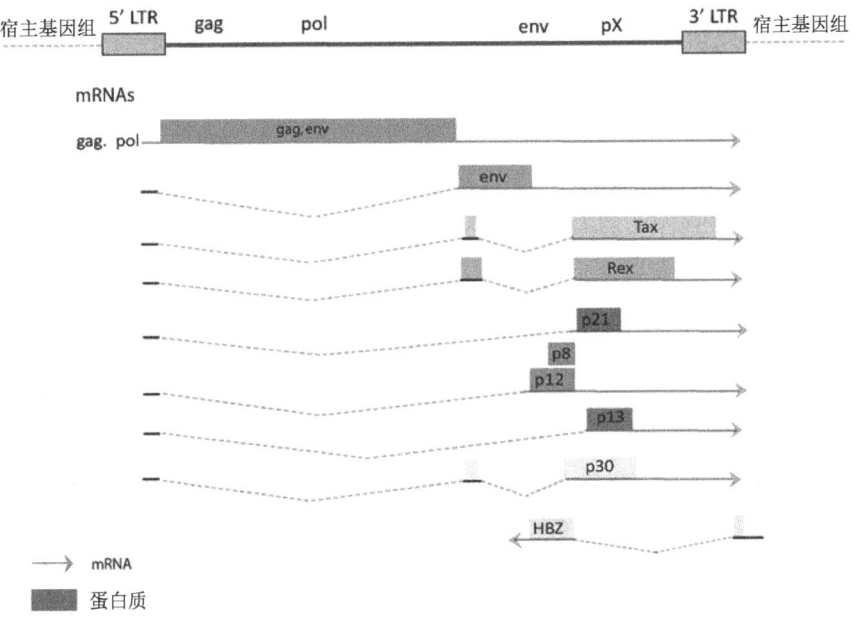

图 13-3　HTLV-1 原病毒基因组中多种剪接转录本的表达产物及其编码的阅读框。此模式图引自 Matsuoka 和 Jeang（2007），并进行了修改。

分别编码 Rex 蛋白和 Tax 蛋白，3′端的 LTR 转录生成反义 mRNA，编码 HTLV-1 的碱性亮氨酸拉链（HBZ）蛋白。下面，我们将简要讨论 Tax 和 HBZ 分别在诱导及维持白血病发生发展中的作用（Matsuoka and Jeang 2007）。

3 Tax 的表达决定 HTLV-1 感染细胞的命运

病毒癌蛋白 Tax 的表达可以使 T 细胞永生化（Grassmann et al. 1992）、使啮齿类动物细胞发生转化（Tanaka et al. 1990），以及在小鼠模型中诱导肿瘤发生（Hinrichs et al. 1987；Nerenberg et al. 1987；Green et al. 1989；Iwakura et al. 1991；Kwon et al. 2005；Hasegawa et al. 2006；Fu et al. 2011）。最近，Banerjee 等报道了人的细胞转化成白血病细胞。利用免疫缺陷的 NOD/SCID 小鼠，他们证明在注射了表达 Tax 的 CD34$^+$造血干细胞的小鼠体内检测到 CD4$^+$淋巴细胞（Banerjee et al. 2010），这提示 CD34$^+$造血祖干细胞可能是 Tax 转化的靶细胞之一，而不是目前认为的、或者可能也包括成熟的 CD4$^+$或 CD8$^+$ T 细胞。

当转化细胞生长的速度比非转化细胞快很多时，会导致肿瘤的产生。肿瘤细胞的遗传改变（染色体发生断裂损伤或非整倍性）可发生累积，并通过使细胞周期检测点失效促使这些异常改变的效应增强。肿瘤细胞还必须逃避宿主的免疫反应，以使其有效地发挥作用（Hanahan and Weinberg 2000，2011）。

在过去的 25 年中，从多个实验室获得的数据已经开始揭示出 Tax 癌蛋白在其将正常细胞转化成白血病细胞的过程中如何促使 HTLV-1 感染细胞保持生长优势、如何触发 DNA 损伤的累积以及抑制细胞周期检测点（图 13-4）。

3.1 Tax 促进 HTLV-1 感染细胞的存活和增殖

3.1.1 Tax 与细胞凋亡和衰老

如同其他肿瘤基因，Tax 具有促进细胞增殖和存活的特性（Schmitt et al. 1998；Xiao et al. 2001；Iwanaga et al. 2008）。令人感到奇怪的是，有报道称该蛋白质的表达也可以促进细胞的凋亡（Yamada et al. 1994；Chlichlia et al. 1995；Fujita and Shiku 1995；Chen et al. 1997；Hall et al. 1998；Kao et al. 2000；Nicot and Harrod 2000）和衰老（Kinjo et al. 2010；Yang et al. 2011；Zhi et al. 2011）。如果把细胞作为一个整体，可以认为 Tax 在引起细胞生长、死亡和衰老的过程中分别触发单一的信号转导事件，这样就能理解上述相互矛盾的结论。因此，在正常的有利细胞生长的生理条件下，刺激细胞生长的 Tax 信号能够促进细胞增殖。然而，在不利于细胞生长的条件下，同样的 Tax 刺激细胞增殖信号可能是启动了促细胞代谢程序，导致细胞进入了凋亡或衰老程序（Kasai and Jeang 2004）。另一个观点是，Tax

第 13 章　HTLV-1 与白血病：成人 T 细胞白血病发生中的病毒-细胞相互作用

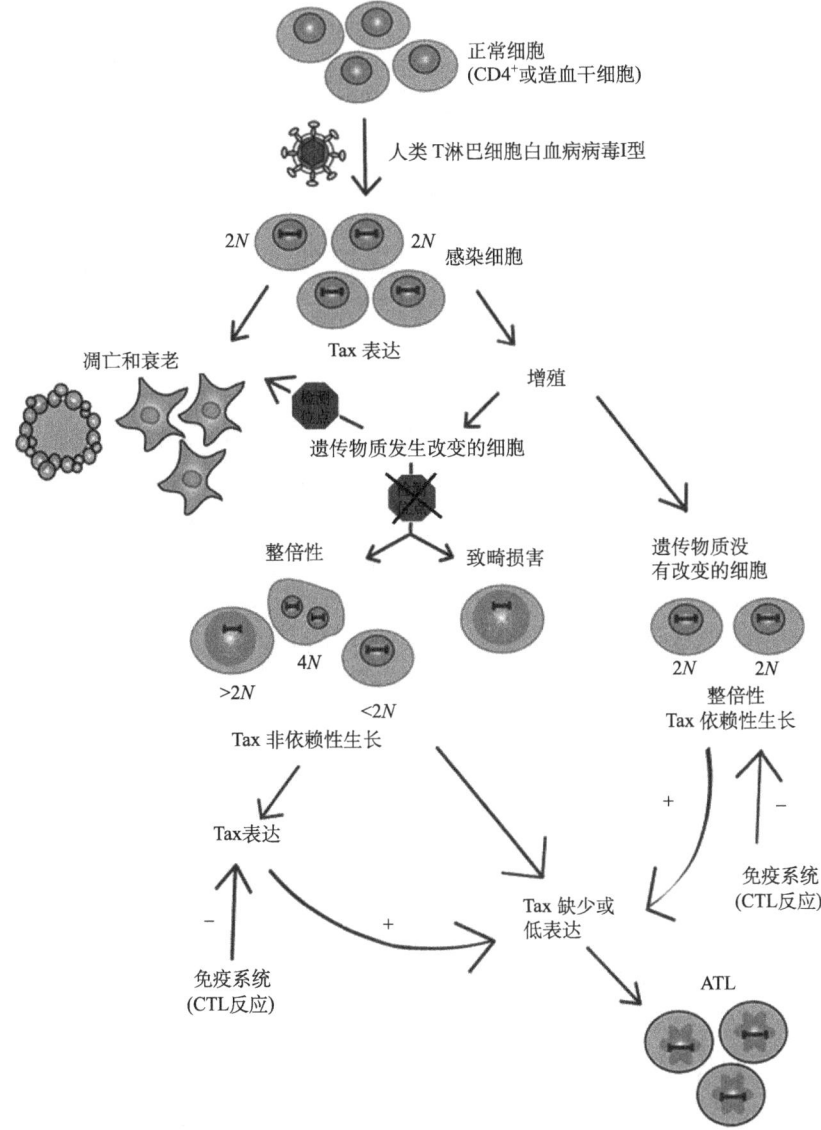

图 13-4　导致正常的造血细胞转化成 ATL 细胞的多步骤过程。这一过程包含 Tax 诱导 ATL 白血病生成的观点。本模式图引自 Matsuoka 和 Jeang（2011），并做了修改。

信号总是趋向于促细胞分化。依据细胞所处的条件决定细胞是增殖还是凋亡或衰老；同样，依据被感染细胞的状态可以引起两种不同的结果（增殖或凋亡/衰老）（Jeang 2010；Boxus and Willems 2012）。由于在 HTLV-1 感染的人中某些个体最终会患白血病和 T 细胞增生，因此，很明显，Tax 在 HTLV-1 感染的这些人体内的主要作用是促细胞增殖和抗凋亡/衰老（Copeland et al. 1994；Kishi et al. 1997；Arai et al. 1998；Mulloy et al. 1998；Kawakami et al. 1999）；而另一些人，虽然感染了 HTLV-1，但没有发展成 ATL，这可能是细胞凋亡/衰老反应占主要的缘故。在白血病生成的过程中 Tax 对一些因子，如 p53（Mulloy et al. 1998；Haoudi and Semmes 2003；Jung et al. 2008）和 NF-κB 的作用能在转化细胞中激活抗凋亡基因和抑制前凋亡基因（Kawakami et al. 1999；Tsukahara et al. 1999；Nicot et al. 2000；Mori et al. 2001；Pise-Masison et al. 2002；Krueger et al. 2006；Okamoto et al. 2006；Waldele et al. 2006）。

3.1.2　Tax 与 NF-κB

NF-κB 是 HTLV-1 作用的一个主要的细胞存活因子。NF-κB 在肿瘤细胞中持续保持活性，对其活性进行抑制可以抑制肿瘤细胞的生长（Chaturvedi et al. 2011；Perkins 2012）。尽管在正常的细胞（包括 T 细胞）中 NF-κB 活性受到严格的控制，但在转化细胞和 HTLV-1 感染的未转化细胞中可持续保持活性（Watanabe et al. 2005；Qu and Xiao 2011）。

转录因子 NF-κB 家族有 5 个紧密相关的 DNA 结合蛋白，即 RelA（p65）、RelB、c-Rel、NF-κB1/p50 和 NF-κB2/p52，这些蛋白质能形成多种同源的或异源的二聚体，能调节启动子中含 κB 结合模式基因的转录。静止或未受刺激的细胞在其细胞质中通过 kappa B 抑制因子（IκB）蛋白，如 IκBα 和 p100，阻止 NF-κB 形成二聚体。在激活状态下，IκB 被降解（经典或称标准通路）或 p100 被处理后生成 p52（非经典通路），导致 NF-κB 被激活的地点发生转移，由细胞质转移到细胞核，从而激活 NF-κB（Qu and Xiao 2011；Rauch and Ratner 2011）。在经典通路下，IκBα 需要通过对 IκB 激酶（IKK）复合物进行磷酸化，该激酶复合物由两个催化亚单位——IKKα（IKK1）和 IKKβ（IKK2）以及一个调节亚单位 IKKγ（NEMO）组成。这种磷酸化过程导致 IκBα 的快速泛素化和被蛋白酶体降解，使得 RelA（p65）和其他的 NF-κB 成员定位到细胞核，从而诱导基因表达。在 NF-κB 非经典通路下，IKKγ 能特异性地与 p100 形成复合物，使 p100 磷酸化，导致 p100 泛素化，加工成 p52，p52 与 NF-κB 结合蛋白连接，并转位至胞核，从而诱导或抑制基因的表达（Qu and Xiao 2011）。

许多研究结果表明，Tax 可以在 HTLV-1 感染细胞中同时激活 NF-κB 的经典和非经典通路（Xiao et al. 2001；Iha et al. 2003；Qu and Xiao 2011）。Tax 通过结合 IKKγ 而持续激活 IKK，导致 IκBα 降解（经典通路）（Chu et al. 1999；Harhaj and Sun 1999；Jin et al. 1999；Xiao et al. 2000）；Tax 也可以促进 IKKα-IKKγ-p100 复合物的形成，随后该复合物加工处理 NF-κB p100 前体蛋白，形成具有活性的 p52（非经典通路）（Xiao et al. 2001）。Tax 也可以结合到 NF-κB 上，增强其稳

定性和活性（Hirai et al. 1992；Suzuki et al. 1993；Suzuki et al. 1994），并使 NF-κB 抑制因子失活（Maggirwar et al. 1995；Suzuki et al. 1995；Good and Sun 1996；McKinsey et al. 1996；Petropoulos et al. 1996）。

最近，利用两种不同的 Tax 转基因小鼠模型，两个相互独立的小组研究表明 Tax 能诱导肿瘤形成依赖 NF-κB 通路，包括经典和非经典通路（Kwon et al. 2005；Fu et al. 2011）。第一个研究采用的是表达野生型 Tax 和不能激活 NF-κB 通路的突变型 Tax 的小鼠模型。表达野生型 Tax 的小鼠模型患有致死性皮肤病，该病与感染 HTLV-1 的白血病早期患者的皮肤病具有相似的特征（Kwon et al. 2005）。第二个研究发现在表达 Tax 转基因小鼠模型中敲除 NF-κB2 基因后，可以显著推迟肿瘤的发生（Fu et al. 2011）。

3.1.3 Tax 与细胞周期

整个细胞周期含受到严格控制，会受到细胞周期蛋白（cyclin）和细胞周期蛋白依赖性激酶（CDK）之间相互作用的调节。Tax 在细胞周期的不同阶段，特别是在 G_1 期中，使感染细胞的细胞周期进程发生异常。

Tax 利用几种机制增加 cyclin D/CDK4、cyclin D/CDK6 和 cyclin E/CDK6 复合物的形成，使细胞加速通过 G_1 期（Marriott and Semmes 2005）。首先，Tax 在转录方面能激活 cyclin D2（Akagi et al. 1996；Santiago et al. 1999；Iwanaga et al. 2001）和 E（Iwanaga et al. 2001）、CDK2 和 4（Iwanaga et al. 2001），抑制 CKI，如 $p18^{INK4C}$、$p19^{INK4D}$ 和 $p27^{KIPI}$（Suzuki et al. 1999；Iwanaga et al. 2001）；而且 Tax 能直接结合到 CDK4（Haller et al. 2002；Fraedrich et al. 2005）和 $p16^{INK4a}$ 上，阻止具有抑制功能的 $p16^{INK4a}$ 分子结合到 CDK4 和 CDK6 上（Low et al. 1997）。最后，Tax 结合到视网膜母细胞瘤（RB）蛋白上，该蛋白质是 cyclin D/CDK4/CDK6 和 E/CDK6 复合物作用的底物。Tax 的结合触发 RB 经蛋白酶体途径降解，使结合在 RB 上的转录因子（E2F1）得以释放，受 E2F1 调控的基因发生转录，表达细胞由 G_1 期进入 S 期所必需的因子（Kehn et al. 2005）。也有报道称 Tax 的表达可以直接激活 E2F1 基因的转录（Mori 1997；Lemasson et al. 1998；Ohtani et al. 2000）。

Tax 的另一个基本特性是能抑制 G_1/S 检测点，导致即使 DNA 存在损伤的情况下细胞周期进程仍继续进行（Marriott and Semmes 2005）。据此，Tax 能抑制 p53 的活性，因为 p53 蛋白的功能是在细胞 G_1/S 期转换中监视 DNA 结构的完整性（Tabakin-Fix et al. 2006）。

3.2 Tax 表达细胞中 DNA 损伤的累积

HTLV-1 感染的细胞遗传物质不稳定，导致细胞出现 8 个生物学改变，这些改变在随后 ATL 形成过程中被利用（Hanahan and Weinberg 2000，2011）。遗传物质不稳定主要包括两种类型，分别为 DNA 修复能力和 DNA 整倍性的丧失。实际上，Tax 能够干扰细胞进行正常的 DNA 修复和染色体分离的进程（Majone et al. 1993；Saggioro et al. 1994，1996；Lemoine and Marriott 2002）。

3.2.1 Tax 与染色体断裂损伤

在 ATL 细胞中可发生染色体断裂损伤（Marriott et al. 2002）。Tax 通过增加活性氧自由基（Kinjo et al. 2010）和/或抑制 p53 的检查点功能（Tabakin-Fix et al. 2006），直接导致 DNA 的损伤。

有两种主要假设解释 Tax 阻断 p53 蛋白功能的机制。一种模型是 Tax 与 p53 竞争性地与转录共激活因子 CREB 结合蛋白——CBP/p300 结合（Ariumi et al. 2000）；另一种模型认为，NF-κB 被 Tax 激活是 p53 被 Tax 灭活所必需的（Miyazato et al. 2005）。更多的新数据表明这两种模式都不能很令人满意地解释 Tax 对 p53 功能的失活作用，目前尚不能全面回答 Tax 如何使 p53 功能失活的机制。

3.2.2 Tax 与染色体的非整倍性

大多数癌细胞（包括 ATL 细胞）的染色体数目具有非整倍性。已经有人提出细胞染色体的非整倍性是细胞转化的原因之一。已经证明 Tax 可以通过几种机制诱导细胞的染色体发生非整倍性。Tax 能直接以两种方式促使染色体分离时发生错误。一种方式是 Tax 可以引起细胞发生多极点的有丝分裂（Peloponese et al. 2005；Ching et al. 2006；Nitta et al. 2006）。Tax 也能通过细胞中的 TAX1BP2 蛋白而诱导中心体异常增殖，TAX1BP2 蛋白具有抑制纺锤体过度倍增的作用（Ching 2006）。另一种方式是在有丝分裂期间，Tax 作用于 RANBP1，使其断裂，形成多个有丝分裂极点，促使细胞发生多极分裂（Peloponese et al. 2005）。而且 Tax 也能通过结合并激活促有丝分裂后期复合物/细胞周期体（APC/C）促进细胞过早分裂。最后，由于 Tax 介导的关键主轴组装检测位点蛋白——Mad1 功能的失活，导致表达 Tax 的细胞在有丝分裂期间丧失了"染色体整倍性"检测和校正（Liu et al. 2005；Jin et al.1998）。

4 ATL

4.1 Tax 表达的缺失与对宿主免疫监测的逃避

当 HTLV-1 的毒力与宿主的免疫系统处于一种平衡，就会发生 HTLV-1 的慢性感染。HTLV-1 需要表达 Tax 以使细胞发生转化，但是 Tax 也是宿主细胞毒性

T淋巴细胞（CTL）的主要靶分子（Jacobson et al. 1990；Kannagi et al. 1991；Elovaara et al. 1993；Yamano et al. 2002）。因此，从生物学角度来说，HTLV-1 不得不进化一个适当的程序控制 Tax 的表达，以便逃避宿主免疫系统的监测。目前的观点是在病毒感染的早期，需要 Tax 启动细胞发生转化的级联事件。另一方面，表达 Tax 的细胞会立即被作为外来的异源物质而被宿主的免疫系统（CTL）识别和清除。由此，需要在细胞表达 Tax 量方面和该细胞被 CTL 杀伤的敏感性方面达到一种平衡。在病毒感染的早期，当细胞表达 Tax 的优势超过 CTL 的杀伤作用时，就可以在感染细胞中表达 Tax；在感染后期，可能就会出现相反的情况，这就可以解释大多数 HTLV-1 感染的表达 Tax 的细胞悄悄地发生了转化。因此，目前认为，尽管在感染早期需要 Tax 启动细胞的转化，然而一旦细胞发生了转化，就不再需要 Tax 维持细胞的转化。只要存在和需要逃避 CTL 的杀伤情形，就不奇怪为什么在病毒感染晚期的 ATL 细胞中，超过 60%的细胞检测不到 Tax 转录子（Takeda et al. 2004；Taniguchi et al. 2005；Miyazaki et al. 2007）。尽管还不完全了解 Tax 是如何沉默表达的，但可能与 Tax 基因遗传信息发生改变（Furukawa et al. 2001；Takeda et al. 2004）、5′LTR 中病毒启动子发生表观遗传学改变（DNA 的甲基化和组蛋白的修饰）（Koiwa et al. 2002；Takeda et al. 2004；Taniguchi et al. 2005）和/或 5′LTR 序列的缺失（Tamiya et al. 1996）有关。

4.2 HBZ 的表达

细胞如何获得 Tax 非依赖性增殖的机制还不完全清楚。一个解释是，在 HTLV-1 感染细胞中经过一定时期宿主染色体改变的积累，使这些细胞具有足够的病毒非依赖性转化/生长特性；另一个解释是病毒的 HBZ 转录子/蛋白的表达。实际上，在 ATL 细胞中，HBZ 的 mRNA 高度表达（Murata et al. 2006；Satou et al.2006；Miyazaki et al. 2007）。利用体外模型，在感染细胞中，HBZ 的表达晚于 Tax 的表达，并且在一定时期内其表达持续增加（Li et al. 2009）。不同于 Tax，在 ATL 细胞中，HBZ 的序列没有发生突变（Fan et al. 2010），在 3′LTR 中的启动子保持不变（Taniguchi et al. 2005；Fan et al. 2010）。尽管 HBZ 是一种免疫原蛋白，HBZ 特异的 CTL 似乎不能有效清除 HTLV-1 感染的细胞（Suemori et al. 2009）。在感染的后期，HBZ 进一步促进病毒感染细胞的增殖（Satou et al. 2006），而沉默其表达能增强病毒感染细胞逃避宿主免疫监测（Gaudray et al. 2002）。Tax 和 HBZ 这种互补的表达模式表明，Tax 和 HBZ 分别在病毒感染的早期及晚期发挥作用，Tax 启动细胞的转化，而 HBZ 维持被转化 ATL 细胞的表型。

5 小结

尽管在 ATL 白血病发生方面的研究取得了很大的进展，但一些问题仍然有待解决。第一，病毒或 Tax 转化真正的靶细胞是什么？目前，只有人的 $CD34^+$ 造血祖干细胞被 Tax 成功转化，而其他分化的人类原代细胞还不能被 Tax 介导转化。因此，还不清楚在祖细胞和分化的人类细胞之间控制着 Tax 诱导的转化的细胞因素有何差异？第二，Tax 是如何使 p53 功能完全失活的？如上所提到的，目前有关 Tax 使 p53 功能失活的假设还不能令人满意。第三，需要什么因子启动和维持 ATL？可以预计，在未来的若干年，将在这些问题和其他一些问题上取得进展。

（邵卫星 译）

参 考 文 献

Akagi T, Ono H et al (1996) Expression of cell-cycle regulatory genes in HTLV-I infected T-cell lines: possible involvement of Tax1 in the altered expression of cyclin D2, p18Ink4 and p21Waf1/Cip1/Sdi1. Oncogene 12(8):1645–1652

Akagi T, Yoshino T et al (1988) Isolation of virus-producing transformants from human gastric cancer cell line, HGC-27, infected with human T-cell leukemia virus type I. Jpn J Cancer Res 79(7):836–842

Arai M, Kannagi M et al (1998) Expression of FAP-1 (Fas-associated phosphatase) and resistance to Fas-mediated apoptosis in T cell lines derived from human T cell leukemia virus type 1-associated myelopathy/tropical spastic paraparesis patients. AIDS Res Hum Retroviruses 14(3):261–267

Ariumi Y, Kaida A et al (2000) HTLV-1 tax oncoprotein represses the p53-mediated trans-activation function through coactivator CBP sequestration. Oncogene 19(12):1491–1499

Banerjee P, Sieburg M et al (2008) Human T-cell lymphotropic virus type 1 infection of CD34+hematopoietic progenitor cells induces cell cycle arrest by modulation of p21(cip1/waf1) and survivin. Stem Cells 26(12):3047–3058

Banerjee P, Tripp A et al (2010) Adult T-cell leukemia/lymphoma development in HTLV-1-infected humanized SCID mice. Blood 115(13):2640–2648

Boxus M, Willems L (2012) How the DNA damage response determines the fate of HTLV-1 Tax-expressing cells. Retrovirology 9:2

Cavrois M, Gessain A et al (1996a) Proliferation of HTLV-1 infected circulating cells in vivo in all asymptomatic carriers and patients with TSP/HAM. Oncogene 12(11):2419–2423

Cavrois M, Leclercq I et al (1998) Persistent oligoclonal expansion of human T-cell leukemia virus type 1-infected circulating cells in patients with Tropical spastic paraparesis/HTLV-1 associated myelopathy. Oncogene 17(1):77–82

Cavrois M, Wain-Hobson S et al (1996b) Adult T-cell leukemia/lymphoma on a background of clonally expanding human T-cell leukemia virus type-1-positive cells. Blood 88(12):4646–4650

Chaturvedi MM, Sung B et al (2011) NF-kappaB addiction and its role in cancer: 'one size does not fit all'. Oncogene 30(14):1615–1630

Chen X, Zachar V et al (1997) Role of the Fas/Fas ligand pathway in apoptotic cell death induced by the human T cell lymphotropic virus type I Tax transactivator. J Gen Virol 78(Pt 12):3277–3285

Ching YP, Chan SF et al (2006) The retroviral oncoprotein Tax targets the coiled-coil centrosomal protein TAX1BP2 to induce centrosome overduplication. Nat Cell Biol 8(7):717–724

Chlichlia K, Moldenhauer G et al (1995) Immediate effects of reversible HTLV-1 tax function: T- cell activation and apoptosis. Oncogene 10(2):269–277

Chu ZL, Shin YA et al (1999) IKKgamma mediates the interaction of cellular IkappaB kinases with the tax transforming protein of human T cell leukemia virus type 1. J Biol Chem 274(22): 15297–15300

Clapham P, Nagy K et al (1983) Productive infection and cell-free transmission of human T-cell leukemia virus in a nonlymphoid cell line. Science 222(4628):1125–1127

Copeland KF, Haaksma AG et al (1994) Inhibition of apoptosis in T cells expressing human T cell leukemia virus type I Tax. AIDS Res Hum Retroviruses 10(10):1259–1268

Elovaara I, Koenig S et al (1993) High human T cell lymphotropic virus type 1 (HTLV-1)- specific precursor cytotoxic T lymphocyte frequencies in patients with HTLV-1-associated neurological disease. J Exp Med 177(6):1567–1573

Etoh K, Tamiya S et al (1997) Persistent clonal proliferation of human T-lymphotropic virus type I-infected cells in vivo. Cancer Res 57(21):4862–4867

Fan J, Ma G et al (2010) APOBEC3G generates nonsense mutations in human T-cell leukemia virus type 1 proviral genomes in vivo. J Virol 84(14):7278–7287

Feuer G, Fraser JK et al (1996) Human T-cell leukemia virus infection of human hematopoietic progenitor cells: maintenance of virus infection during differentiation in vitro and in vivo. J Virol 70(6):4038–4044

Fraedrich K, Muller B et al (2005) The HTLV-1 Tax protein binding domain of cyclin-dependent kinase 4 (CDK4) includes the regulatory PSTAIRE helix. Retrovirology 2:54

Fu J, Qu Z et al (2011) The tumor suppressor gene WWOX links the canonical and noncanonical NF-kappaB pathways in HTLV-I Tax-mediated tumorigenesis. Blood 117(5):1652–1661

Fujita M, Shiku H (1995) Differences in sensitivity to induction of apoptosis among rat fibroblast cells transformed by HTLV-I tax gene or cellular nuclear oncogenes. Oncogene 11(1):15–20

Fukumoto R, Andresen V et al (2009) In vivo genetic mutations define predominant functions of the human T-cell leukemia/lymphoma virus p12I protein. Blood 113(16):3726–3734

Furukawa Y, Kubota R et al (2001) Existence of escape mutant in HTLV-I tax during the development of adult T-cell leukemia. Blood 97(4):987–993

Gallo RC (2005) History of the discoveries of the first human retroviruses: HTLV-1 and HTLV-2. Oncogene 24(39):5926–5930

Gaudray G, Gachon F et al (2002) The complementary strand of the human T-cell leukemia virus type 1 RNA genome encodes a bZIP transcription factor that down-regulates viral transcription. J Virol 76(24):12813–12822

Gessain A (2011) Human retrovirus HTLV-1: descriptive and molecular epidemiology, origin, evolution, diagnosis and associated diseases. Bull Soc Pathol Exot 104(3):167–180

Ghez D, Lepelletier Y et al (2006) Neuropilin-1 is involved in human T-cell lymphotropic virus type 1 entry. J Virol 80(14):6844–6854

Goncalves DU, Proietti FA et al (2010) Epidemiology, treatment, and prevention of human T-cell leukemia virus type 1-associated diseases. Clin Microbiol Rev 23(3):577–589

Good L, Sun SC (1996) Persistent activation of NF-kappa B/Rel by human T-cell leukemia virus type 1 tax involves degradation of I kappa B beta. J Virol 70(5):2730–2735

Grant C, Barmak K et al (2002) Human T cell leukemia virus type I and neurologic disease: events in bone marrow, peripheral blood, and central nervous system during normal immune surveillance and neuroinflammation. J Cell Physiol 190(2):133–159

Grassmann R, Berchtold S et al (1992) Role of human T-cell leukemia virus type 1 X region proteins in immortalization of primary human lymphocytes in culture. J Virol 66(7):4570–4575

Green JE, Hinrichs SH et al (1989) Exocrinopathy resembling Sjogren's syndrome in HTLV-1 tax transgenic mice. Nature 341(6237):72–74

Hall AP, Irvine J et al (1998) Tumours derived from HTLV-I tax transgenic mice are characterized by enhanced levels of apoptosis and oncogene expression. J Pathol 186(2):209–214

Haller K, Wu Y et al (2002) Physical interaction of human T-cell leukemia virus type 1 Tax with cyclin-dependent kinase 4 stimulates the phosphorylation of retinoblastoma protein. Mol Cell Biol 22(10):3327–3338

Hanahan D, Weinberg RA (2000) The hallmarks of cancer. Cell 100(1):57–70

Hanahan D, Weinberg RA (2011) Hallmarks of cancer: the next generation. Cell 144(5):646–674

Haoudi A, Semmes OJ (2003) The HTLV-1 tax oncoprotein attenuates DNA damage induced G1 arrest and enhances apoptosis in p53 null cells. Virology 305(2):229–239

Harhaj EW, Sun SC (1999) IKKgamma serves as a docking subunit of the IkappaB kinase (IKK) and mediates interaction of IKK with the human T-cell leukemia virus Tax protein. J Biol Chem 274(33):22911–22914

Hasegawa H, Sawa H et al (2006) Thymus-derived leukemia-lymphoma in mice transgenic for the Tax gene of human T-lymphotropic virus type I. Nat Med 12(4):466–472

Hayami M, Tsujimoto H et al (1984) Transmission of adult T-cell leukemia virus from lymphoid cells to non-lymphoid cells associated with cell membrane fusion. Gann 75(2):99–102

Hinrichs SH, Nerenberg M et al (1987) A transgenic mouse model for human neurofibromatosis. Science 237(4820):1340–1343

Hinuma Y, Nagata K et al (1981) Adult T-cell leukemia: antigen in an ATL cell line and detection of antibodies to the antigen in human sera. Proc Natl Acad Sci USA 78(10):6476–6480

Hirai H, Fujisawa J et al (1992) Transcriptional activator Tax of HTLV-1 binds to the NF-kappa B precursor p105. Oncogene 7(9):1737–1742

Hiramatsu K, Masuda M et al (1986) Mode of transmission of human T-cell leukemia virus type I (HTLV I) in a human promyelocytic leukemia HL60 cell. Int J Cancer 37(4):601–606

Ho DD, Rota TR et al (1984) Infection of human endothelial cells by human T-lymphotropic virus type I. Proc Natl Acad Sci USA 81(23):7588–7590

Igakura T, Stinchcombe JC et al (2003) Spread of HTLV-I between lymphocytes by virus-induced polarization of the cytoskeleton. Science 299(5613):1713–1716

Iha H, Kibler KV et al (2003) Segregation of NF-kappaB activation through NEMO/IKKgamma by Tax and TNFalpha: implications for stimulus-specific interruption of oncogenic signaling. Oncogene 22(55):8912–8923

Iwakura Y, Tosu M et al (1991) Induction of inflammatory arthropathy resembling rheumatoid arthritis in mice transgenic for HTLV-I. Science 253(5023):1026–1028

Iwanaga R, Ohtani K et al (2001) Molecular mechanism of cell cycle progression induced by the oncogene product Tax of human T-cell leukemia virus type I. Oncogene 20(17):2055–2067

Iwanaga R, Ozono E et al (2008) Activation of the cyclin D2 and cdk6 genes through NF-kappaB is critical for cell-cycle progression induced by HTLV-I Tax. Oncogene 27(42):5635–5642

Jacobson S, Shida H et al (1990) Circulating CD8+ cytotoxic T lymphocytes specific for HTLV-I pX in patients with HTLV-I associated neurological disease. Nature 348(6298):245–248

Jeang KT (2010) HTLV-1 and adult T-cell leukemia: insights into viral transformation of cells 30 years after virus discovery. J Formos Med Assoc 109(10):688–693

Jin DY, Spencer F et al (1998) Human T cell Leukemia virus type 1 oncoprotein Tax targets the human mitotic checkpoint protein MAD1. Cell 93(1):81–91

Jin DY, Giordano V et al (1999) Role of adapter function in oncoprotein-mediated activation of NF-kappaB. Human T-cell leukemia virus type I Tax interacts directly with IkappaB kinase gamma. J Biol Chem 274(25):17402–17405

Jones KS, Akel S et al (2005) Induction of human T cell leukemia virus type I receptors on quiescent naive T lymphocytes by TGF-beta. J Immunol 174(7):4262–4270

Jones KS, Lambert S et al (2011) Molecular aspects of HTLV-1 entry: functional domains of the HTLV-1 surface subunit (SU) and their relationships to the entry receptors. Viruses 3(6):794–810

Jones KS, Petrow-Sadowski C et al (2008) Cell-free HTLV-1 infects dendritic cells leading to transmission and transformation of CD4(+) T cells. Nat Med 14(4):429–436

Jung KJ, Dasgupta A et al (2008) Small-molecule inhibitor which reactivates p53 in human T-cell leukemia virus type 1-transformed cells. J Virol 82(17):8537–8547

Kannagi M, Harada S et al (1991) Predominant recognition of human T cell leukemia virus type I (HTLV-I) pX gene products by human CD8+ cytotoxic T cells directed against HTLV-I-infected cells. Int Immunol 3(8):761–767

Kao SY, Lemoine FJ et al (2000) HTLV-1 Tax protein sensitizes cells to apoptotic cell death induced by DNA damaging agents. Oncogene 19(18):2240–2248

Kasai T, Jeang KT (2004) Two discrete events, human T-cell leukemia virus type I Tax oncoprotein expression and a separate stress stimulus, are required for induction of apoptosis in T-cells. Retrovirology 1:7

Kawakami A, Nakashima T et al (1999) Inhibition of caspase cascade by HTLV-I tax through induction of NF-kappaB nuclear translocation. Blood 94(11):3847–3854

Kehn K, Fuente Cde L et al (2005) The HTLV-I Tax oncoprotein targets the retinoblastoma protein for proteasomal degradation. Oncogene 24(4):525–540

Kinjo T, Ham-Terhune J et al (2010) Induction of reactive oxygen species by human T-cell leukemia virus type 1 tax correlates with DNA damage and expression of cellular senescence marker. J Virol 84(10):5431–5437

Kishi S, Saijyo S et al (1997) Resistance to fas-mediated apoptosis of peripheral T cells in human T lymphocyte virus type I (HTLV-I) transgenic mice with autoimmune arthropathy. J Exp Med 186(1):57–64

Koiwa T, Hamano-Usami A et al (2002) 5^0-long terminal repeat-selective CpG methylation of latent human T-cell leukemia virus type 1 provirus in vitro and in vivo. J Virol 76(18):9389–9397

Koyanagi Y, Itoyama Y et al (1993) In vivo infection of human T-cell leukemia virus type I in non-T cells. Virology 196(1):25–33

Krueger A, Fas SC et al (2006) HTLV-1 Tax protects against CD95-mediated apoptosis by induction of the cellular FLICE-inhibitory protein (c-FLIP). Blood 107(10):3933–3939

Kwon H, Ogle L et al (2005) Lethal cutaneous disease in transgenic mice conditionally expressing type I human T cell leukemia virus Tax. J Biol Chem 280(42):35713–35722 Lambert S,

Bouttier M et al (2009) HTLV-1 uses HSPG and neuropilin-1 for entry by molecular mimicry of VEGF165. Blood 113(21):5176–5185

Lemasson I, Thebault S et al (1998) Activation of E2F-mediated transcription by human T-cell leukemia virus type I Tax protein in a p16(INK4A)-negative T-cell line. J Biol Chem 273(36):23598–23604

Lemoine FJ, Marriott SJ (2002) Genomic instability driven by the human T-cell leukemia virus type I (HTLV-I) oncoprotein, Tax. Oncogene 21(47):7230–7234

LeVasseur RJ, Southern SO et al (1998) Mammary epithelial cells support and transfer productive human T-cell lymphotropic virus infections. J Hum Virol 1(3):214–223

Li M, Kesic M et al (2009) Kinetic analysis of human T-cell leukemia virus type 1 gene expression in cell culture and infected animals. J Virol 83(8):3788–3797

Liu B, Hong S et al (2005) HTLV-I Tax directly binds the Cdc20-associated anaphase-promoting complex and activates it ahead of schedule. Proc Natl Acad Sci USA 102(1):63–68

Low KG, Dorner LF et al (1997) Human T-cell leukemia virus type 1 Tax releases cell cycle arrest induced by p16INK4a. J Virol 71(3):1956–1962

Macatonia SE, Cruickshank JK et al (1992) Dendritic cells from patients with tropical spastic paraparesis are infected with HTLV-1 and stimulate autologous lymphocyte proliferation. AIDS Res Hum Retroviruses 8(9):1699–1706

Maggirwar SB, Harhaj E et al (1995) Activation of NF-kappa B/Rel by Tax involves degradation of I kappa B alpha and is blocked by a proteasome inhibitor. Oncogene 11(5):993–998 Mahieux R, Gessain A (2005) New human retroviruses: HTLV-3 and HTLV-4. Med Trop (Mars) 65(6):525–528

Mahieux R, Gessain A (2009) The human HTLV-3 and HTLV-4 retroviruses: new members of the HTLV family. Pathol Biol (Paris) 57(2):161–166

Majone F, Semmes OJ et al (1993) Induction of micronuclei by HTLV-I Tax: a cellular assay for function. Virology 193(1):456–459

Manel N, Kim FJ et al (2003) The ubiquitous glucose transporter GLUT-1 is a receptor for HTLV. Cell 115(4):449–459

Marriott SJ, Lemoine FJ et al (2002) Damaged DNA and miscounted chromosomes: human T cell leukemia virus type I tax oncoprotein and genetic lesions in transformed cells. J Biomed Sci 9(4):292–298

Marriott SJ, Semmes OJ (2005) Impact of HTLV-I Tax on cell cycle progression and the cellular DNA damage repair response. Oncogene 24(39):5986–5995

Matsuoka M, Jeang KT (2007) Human T-cell leukaemia virus type 1 (HTLV-1) infectivity and cellular transformation. Nat Rev Cancer 7(4):270–280

Matsuoka M, Jeang KT (2011) Human T-cell leukemia virus type 1 (HTLV-1) and leukemic transformation: viral infectivity, Tax, HBZ and therapy. Oncogene 30(12):1379–1389

Matsuura E, Yamano Y et al (2010) Neuroimmunity of HTLV-I Infection. J Neuroimmune Pharmacol 5(3):310–325

McKinsey TA, Brockman JA et al (1996) Inactivation of IkappaBbeta by the tax protein of human T-cell leukemia virus type 1: a potential mechanism for constitutive induction of NF- kappaB. Mol Cell Biol 16(5):2083–2090

Miyazaki M, Yasunaga J et al (2007) Preferential selection of human T-cell leukemia virus type 1 provirus lacking the 5^0 long terminal repeat during oncogenesis. J Virol 81(11):5714–5723

Miyazato A, Sheleg S et al (2005) Evidence for NF-kappaB- and CBP-independent repression of p53's transcriptional activity by human T-cell leukemia virus type 1 Tax in mouse embryo and primary human fibroblasts. J Virol 79(14):9346–9350

Miyoshi I, Kubonishi I et al (1981) Type C virus particles in a cord T-cell line derived by co-cultivating normal human cord leukocytes and human leukaemic T cells. Nature 294(5843):770–771

Mori N (1997) High levels of the DNA-binding activity of E2F in adult T-cell leukemia and human T-cell leukemia virus type I-infected cells: possible enhancement of DNA-binding of E2F by the human T-cell leukemia virus I transactivating protein, Tax. Eur J Haematol 58(2):114–120

Mori N, Fujii M et al (2001) Human T-cell leukemia virus type I tax protein induces the expression of anti-apoptotic gene Bcl-xL in human T-cells through nuclear factor-kappaB and c-AMP responsive element binding protein pathways. Virus Genes 22(3):279–287

Mortreux F, Kazanji M et al (2001) Two-step nature of human T-cell leukemia virus type 1 replication in experimentally infected squirrel monkeys (*Saimiri sciureus*). J Virol 75(2):1083–1089

Moules V, Pomier C et al (2005) Fate of premalignant clones during the asymptomatic phase preceding lymphoid malignancy. Cancer Res 65(4):1234–1243

Mulloy JC, Kislyakova T et al (1998) Human T-cell lymphotropic/leukemia virus type 1 Tax abrogates p53-induced cell cycle arrest and apoptosis through its CREB/ATF functional domain. J Virol 72(11):8852–8860

Murata K, Hayashibara T et al (2006) A novel alternative splicing isoform of human T-cell leukemia virus type 1 bZIP factor (HBZ-SI) targets distinct subnuclear localization. J Virol 80(5):2495–2505

Nagai M, Brennan MB et al (2001) CD8(+) T cells are an in vivo reservoir for human T-cell lymphotropic virus type I. Blood 98(6):1858–1861

Nejmeddine M, Barnard AL et al (2005) Human T-lymphotropic virus, type 1, tax protein triggers microtubule reorientation in the virological synapse. J Biol Chem 280(33):29653–29660

Nerenberg M, Hinrichs SH et al (1987) The tat gene of human T-lymphotropic virus type 1 induces mesenchymal tumors in transgenic mice. Science 237(4820):1324–1329

Nicot C, Harrod R (2000) Distinct p300-responsive mechanisms promote caspase-dependent apoptosis by human T-cell lymphotropic virus type 1 Tax protein. Mol Cell Biol 20(22):8580–8589

Nicot C, Mahieux R et al (2000) Bcl-X(L) is up-regulated by HTLV-I and HTLV-II in vitro and in ex vivo ATLL samples. Blood 96(1):275–281

Nitta T, Kanai M et al (2006) Centrosome amplification in adult T-cell leukemia and human T- cell leukemia virus type 1 Tax-induced human T cells. Cancer Sci 97(9):836–841

Ohtani K, Iwanaga R et al (2000) Cell type-specific E2F activation and cell cycle progression induced by the oncogene product Tax of human T-cell leukemia virus type I. J Biol Chem 275(15):11154–11163

Okamoto K, Fujisawa J et al (2006) Human T-cell leukemia virus type-I oncoprotein Tax inhibits Fas-mediated apoptosis by inducing cellular FLIP through activation of NF-kappaB. Genes Cells 11(2):177–191

Ono A, Miura T et al (1994) Subtype analysis of HTLV-1 in patients with HTLV-1 uveitis. Jpn J Cancer Res 85(8):767–770

Pais-Correia AM, Sachse M et al (2010) Biofilm-like extracellular viral assemblies mediate HTLV-1 cell-to-cell transmission at virological synapses. Nat Med 16(1):83–89

Peloponese JM Jr, Haller K et al (2005) Abnormal centrosome amplification in cells through the targeting of Ran-binding protein-1 by the human T cell leukemia virus type-1 Tax oncoprotein. Proc Natl Acad Sci USA 102(52):18974–18979

Perkins ND (2012) The diverse and complex roles of NF-kappaB subunits in cancer. Nat Rev Cancer 12(2):121–132

Petropoulos L, Lin R et al (1996) Human T cell leukemia virus type 1 tax protein increases NF-kappa B dimer formation and antagonizes the inhibitory activity of the I kappa B alpha regulatory protein. Virology 225(1):52–64

Pinon JD, Klasse PJ et al (2003) Human T-cell leukemia virus type 1 envelope glycoprotein gp46 interacts with cell surface heparan sulfate proteoglycans. J Virol 77(18):9922–9930

Pise-Masison CA, Radonovich M et al (2002) Transcription profile of cells infected with human T-cell leukemia virus type I compared with activated lymphocytes. Cancer Res 62(12):3562–3571

Poiesz BJ, Ruscetti FW et al (1980) Detection and isolation of type C retrovirus particles from fresh and cultured lymphocytes of a patient with cutaneous T-cell lymphoma. Proc Natl Acad Sci USA 77(12):7415–7419

Pomier C, Alcaraz MT et al (2008) Early and transient reverse transcription during primary deltaretroviral infection of sheep. Retrovirology 5:16

Proietti FA, Carneiro-Proietti AB et al (2005) Global epidemiology of HTLV-I infection and associated diseases. Oncogene 24(39):6058–6068

Qu Z, Xiao G (2011) Human T-cell lymphotropic virus: a model of NF-kappaB-associated tumorigenesis. Viruses 3(6):714–749

Rauch DA, Ratner L (2011) Targeting HTLV-1 activation of NFkappaB in mouse models and ATLL patients. Viruses 3(6):886–900

Saggioro D, Majone F et al (1994) Tax protein of human T-lymphotropic virus type I triggers DNA damage. Leuk Lymphoma 12(3–4):281–286

Santiago F, Clark E et al (1999) Transcriptional up-regulation of the cyclin D2 gene and acquisition of new cyclin-dependent kinase partners in human T-cell leukemia virus type 1- infected cells. J Virol 73(12):9917–9927

Satou Y, Yasunaga J et al (2006) HTLV-I basic leucine zipper factor gene mRNA supports proliferation of adult T cell leukemia cells. Proc Natl Acad Sci USA 103(3):720–725

Schmitt I, Rosin O et al (1998) Stimulation of cyclin-dependent kinase activity and G1- to S- phase transition in human lymphocytes by the human T-cell leukemia/lymphotropic virus type 1 Tax protein. J Virol 72(1):633–640

Semmes OJ, Majone F et al (1996) HTLV-I and HTLV-II Tax: differences in induction of micronuclei in cells and transcriptional activation of viral LTRs. Virology 217(1):373–379

Suemori K, Fujiwara H et al (2009) HBZ is an immunogenic protein, but not a target antigen for human T-cell leukemia virus type 1-specific cytotoxic T lymphocytes. J Gen Virol 90(Pt 8):1806–1811

Suzuki T, Hirai H et al (1993) A trans-activator Tax of human T-cell leukemia virus type 1 binds to NF-kappa B p50 and serum response factor (SRF) and associates with enhancer DNAs of the NF-kappa B site and CArG box. Oncogene 8(9):2391–2397

Suzuki T, Hirai H et al (1995) Tax protein of HTLV-1 destabilizes the complexes of NF-kappa B and I kappa B-alpha and induces nuclear translocation of NF-kappa B for transcriptional activation. Oncogene 10(6):1199–1207

Suzuki T, Hirai H et al (1994) Tax protein of HTLV-1 interacts with the Rel homology domain of NF-kappa B p65 and c-Rel proteins bound to the NF-kappa B binding site and activates transcription. Oncogene 9(11):3099–3105

Suzuki T, Narita T et al (1999) Down-regulation of the INK4 family of cyclin-dependent kinase inhibitors by tax protein of HTLV-1 through two distinct mechanisms. Virology 259(2):384–391

Tabakin-Fix Y, Azran I et al (2006) Functional inactivation of p53 by human T-cell leukemia virus type 1 Tax protein: mechanisms and clinical implications. Carcinogenesis 27(4):673–681

Takatsuki K (2005) Discovery of adult T-cell leukemia. Retrovirology 2:16

Takeda S, Maeda M et al (2004) Genetic and epigenetic inactivation of tax gene in adult T-cell leukemia cells. Int J Cancer 109(4):559–567

Tamiya S, Matsuoka M et al (1996) Two types of defective human T-lymphotropic virus type I provirus in adult T-cell leukemia. Blood 88(8):3065–3073

Tanaka A, Takahashi C et al (1990) Oncogenic transformation by the tax gene of human T-cell leukemia virus type I in vitro. Proc Natl Acad Sci USA 87(3):1071–1075

Taniguchi Y, Nosaka K et al (2005) Silencing of human T-cell leukemia virus type I gene transcription by epigenetic mechanisms. Retrovirology 2:64

Tripp A, Banerjee P et al (2005) Induction of cell cycle arrest by human T-cell lymphotropic virus type 1 Tax in hematopoietic progenitor (CD34+) cells: modulation of p21cip1/waf1 and p27kip1 expression. J Virol 79(22):14069–14078

Tripp A, Liu Y et al (2003) Human T-cell leukemia virus type 1 tax oncoprotein suppression of multilineage hematopoiesis of CD34+ cells in vitro. J Virol 77(22):12152–12164

Tsukahara T, Kannagi M et al (1999) Induction of Bcl-x(L) expression by human T-cell leukemia virus type 1 Tax through NF-kappaB in apoptosis-resistant T-cell transfectants with Tax. J Virol 73(10):7981–7987

Van Prooyen N, Gold H et al (2010) Human T-cell leukemia virus type 1 p8 protein increases cellular conduits and virus transmission. Proc Natl Acad Sci USA 107(48):20738–20743

Waldele K, Silbermann K et al (2006) Requirement of the human T-cell leukemia virus (HTLV-tax-stimulated HIAP-1 gene for the survival of transformed lymphocytes. Blood 107(11):4491–4499

Watanabe M, Ohsugi T et al (2005) Dual targeting of transformed and untransformed HTLV-1-infected T cells by DHMEQ, a potent and selective inhibitor of NF-kappaB, as a strategy for chemoprevention and therapy of adult T-cell leukemia. Blood 106(7):2462–2471

Watanabe T (2011) Current status of HTLV-1 infection. Int J Hematol 94(5):430–434 Watanabe T, Seiki M et al (1983) Retrovirus terminology. Science 222(4629):1178

Wattel E, Cavrois M et al (1996) Clonal expansion of infected cells: a way of life for HTLV-I. J Acquir Immune Defic Syndr Hum Retrovirol 13(Suppl 1):S92–S99

Wattel E, Vartanian JP et al (1995) Clonal expansion of human T-cell leukemia virus type I-infected cells in asymptomatic and symptomatic carriers without malignancy. J Virol 69(5):2863–2868

Xiao G, Cvijic ME et al (2001) Retroviral oncoprotein Tax induces processing of NF-kappaB2/p100 in T cells: evidence for the involvement of IKKalpha. EMBO J 20(23):6805–6815

Xiao G, Harhaj EW et al (2000) Domain-specific interaction with the I kappa B kinase (IKK)regulatory subunit IKK gamma is an essential step in tax-mediated activation of IKK. J

Biol Chem 275(44):34060–34067

Yamada T, Yamaoka S et al (1994) The human T-cell leukemia virus type I Tax protein induces apoptosis which is blocked by the Bcl-2 protein. J Virol 68(5):3374–3379

Yamano Y, Nagai M et al (2002) Correlation of human T-cell lymphotropic virus type 1 (HTLV-mRNA with proviral DNA load, virus-specific CD8(+) T cells, and disease severity in HTLV-1-associated myelopathy (HAM/TSP). Blood 99(1):88–94

Yang L, Kotomura N et al (2011) Complex cell cycle abnormalities caused by human T-lymphotropic virus type 1 Tax. J Virol 85(6):3001–3009

Yasunaga J, Matsuoka M (2011) Molecular mechanisms of HTLV-1 infection and pathogenesis. Int J Hematol 94(5):435–442

Yoshida M, Miyoshi I et al (1982) Isolation and characterization of retrovirus from cell lines of human adult T-cell leukemia and its implication in the disease. Proc Natl Acad Sci USA 79(6):2031–2035

Zane L, Sibon D et al (2009) Clonal expansion of HTLV-1 infected cells depends on the CD4 versus CD8 phenotype. Front Biosci 14:3935–3941

Zhi H, Yang L et al (2011) NF-kappaB hyper-activation by HTLV-1 tax induces cellular senescence, but can be alleviated by the viral anti-sense protein HBZ. PLoS Pathog 7(4):e1002025

第14章 人类嗜T淋巴细胞病毒1型感染与成人T细胞白血病/淋巴瘤的预防

Makoto Yoshimitsu, Yohann White 和 Naomichi Arima

摘　要　成人T细胞白血病/淋巴瘤（ATLL）是长期慢性感染人类嗜T淋巴细胞病毒1型（HTLV-1）后逐渐形成的一种高度侵袭性外周T细胞恶性肿瘤。虽然最近在化疗、异体造血干细胞移植（alloHSCT）以及支持疗法方面取得了一定进展，但是，ATLL患者在血液系统恶性肿瘤患者中，仍为预后最为不良的一种，在更具侵犯性的ATLL亚型中，3年总体存活率仅为24%。HTLV-1是一种人逆转录病毒，世界上大约有1000万~2000万人感染，特别是在日本南部和东南部、加勒比地区、南美洲高原地带、美拉尼西亚和赤道非洲地区。虽然人类高频率感染，但只有2%~5%的HTLV-1感染者发展成ATLL。目前已知有三种主要的病毒传播途径：①通过母乳喂养的母-婴传播；②性传播，主要是男性传播给女性；③血液传播。虽然白血病的发生机制尚未被完全阐明，但是，多重因素（如病毒、宿主细胞和免疫因子）影响ATLL的进程。目前没有针对HTLV-1的预防性疫苗，阻断HTLV-1传播是公认的预防ATLL的主要措施。业已证实，母乳喂养替代方法对通过预防母-婴传播从而降低HTLV-1感染具有显著作用。不过，公共健康部门应考虑营养不良的风险，特别是在发展中国家，营养不良是婴儿死亡的重要原因。

关键词　HTLV-1，ATLL，ATL，母乳喂养，输血

M. Yoshimitsu (✉) _ N. Arima
Department of Hematology and Immunology, Kagoshima University Hospital,
8-35-1 Sakuragaoka, Kagoshima, 890-8520, Japan
e-mail: myoshimi@m.kufm.kagoshima-u.ac.jp

Y. White _ N. Arima
Division of Hematology and Immunology, Center for Chronic Viral Diseases, Graduate School of Medical and Dental Sciences, 8-35-1 Sakuragaoka, Kagoshima, 890-8544, Japan

1 引言

人类嗜 T 淋巴细胞病毒 1 型（HTLV-1）首次被发现作为人类逆转录病毒，与 T 细胞血液恶性肿瘤和成人 T 细胞白血病/淋巴瘤有关（Poiesz et al. 1980；Yoshida et al. 1982）。该病毒通过与含 HTLV-1 感染细胞的体液接触后传播，大多通过哺乳引起母-婴传播或通过输血传播。成人 T 细胞白血病/淋巴瘤（ATLL）通过在少数感染 HTLV-1 的人体中持续增殖一段时间后发展，故 ATLL 的预防策略应基于阻断 HTLV-1 的传播。首先，在 HTLV-1 流行区，通过在供血者中筛选 HTLV-1，以及限制携带 HTLV-1 母亲的母乳喂养一直是主要的公共卫生措施。第二种策略是预防 HTLV-1 携带者发展成 ATLL，虽然该种方法直接，但因缺乏有效的方式而未被实施。大约 90%的 HTLV-1 携带者在其一生中表现为健康未感染状态，且没有发展成 ATLL 的明显迹象。另外，基于目前我们对与 HTLV-1 相关的免疫紊乱疾病[包括 HTLV-1 相关脊髓病/热带痉挛性截瘫（HAM/TSP）]所拥有的有限知识，预防策略（如免疫接种）理论上可成为预防措施。

2 HTLV-1 感染的流行病学

2.1 全球概况

估计全球有近 2000 万人感染 HTLV-1（de The and Kazanji 1996）。其中，只有不到 10%的患者在其生命过程中发展成 HTLV-1 相关疾病，包括成人 T 细胞白血病/淋巴瘤。在过去的三十多年中，有一些研究调查了该病毒的地域和种族流行病学分布情况（Goncalves et al. 2010；Sonoda et al. 2011），结果表明，日本西南部、非洲部分地区、加勒比地区、中美洲和南美洲地区是流行地区。在欧洲和北美，HTLV-1 感染主要在来自流行地区国家的移民中被发现。

2.2 日本

最近一项血清流行病学研究显示，在日本，估计至少有 108 万 HTLV-1 携带者（Satake et al. 2012）。这比 1988 年所报道的低 10%。估计流行率在男性为 0.66%，在女性为 1.02%。

3 传播模式和临床转归

感染 HTLV-1 的主要模式已被揭示，即：①母-婴传播，主要通过母乳喂养

（Kinoshita et al. 1987；Yamanouchi et al. 1985）；②性传播，主要是从男性传染给女性（Murphy et al. 1989；Tajima et al. 1982）；③通过血细胞成分的血液传播（Okochi and Sato 1984）。研究表明，感染的模式与表现的 HTLV-1 疾病类型之间存在相关性。ATLL 主要与经母乳喂养获得感染有关，HAT/TSP 与输血感染有关（Osame et al. 1990）。因患者输血感染而造成 ATLL 的报道很少见（Chen et al. 1989）。母-婴传播的风险在母乳喂养期间大约为 20%（Hino et al. 1985），而在怀孕或分娩期间的估计值小于 5%（Fujino and Nagata 2000）。ATLL 的发展可能与因垂直传播获得 HTLV-1 持续感染有关。

4　成人 T 细胞白血病/淋巴瘤的流行病学

只有一小部分 HTLV-1 携带者经过较长的潜伏期之后发展成 ATLL。虽然该病在世界范围内分布，但除日本外，有关 ATLL 发生和流行程度的数据很少。而且，已有的报道可能低估了淋巴瘤亚型的流行程度，特别是，因在临床上与其他 T 细胞淋巴瘤相似，以及有限的诊断能力等原因。在日本人群中，ATLL 携带者在男性中为 4.5%~7.3%，在女性中为 2.6%~3.5%（Koga et al. 2010；Kondo et al. 1989；Tokudome et al. 1989）。据报道，日本人群主要在 50 多岁时发展成 ATLL（Takatsuki et al. 1996）；而在牙买加和巴西，患者在 40 多岁时开始呈现疾病症状，表明其他一些免疫或宿主遗传因素在 ATLL 的致病中发挥作用（Gibbs et al. 1987；Pombo de Oliveira et al. 1995）。

5　HTLV-1 的传播机制

在体外，HTLV-1 能够感染不同种类的细胞类型（Koyanagi et al. 1993；Sommerfelt et al. 1988），因此，其受体被认为是广泛表达的分子。葡萄糖转运体 1（GLUT1）、类肝素硫酸蛋白聚糖（HSPG）和神经纤毛蛋白-1 已被报道参与病毒囊膜与宿主细胞膜之间的相互作用，以及病毒进入靶细胞（Jones et al. 2005；Lambert et al. 2009；Manel et al. 2003）。当前的模型假设 HTLV-1 粒子首先与 HSPG 接触，随后通过神经纤毛蛋白-1 将 HTLV-1/HSPG 复合体纳入，最后与 GLUT1 作用。HSPG/神经纤毛蛋白-1/GLUT1 复合体的形成对病毒囊膜与宿主细胞的融合以及病毒穿入细胞是必需的。在体外，无细胞的 HTLV-1 粒子对大多数类型细胞的感染性很差，包括其主要靶细胞，即 CD4 T 细胞。直接的细胞-细胞接触似乎对 HTLV-1 感染是必需的，这对骨髓和浆细胞样树突状细胞（DC）是例外，因它们对无细胞的 HTLV-1 病毒粒子感染敏感（Jones et al. 2008）。因此，DC 在病毒传播中发挥作用，可能在乳汁与婴儿肠道黏膜之间的接触中促进扩散。HTLV-1

通过细胞-细胞传播的三个主要机制已被提出：①HTLV-1 感染淋巴细胞导致微管分子和病毒成分与其他 T 细胞接触时产生极性，形成所谓的病毒性突触（Igakura et al. 2003）；②HTLV-1 感染细胞产生病毒粒子，瞬时储存在含丰富基质成分的细胞外黏附结构中，包括胶原蛋白和聚集蛋白，以及细胞连接蛋白，如 Tetherin 和半乳素 3，它们类似于细菌生物膜。细胞外病毒组件通过接触，迅速黏附到其他细胞上，引起病毒扩散和感染靶细胞（Pais-Correia et al. 2010）；③HTLV-1 pX 区编码的 p8 蛋白通过淋巴细胞功能相关抗原 1 聚合增加与 T 细胞的结合。另外，p8 蛋白诱导 T 细胞间的细胞导管，增强病毒的传播（Van Prooyen et al. 2010）。

6　HTLV-1 传播的预防

ATLL 预后仍然是恶性血液病中最差的一个，虽然有最好的治疗方法，但当前没有疫苗预防 HTLV-1。因此，预防 HTLV-1 的传播是预防 ATLL 的一个重要策略。

6.1　垂直传播的预防

根据追溯性和前瞻性流行病学研究，母-婴传播概率约为 20%（Hino et al. 1985）。通过限制母乳喂养来预防母亲传染给小孩，对 HTLV-1 的感染及其相关疾病具有重要作用。在日本南部长崎市辖区内所做的一个干扰研究中，HTLV-1 感染母亲被劝告避免母乳喂养，结果发现母亲到小孩的传播从 20.3%显著降低到 2.5%。因此，在地方性流行区进行产前筛查 HTLV-1，结合对母亲进行劝告，避免哺乳喂养可能是一个重要的公共卫生策略。虽然母乳喂养少于 6 个月的儿童对 HTLV-1 的感染概率明显低于母乳喂养大于 6 个月的儿童，但与用配方奶喂养组的婴儿相比，其传播风险仍明显较高（Hino 2011）。

即使使用专用奶瓶喂养，仍有 2.5%的婴儿因来自母亲携带的病毒而感染 HTLV-1。HLLV-1 经子宫内传播是罕见的，不过分娩时经胎盘传播似乎仍是一种可能的传播模式，就像所报道的乙型肝炎病毒和丙型肝炎病毒一样。虽然单独的配方奶喂养可减少母-婴间的 HTLV-1 传播，但是，在发展中国家，营养不良的风险又是一个值得注意的重要问题，因营养不良是发展中国家婴儿死亡的一个重要因素。

6.2　水平传播的预防

HTLV-1 同样可通过接触体液、全血或血液成分扩散。因 ATLL 与垂直传播中获得的持续感染、经输血感染有关，因此预防水平传播的目的主要是减少 HTLV-1 携带者的总人群数。

6.3 输血和性传播的预防

自从 1986 年以来,在很多 HTLV-1 地方性流行区域,旨在通过系统性筛查所有献血者来预防与输血有关的 HTLV-1 传播的筛查计划被作为一个公共卫生控制策略得以实施(Inaba et al. 1989;Osame et al. 1990)。在日本南部的鹿儿岛县,通过限制母乳喂养和供血者筛查,使 HTLV-1 携带者从 2.79%降到 0.44%(表 14-1)。报道显示,在 HTLV-1 非流行区,HTLV-1 感染可能集中在选择供体人群,尤其是来自流行地区的移民。对发展中国家来说,进口的筛查检测试剂盒的花费可能太高,所以,有必要开发更低廉的检测工具及供血者筛查程序。在大多数非洲国家,输血仍是 HTLV-1 传播的主要原因。

表 14-1 日本南部鹿儿岛县输血供体中 HTLV-1 携带者的数量变化(1999~2008)

年份	输血供体数量	HTLV-1 携带者数量	所占比例/%
1999	98 644	2 751	2.79
2000	91 456	1 368	1.50
2001	92 281	1 048	1.14
2002	89 458	827	0.92
2003	86 000	686	0.80
2004	82 310	565	0.69
2005	73 792	435	0.59
2006	69 133	388	0.56
2007	69 741	360	0.52
2008	71 226	313	0.44

HTLV-1 的性传播主要是病毒从男性传给女性。应强化防止性传播感染的建议,包括使用避孕套,以及避免有多名及隐性性伴伴。获得 HTLV-1 感染的准确信息和适当的心理咨询是重要的预防策略,因为献血者和性活跃者一般是无症状的,且通常正处于生育年龄。

7 成人 T 细胞白血病/淋巴瘤的病程

7.1 成人 T 细胞白血病/淋巴瘤的致病性

ATLL 的发病机制尚不完全清楚。大量的研究表明,HTLV-1 反式作用因子/转录活化因子(Tax)在病毒感染细胞的转化中起重要作用。Tax 被认为是一种有效的癌蛋白,因为其可导致人类原发性 T 细胞永生化及 Tax 转基因鼠恶性肿瘤。

Tax 通过反式激活 5′端长串联重复（LTR）序列即病毒启动子来增强病毒的复制，激活核因子 kappa-B（NF-κB）信号途径，干扰细胞周期调节子，引起基因组非整倍体改变、DNA 损伤及削弱 DNA 修复。因此，Tax 被认为在 ATLL 的致病中起关键作用（Matsuoka and Jeang 2011）。

HTLV-1 bZIP 因子（HBZ）由 HTLV-1 前病毒的负链编码，在所有 ATLL 细胞中均可发现（Satou et al. 2006）。HBZ 蛋白最初被报道可抑制 Tax 介导的病毒转录，不过，HBZ RNA 同样被发现促进细胞增殖。重要的是，HBZ 转基因鼠可发展为 CD4/叉头框蛋白 3（Foxp3）阳性 T 细胞淋巴瘤，这与人类 ATLL 的免疫表型和临床特征类似。这些研究表明，HBZ 在白血病的发生中是一个关键因素。Tax 与 HBZ 之间相互作用的模型是，启动 HTLV-1 感染细胞的转化需要 Tax，而在 ATLL 中保持转化的表型需要 HBZ（Matsuoka and Jeang 2011）。

7.2 从无症状带毒发展到 ATLL 的决定因素

在很多流行病学和临床研究中，对 HTLV-1 携带者的 ATLL 病程的决定因素进行了研究。在日本人群中，诊断为 ATLL 的平均年龄大约是 65 岁（Yamada et al. 2011），这比在牙买加人群大约在 40 岁中旬出现要大很多，表明其他宿主和环境因素可能参与 ATLL 的致病性（Hanchard 1996）。在 ATLL 病程中，HTLV-1 感染时的年龄同样是一个重要因素，因为通过水平传播获得感染的 HTLV-I 携带者很少发生 ATLL。对包括 HLA 单倍型在内的宿主遗传因素进行了几项研究，观察发现，与普通人群相比，ATLL 患者更可能有 ATLL 家族史。在日本，与无症状 HTLV-1 携带者相比，ATLL 患者在 A*26、HLA-B*4002、HLA-B*4006 和 HLA-B*4801 等位基因的频率上明显更高（Yashiki et al. 2001）。在宫崎，HTLV-1 携带者具有较高的抗 HTLV-1 效价及较低的抗 Tax 反应性，最可能发展成 ATLL（Hisada et al. 1998），且高的 HTLV-1 前病毒滴度是无症状 HTLV-1 携带者发展成 ATLL 的重要风险因素。在日本，对 HTLV-1 携带者进行的一个全国范围的前瞻性研究已率先启动，以此来确定 ATLL 病程的决定因素。1218 个无症状携带者中有 14 个发展成 ATLL，所有这 14 个受试者均有更高水平的基线前病毒载量。受试者体内每 100 个外周血单核细胞中，基线前病毒载量小于 4 个拷贝的均没有 ATLL（Iwanaga et al. 2010）。

8 成人 T 细胞白血病/淋巴瘤患者的预后

8.1 急性和淋巴瘤亚型

即使采用化疗或异体造血干细胞移植（alloHSCT），急性和淋巴瘤亚型的

ATLL 患者的预后仍然很差。在目前一系列最好的化疗中(Tsukasaki et al. 2007)，完全反应(CR)的比率为 40%，3 年总体生存率(OS)为 24%，中位生存时间(MST)为 13 个月。

8.2 慢性和郁积亚型

在先前的一个研究中，对 ATLL 日本患者跟踪研究 7 年，结果慢性和郁积亚型的 4 年生存率分别为 26.9%和 62.8%，慢性亚型的 MST 为 24.3 个月(Shimoyama 1991)。慢性和郁积亚型 ATLL 患者以无痛的临床进程为特征，一般通过观察或"观察等待"进行管理，直至疾病发展为急性，这与慢性淋巴白血病或郁积性骨髓瘤的管理方法相似。不过，最近对无痛型 ATLL 亚型（慢性和郁积亚型）进行长期跟踪的报道显示，其 MST 为 4.1 年，5 年、10 年和 15 年的估算存活率分别为 47.2%、25.4%和 14.1%，该结果比预期的差些。这些研究表明，即使对于无痛型 ATLL 患者，在临床实践中也应仔细观察，需要进一步研究来提高对这些患者的管理。

9 当前的治疗措施

9.1 传统化疗方法

一项 III 期随机对照试验的结果表明，三种方案[长春新碱、环磷酰胺、阿霉素和泼尼松（VCAP）；阿霉素、雷莫司汀和强的松（AMP）；长春地辛、依托泊苷、卡铂和强的松（VECP）]对于初诊的急性、恶性淋巴瘤或情况不妙的 ATLL 慢性亚型患者来说，在 OS、主要研究终点或无发展生存期上，与两周一次使用环磷酰胺、阿霉素、长春新碱和泼尼松（CHOP）相比，并未显示其有利的优势(Tsukasaki et al. 2007)。不过，VCAP-AMP-VECP 组的 CR 比率高于两周一次的 CHOP 组（分别为 40% vs 25%，P=0.020）。VCAP-AMP-VECP 组的 3 年 OS 为 24%，CHOP 组为 13%（P=0.085）。与其他恶性血液病相比，13 个月的 MST 并未显示任何有利的方面。

9.2 异体造血干细胞移植

作为一种有前途的替代治疗方法，异体造血干细胞移植（alloHSCT）已被应用，并在一定比例的 ATLL 患者中能长期地缓解病症（Choi et al. 2011；Hishizawa et al. 2010；Utsunomiya et al. 2001）。近期在日本的一次全国大型回顾性研究中，研究者比较了 386 例 ATLL 患者接受 alloHSCT 治疗的效果。在中期随访 41 个月后，群体的 3 年 OS 为 33%（Hishizawa et al. 2010）。另外一个基于 294 位接受

alloHSCT 治疗的回顾性研究表明，轻中度急性 GVHD 的疾病发展的风险较低，并且对患者生存有利（Kanda et al. 2012），这是移植对抗 ATLL 的标志性效果。在日本，另外一个对 586 个 ATLL 患者接受 alloHSCT 治疗的大型回顾性分析显示，抑髓性预处理（MAC）与减低剂量预处理（RIC）两种方案在 OS 上无显著差异。在接受 RIC 治疗的老年患者中，有向更好 OS 变化的趋势（Ishida et al. 2012）。因为年龄较大和低 CR 率的关系，所以能够接受异体移植的 ATLL 合格患者数量较少。ATLL 患者进行 alloHSCT 治疗的选择标准有待确定。

9.3　α 干扰素（IFN-α）和叠氮脱氧胸苷

最近，对世界上 254 名 ATLL 患者使用叠氮脱氧胸苷（AZT）和干扰素（IFN）的荟萃分析结果表明，用 AZT 和 IFN 对患者进行处理后，患者反应更好，OS 更长（Bazarbachi et al. 2010）。207 名患者接受了 AZT/IFN 治疗，在这些患者中，接受抗病毒治疗的 75 名患者 5 年 OS 率为 46%（$P=0.004$）。对于急性 ATLL，经抗病毒治疗完全缓解症状的患者 5 年生存率为 82%。这些结果表明，用 AZT/IFN 对 ATLL 处理，除淋巴瘤型的 ATLL 外，结果为高度反应和高 CR 率，很大比例的患者存活时间延长。虽然这是个回顾性分析，但是其结果似乎很有前景，将来有必要对 AZT/IFN-α 与常规化疗进行深入比较研究。

9.4　ATLL 的预防

如前所述，ATLL 的预防主要依赖于防止 HTLV-1 传播。另一种策略可能是在 HTLV-1 携带者中预防 ATLL 的发展。尽管在 ATLL 发展之前有持续的带毒状态，但是没有利用此时机开发 ATLL 治疗的干预措施。部分原因是由于大约只有 10%的 HTLV-1 携带者在其一生中最后发展成 HTLV-1 相关疾病。还需要进行谨慎的、在干预期间对副反应可接受性风险效益的分析。

9.5　ATLL 预防的未来展望

9.5.1　HTLV-1 特异性 T 细胞的免疫抑制

垂直传播、高负荷前病毒载量和特异性 HTLV-1 T 细胞免疫应答抑制是 ATLL 发展的重要风险因素。已有报道表明，在慢性和郁积型 ATLL 患者，以及小部分无症状携带者中，检测到的 Tax 特异性细胞毒性 T 淋巴细胞（CTL）对抗原刺激是无反应的（Takamori et al. 2011）。这样的 CTL 功能性受损似乎只是特异性地发生在 HTLV-1，因为其他方面（如巨细胞病毒特异性 CTL）仍完好无损。

在动物模型中，口服接种 HTLV-1 病毒粒子可诱导抵抗 HTLV-1 的 T 细胞耐受（Hasegawa et al. 2003）。由于母乳喂养是 HTLV-1 感染中垂直传播的主要途径，因此，这可能会引起新生儿抵抗 HTLV-1 的 T 细胞耐受。除免疫耐受外，T 细胞耗竭可能是抗原特异性 T 细胞抑制的另外一种机制。据报道，在 Tax 特异性 CTL 中，程序性死亡分子 1（PD-1）表达上调，这提示 Tax 特异性 T 细胞耗竭（Kozako et al. 2009）。

9.5.2 疫苗

在 ATLL 的预防方面，对未感染的个体进行接种来抵抗 HTLV-1 感染并不是一个执行起来很复杂的策略，因为 HTLV-1 携带者在其生命中的前 6 个月通过垂直传播感染，需要经过长期的潜伏后才会发展为 ATLL，而垂直传播可通过阻止母乳喂养而几乎被完全遏制。因此，接种的目的应该是增强无症状携带者 HTLV-1 特异性 T 细胞反应，增强感染和转化细胞的清除，从而防止 ATLL。在 HTLV-1 诱导的大鼠淋巴瘤模型中，靶向于 Tax 的 HTLV-1 疫苗显示出有希望的抗肿瘤效果（Ohashi et al. 2000）。此外，用来源于 HTLV-1 合成肽疫苗免疫的猴子产生了较强的细胞免疫，这些猴子被攻毒后，观察到前病毒滴度显著降低（Kazanji et al. 2006）。这些结果为临床应用疫苗来预防 ATLL 提供了科学依据。不过，在临床应用实现之前，仍有几个障碍需要克服。HTLV-1 合成肽免疫原性低，诱导的抗原特异性 CTL 不足。在先前的报道中，使用甘露糖包裹的脂质体（OML）封装 HLA-A *0201 限制性 HTLV-1 Tax 表位（OML /Tax）可高效诱导 HTLV-1 特异性 T 细胞应答（Kozako et al. 2011）。而且，用 OML/Tax 免疫 HLA-A*0201 转基因小鼠，结果诱导能产生 HTLV-1 特异性 IFN-γ 的 T 细胞，暴露于 MOL/Tax 的 DC 的成熟标记蛋白的表达增强。此外，用来源于 HTLV-1 携带者的 OML/Tax 处理后，有效地诱导了 HTLV-1-Tax 特异性 CD8$^+$ T 细胞的产生。OML/Tax 增加 HTLV-1-Tax 特异性 CD8$^+$ T 细胞数量，平均达到 170 倍。另外，这些 HTLV-1-Tax 特异性 CD8$^+$ T 细胞能有效裂解 HTLV-1 合成肽脉冲处理的 T2-A2 细胞。这些研究结果表明，OML/Tax 可在不需要佐剂的情况下，诱导抗原特异性细胞免疫应答，它可能是一个有效降低 ATLL 发生率的候选疫苗。

更好的预测将有助于鉴别具有高风险发展成 ATLL 的个体，使我们限制低风险个体接受不必要的疫苗接种并发生免疫反应，包括发生如 HAM/TSP 的自身免疫样情况。

10 小结

迄今为止，通过限制 HTLV-1 感染母亲进行母乳喂养一直是预防 HTLV-1 从而延长 ATLL 发生的主要方法。应在流行地区实施 HTLV-1 产前筛查，并提供准确的信息和咨询。此外，筛查献血候选者也被证明可有效预防 HTLV-1 的传播。

应加强预防性传播的建议，包括使用安全套及采取安全的性行为。开发一种安全有效的疫苗可能是保护 HTLV-1 感染携带者、防止其发展成 ATLL 的重要工具。

（刘玉良 译）

参 考 文 献

Bazarbachi A, Plumelle Y, Carlos Ramos J, Tortevoye P, Otrock Z, Taylor G, Gessain A, Harrington W, Panelatti G, Hermine O (2010) Meta-analysis on the use of zidovudine and interferon-alfa in adult T-cell leukemia/lymphoma showing improved survival in the leukemic subtypes. J Clin Oncol 28:4177–4183

Chen YC, Wang CH, Su IJ, Hu CY, Chou MJ, Lee TH, Lin DT, Chung TY, Liu CH, Yang CS (1989) Infection of human T-cell leukemia virus type I and development of human T-cell leukemia lymphoma in patients with hematologic neoplasms: a possible linkage to blood transfusion. Blood 74:388–394

Choi I, Tanosaki R, Uike N, Utsunomiya A, Tomonaga M, Harada M, Yamanaka T, Kannagi M, Okamura J (2011) Long-term outcomes after hematopoietic SCT for adult T-cell leukemia/lymphoma: results of prospective trials. Bone Marrow Transplant 46:116–118

de The G, Kazanji M (1996) An HTLV-I/II vaccine: from animal models to clinical trials? J Acquir Immune Defic Syndr Hum Retrovirol 13(Suppl 1):S191–S198

Fujino T, Nagata Y (2000) HTLV-I transmission from mother to child. J Reprod Immunol 47:197–206

Gibbs WN, Lofters WS, Campbell M, Hanchard B, LaGrenade L, Cranston B, Hendriks J, Jaffe ES, Saxinger C, Robert-Guroff M et al (1987) Non-hodgkin lymphoma in Jamaica and its relation to adult T-cell leukemia-lymphoma. Ann Intern Med 106:361–368

Goncalves DU, Proietti FA, Ribas JG, Araujo MG, Pinheiro SR, Guedes AC, Carneiro-Proietti AB (2010) Epidemiology, treatment, and prevention of human T-cell leukemia virus type 1-associated diseases. Clin Microbiol Rev 23:577–589

Hanchard B (1996) Adult T-cell leukemia/lymphoma in Jamaica: 1986–1995. J Acquir Immune Defic Syndr Hum Retrovirol 13(Suppl 1):S20–S25

Hasegawa A, Ohashi T, Hanabuchi S, Kato H, Takemura F, Masuda T, Kannagi M (2003) Expansion of human T-cell leukemia virus type 1 (HTLV-1) reservoir in orally infected rats: inverse correlation with HTLV-1-specific cellular immune response. J Virol 77:2956–2963

Hino S (2011) Establishment of the milk-borne transmission as a key factor for the peculiar endemicity of human T-lymphotropic virus type 1 (HTLV-1): the ATL prevention program Nagasaki. Proc Jpn Acad Ser B Phys Biol Sci 87:152–166

Hino S, Yamaguchi K, Katamine S, Sugiyama H, Amagasaki T, Kinoshita K, Yoshida Y, Doi H, Tsuji Y,

Miyamoto T (1985) Mother-to-child transmission of human T-cell leukemia virus type-I. Jpn J Cancer Res 76:474–480

Hisada M, Okayama A, Shioiri S, Spiegelman DL, Stuver SO, Mueller NE (1998) Risk factors for adult T-cell leukemia among carriers of human T-lymphotropic virus type I. Blood 92:3557–3561

Hishizawa M, Kanda J, Utsunomiya A, Taniguchi S, Eto T, Moriuchi Y, Tanosaki R, Kawano F, Miyazaki Y, Masuda M et al (2010) Transplantation of allogeneic hematopoietic stem cells for adult T-cell leukemia: a nationwide retrospective study. Blood 116:1369–1376

Igakura T, Stinchcombe JC, Goon PK, Taylor GP, Weber JN, Griffiths GM, Tanaka Y, Osame M, Bangham CR (2003) Spread of HTLV-I between lymphocytes by virus-induced polarization of the cytoskeleton. Science 299:1713–1716

Inaba S, Sato H, Okochi K, Fukada K, Takakura F, Tokunaga K, Kiyokawa H, Maeda Y (1989) Prevention of transmission of human T-lymphotropic virus type 1 (HTLV-1) through transfusion, by donor screening with antibody to the virus. One-year experience. Transfusion 29:7–11

Ishida T, Hishizawa M, Kato K, Tanosaki R, Fukuda T, Taniguchi S, Eto T, Takatsuka Y, Miyazaki Y, Moriuchi Y et al (2012) Allogeneic hematopoietic stem cell transplantation for adult T-cell leukemia-lymphoma with special emphasis on preconditioning regimen: a nationwide retrospective study. Blood 120:1734–1741

Iwanaga M, Watanabe T, Utsunomiya A, Okayama A, Uchimaru K, Koh KR, Ogata M, Kikuchi H, Sagara Y, Uozumi K et al (2010) Human T-cell leukemia virus type I (HTLV-1) proviral load and disease progression in asymptomatic HTLV-1 carriers: a nationwide prospective study in Japan. Blood 116:1211–1219

Jones KS, Petrow-Sadowski C, Bertolette DC, Huang Y, Ruscetti FW (2005) Heparan sulfate proteoglycans mediate attachment and entry of human T-cell leukemia virus type 1 virions into CD4+ T cells. J Virol 79:12692–12702

Jones KS, Petrow-Sadowski C, Huang YK, Bertolette DC, Ruscetti FW (2008) Cell-free HTLV-1 infects dendritic cells leading to transmission and transformation of CD4(+) T cells. Nat Med 14:429–436

Kanda J, Hishizawa M, Utsunomiya A, Taniguchi S, Eto T, Moriuchi Y, Tanosaki R, Kawano F, Miyazaki Y, Masuda M et al (2012) Impact of graft-versus-host disease on outcomes after allogeneic hematopoietic cell transplantation for adult T-cell leukemia: a retrospective cohort study. Blood 119:2141–2148

Kazanji M, Heraud JM, Merien F, Pique C, de The G, Gessain A, Jacobson S (2006) Chimeric peptide vaccine composed of B- and T-cell epitopes of human T-cell leukemia virus type 1 induces humoral and cellular immune responses and reduces the proviral load in immunized squirrel monkeys (*Saimiri sciureus*). J Gen Virol 87:1331–1337

Kinoshita K, Amagasaki T, Hino S, Doi H, Yamanouchi K, Ban N, Momita S, Ikeda S, Kamihira S,

Ichimaru M et al (1987) Milk-borne transmission of HTLV-I from carrier mothers to their children. Jpn J Cancer Res 78:674–680

Koga Y, Iwanaga M, Soda M, Inokuchi N, Sasaki D, Hasegawa H, Yanagihara K, Yamaguchi K, Kamihira S, Yamada Y (2010) Trends in HTLV-1 prevalence and incidence of adult T-cell leukemia/lymphoma in Nagasaki, Japan. J Med Virol 82:668–674

Kondo T, Kono H, Miyamoto N, Yoshida R, Toki H, Matsumoto I, Hara M, Inoue H, Inatsuki A, Funatsu T et al (1989) Age- and sex-specific cumulative rate and risk of ATLL for HTLV-I carriers. Int J Cancer 43:1061–1064

Koyanagi Y, Itoyama Y, Nakamura N, Takamatsu K, Kira J, Iwamasa T, Goto I, Yamamoto N (1993) In vivo infection of human T-cell leukemia virus type I in non-T cells. Virology 196:25–33

Kozako T, Yoshimitsu M, Fujiwara H, Masamoto I, Horai S, White Y, Akimoto M, Suzuki S, Matsushita K, Uozumi K et al (2009) PD-1/PD-L1 expression in human T-cell leukemia virus type 1 carriers and adult T-cell leukemia/lymphoma patients. Leukemia 23:375–382

Kozako T, Hirata S, Shimizu Y, Satoh Y, Yoshimitsu M, White Y, Lemonnier F, Shimeno H, Soeda S, Arima N (2011) Oligomannose-coated liposomes efficiently induce human T-cell leukemia virus-1-specific cytotoxic T lymphocytes without adjuvant. FEBS J 278:1358–1366

Lambert S, Bouttier M, Vassy R, Seigneuret M, Petrow-Sadowski C, Janvier S, Heveker N, Ruscetti FW, Perret G, Jones KS et al (2009) HTLV-1 uses HSPG and neuropilin-1 for entry by molecular mimicry of VEGF165. Blood 113:5176–5185

Manel N, Kim FJ, Kinet S, Taylor N, Sitbon M, Battini JL (2003) The ubiquitous glucose transporter GLUT-1 is a receptor for HTLV. Cell 115:449–459

Matsuoka M, Jeang KT (2011) Human T-cell leukemia virus type 1 (HTLV-1) and leukemic transformation: viral infectivity, Tax, HBZ and therapy. Oncogene 30:1379–1389

Murphy EL, Figueroa JP, Gibbs WN, Brathwaite A, Holding-Cobham M, Waters D, Cranston B, Hanchard B, Blattner WA (1989) Sexual transmission of human T-lymphotropic virus type I (HTLV-I). Ann Intern Med 111:555–560

Ohashi T, Hanabuchi S, Kato H, Tateno H, Takemura F, Tsukahara T, Koya Y, Hasegawa A, Masuda T, Kannagi M (2000) Prevention of adult T-cell leukemia-like lymphoproliferative disease in rats by adoptively transferred T cells from a donor immunized with human T-cell leukemia virus type 1 Tax-coding DNA vaccine. J Virol 74:9610–9616

Okochi K, Sato H (1984) Transmission of ATLV (HTLV-I) through blood transfusion. Princess Takamatsu Symp 15:129–135

Osame M, Janssen R, Kubota H, Nishitani H, Igata A, Nagataki S, Mori M, Goto I, Shimabukuro H, Khabbaz R et al (1990) Nationwide survey of HTLV-I-associated myelopathy in Japan: association with blood transfusion. Ann Neurol 28:50–56

Pais-Correia AM, Sachse M, Guadagnini S, Robbiati V, Lasserre R, Gessain A, Gout O, Alcover A,

Thoulouze MI (2010) Biofilm-like extracellular viral assemblies mediate HTLV-1 cell-to- cell transmission at virological synapses. Nat Med 16:83–89

Poiesz BJ, Ruscetti FW, Gazdar AF, Bunn PA, Minna JD, Gallo RC (1980) Detection and isolation of type C retrovirus particles from fresh and cultured lymphocytes of a patient with cutaneous T-cell lymphoma. Proc Natl Acad Sci USA 77:7415–7419

Pombo de Oliveira MS, Matutes E, Schulz T, Carvalho SM, Noronha H, Reaves JD, Loureiro P, Machado C, Catovsky D (1995) T-cell malignancies in Brazil. Clinico-pathological and molecular studies of HTLV-I-positive and -negative cases. Int J Cancer 60:823–827

Satake M, Yamaguchi K, Tadokoro K (2012) Current prevalence of HTLV-1 in Japan as determined by screening of blood donors. J Med Virol 84:327–335

Satou Y, Yasunaga J, Yoshida M, Matsuoka M (2006) HTLV-I basic leucine zipper factor gene mRNA supports proliferation of adult T cell leukemia cells. Proc Natl Acad Sci USA 103:720–725

Shimoyama M (1991) Diagnostic criteria and classification of clinical subtypes of adult T-cell leukaemia-lymphoma. A report from the Lymphoma Study Group (1984–87). Br J Haematol 79:428–437

Sommerfelt MA, Williams BP, Clapham PR, Solomon E, Goodfellow PN, Weiss RA (1988) Human T cell leukemia viruses use a receptor determined by human chromosome 17. Science 242:1557–1559

Sonoda S, Li HC, Tajima K (2011) Ethnoepidemiology of HTLV-1 related diseases: ethnic determinants of HTLV-1 susceptibility and its worldwide dispersal. Cancer Sci 102:295–301

Tajima K, Tominaga S, Suchi T, Kawagoe T, Komoda H, Hinuma Y, Oda T, Fujita K (1982) Epidemiological analysis of the distribution of antibody to adult T-cell leukemia-virus-associated antigen: possible horizontal transmission of adult T-cell leukemia virus. Gann 73:893–901

Takamori A, Hasegawa A, Utsunomiya A, Maeda Y, Yamano Y, Masuda M, Shimizu Y, Tamai Y, Sasada A, Zeng N et al (2011) Functional impairment of Tax-specific but not cytomegalovirus-specific CD8+ T lymphocytes in a minor population of asymptomatic human T-cell leukemia virus type 1-carriers. Retrovirology 8:100

Takasaki Y, Iwanaga M, Imaizumi Y, Tawara M, Joh T, Kohno T, Yamada Y, Kamihira S, Ikeda S, Miyazaki Y et al (2010) Long-term study of indolent adult T-cell leukemia-lymphoma. Blood 115:4337–4343

Takatsuki K, Matsuoka M, Yamaguchi K (1996) Adult T-cell leukemia in Japan. J Acquir Immune Defic Syndr Hum Retrovirol 13(Suppl 1):S15–S19

Tokudome S, Tokunaga O, Shimamoto Y, Miyamoto Y, Sumida I, Kikuchi M, Takeshita M, Ikeda T, Fujiwara K, Yoshihara M et al (1989) Incidence of adult T-cell leukemia/lymphoma among human T-lymphotropic virus type I carriers in Saga, Japan. Cancer Res 49:226–228

Tsukasaki K, Utsunomiya A, Fukuda H, Shibata T, Fukushima T, Takatsuka Y, Ikeda S, Masuda M,

Nagoshi H, Ueda R et al (2007) VCAP-AMP-VECP compared with biweekly CHOP for adult T-cell leukemia-lymphoma: Japan Clinical Oncology Group Study JCOG9801. J Clin Oncol 25:5458–5464

Utsunomiya A, Miyazaki Y, Takatsuka Y, Hanada S, Uozumi K, Yashiki S, Tara M, Kawano F, Saburi Y, Kikuchi H et al (2001) Improved outcome of adult T cell leukemia/lymphoma with allogeneic hematopoietic stem cell transplantation. Bone Marrow Transplant 27:15–20

Van Prooyen N, Gold H, Andresen V, Schwartz O, Jones K, Ruscetti F, Lockett S, Gudla P, Venzon D, Franchini G (2010) Human T-cell leukemia virus type 1 p8 protein increases cellular conduits and virus transmission. Proc Natl Acad Sci USA 107:20738–20743

Yamada Y, Atogami S, Hasegawa H, Kamihira S, Soda M, Satake M, Yamaguchi K (2011) Nationwide survey of adult T-cell leukemia/lymphoma (ATL) in Japan. Rinsho Ketsueki 52:1765–1771

Yamanouchi K, Kinoshita K, Moriuchi R, Katamine S, Amagasaki T, Ikeda S, Ichimaru M, Miyamoto T, Hino S (1985) Oral transmission of human T-cell leukemia virus type-I into a common marmoset (*Callithrix jacchus*) as an experimental model for milk-borne transmis- sion. Jpn J Cancer Res 76:481–487

Yashiki S, Fujiyoshi T, Arima N, Osame M, Yoshinaga M, Nagata Y, Tara M, Nomura K, Utsunomiya A, Hanada S et al (2001) HLA-A*26, HLA-B*4002, HLA-B*4006, and HLA-B*4801 alleles predispose to adult T cell leukemia: the limited recognition of HTLV type 1 tax peptide anchor motifs and epitopes to generate anti-HTLV type 1 tax CD8(+) cytotoxic T lymphocytes. AIDS Res Hum Retroviruses 17:1047–1061

Yoshida M, Miyoshi I, Hinuma Y (1982) Isolation and characterization of retrovirus from cell lines of human adult T-cell leukemia and its implication in the disease. Proc Natl Acad Sci USA 79:2031–2035

第 15 章 人疱疹病毒 8 型分子生物学：病毒致病性和复制相关的新功能及病毒-宿主相互作用

Emily Cousins 和 John Nicholas

摘　要　人疱疹病毒 8 型（human herpesvirus 8，HHV-8），又叫卡波西肉瘤相关疱疹病毒（Kaposi's sarcoma-associated herpesvirus，KSHV），是第二种被鉴定的人类 γ-疱疹病毒。HHV-8 像 EB 病毒一样，与 B 细胞肿瘤有关联，尤其是原发性渗出性淋巴瘤、多中心 Castleman 病和内皮细胞来源的卡波西肉瘤（Kaposi's sarcoma，KS）。HHV-8 病毒除了有核心保守的疱疹病毒和 γ-疱疹病毒的基因外（这些对于病毒的基本生物学功能是必需的），它还拥有多种辅助基因和编码的蛋白质。HHV-8 的辅助蛋白不仅具有从其细胞蛋白同源物推导而来的活性，还有一些新的、未知的活性，这些功能揭示了病毒与宿主之间的相互作用有助于病毒复制或潜伏感染的机制，也可能有助于病毒相关肿瘤的发生。这些蛋白质包括：病毒白细胞介素 6（vIL-6）、病毒趋化因子（vCCL）、病毒 G 蛋白偶联受体（vGPCR）、病毒干扰素调节因子（vIRF）、FLICE 同系物病毒抗凋亡蛋白（FADD 样 IL-1 转化酶）抑制蛋白（FLIP）和生存素类似物。其他 HHV-8 蛋白，例如，开放阅读框 K1 和 K15 编码的信号膜受体，与宿主细胞膜以一种独特的方式相互作用，这提示可能与病毒的致病性有关。此外，HHV-8 编码的一套 microRNA 也能调节多个宿主蛋白的表达，为病毒在宿主内持久性感染和 HHV-8 诱导肿瘤提供了证据。在这里，作者阐述了在病毒生物学和病毒相关疾病中，这种病毒与宿主之间新型的相互作用及其潜在功能的分子生物学机制。

E. Cousins ＿ J. Nicholas (✉)
Department of Oncology, Sidney Kimmel Comprehensive Cancer Center at Johns Hopkins,
1650 Orleans Street, Baltimore, MD 21287, USA
e-mail: nichojo@jhmi.edu

E. Cousins
e-mail: ecousins@jhmi.edu

1 引言

人疱疹病毒 8 型（human herpesvirus 8，HHV-8）属于第 2 亚家族 γ（γ-2）-疱疹病毒，与 γ-1 亚家族的 EB 病毒有一定的关系。γ 疱疹病毒一个重要的方面是它们与自然界或动物模型中的肿瘤形成有关。HHV-8 与 B 细胞来源的原发性渗出性淋巴瘤（primary effusion lymphoma，PEL）、多中心 Castleman 病（MCD）、内皮细胞来源的卡波西肉瘤（Kaposi's sarcoma，KS）的发生有关（Arvanitakis et al. 1996；Carbone et al. 2000；Chang and Moore 1996；Gaidano et al. 1997）。EBV 与多种 B 细胞瘤有关，如伯基特淋巴瘤、霍奇金淋巴瘤、移植后淋巴扩增病、表皮鼻咽和肠道癌、T 细胞淋巴瘤和肌肉瘤（Kawa 2000；Okano 2000；Young and Murray 2003）。尽管这些病毒及病毒相关性肿瘤之间有相似性，但是参与病毒生物学和肿瘤相关方面的特定蛋白质功能及活性表现明显不同。实际上，HHV-8 的多种蛋白质在 γ 疱疹病毒、疱疹病毒，甚至一般的病毒中，以前是没有被鉴定的，这些蛋白质被认为在病毒生物学中起重要作用，主要是参与病毒的致病作用。

其中这样的一个基因是病毒白细胞介素-6（vIL-6）。vIL-6 自发现之初，就被认为是 HHV-8 病毒致病作用的候选因子（Moore et al. 1996；Neipel et al. 1997a；Nicholas et al. 1997）。以前的报道表明，KS 细胞产生的 IL-6，支持 KS 细胞的生长，促进 KS 典型的炎症和血管生成。同时，作为一个重要的 B 细胞生长因子，发现其在 MCD 患者血清中的水平升高（Burger et al. 1994；Ishiyama et al. 1994；Miles et al. 1990；Roth 1991；Yoshizaki et al. 1989）。类似地，病毒趋化因子 vCCL 1-3 的发现，以及它们在实验系统中促血管生成活性表明，这些蛋白质除了在 HHV-8 有效复制过程的免疫逃逸中可能起作用外，它们也可能引起疾病（Boshoff et al. 1997；Stine et al. 2000）。研究发现，趋化因子受体同型物 vGPCR 诱导具有血管生成作用的细胞因子和参与促进 KS 病变的增长（Cannon et al. 2003；Pati et al. 2001；Schwarz and Murphy 2001）。HHV-8 开放阅读框 K1 和 K15 编码的组成型活性膜受体有类似的功能（Brinkmann et al. 2007；Caselli et al. 2007；Samaniego et al. 2001；Wang et al. 2006）。vGPCR 和 K1 也作为致癌基因在动物模型中促进细胞转化和诱导致瘤作用（Bais et al. 1998；Lee et al. 1998b；Yang et al. 2000）。然而，像病毒细胞因子一样，vGPCR 和 K1 主要（或者说完全）在有效裂解复制期表达。因此，任何肿瘤的致病作用可能都是通过旁分泌信号介导的。有充足的证据表明，细胞因子介导的旁分泌信号转导在 KS 中起作用。B 细胞生长也受这条途径的影响，下面将进行讨论。这些病毒蛋白可能参与 HHV-8 相关的致病作用。此外，在这些独特的病毒产物中，有些蛋白质在病毒生物学中的作用只是刚刚开始受到重视。例如，研究表明，vCCL 和 vGPCR 诱导的促生存信号和 vIRF-1 的抗凋亡活性能增强病毒的有效复制。因此，作为正常病毒生物学的功能，例如，抑制感染诱导的凋亡，可能有促进病毒相关肿瘤形成的副作用。这个概念对于病毒肿瘤学家来说是比较熟悉了，但是 HHV-8 所采用的精确机制还是一个很新的领域。

经典的致癌基因和肿瘤抑制基因的活性是由自分泌方式介导的。潜伏期表达的病毒基因对肿瘤疾病有潜在的作用。对 HHV-8 来说，最重要的是潜伏相关核抗原（LANA），它对正在分裂细胞的基本复制和基因组分离活性起重要作用，并且还影响宿主的几条促进细胞存活和扩增的信号途径（Verma et al. 2007）。这些活性明显与肿瘤形成的一些过程有关联。同样，细胞 FLICE 抑制蛋白的病毒类似物 vFLIP 也潜伏表达，对维持细胞的活性至关重要。vFLIP 通过诱导 NF-κB 活性和相关的抗凋亡机制起作用，而不是通过抑制受体介导的 caspase 激活来发挥作用（Chugh et al. 2005；Guasparri et al. 2004）。潜伏基因 v-cyclin（ORF72）和 miRNA 也参与病毒致病作用（Gottwein et al. 2011；Liang et al. 2012；Suffert et al. 2011；Verschuren et al. 2004）。除了这些潜伏期产物外，vIL-6、vIRF-1、vIRF-3、K1 和 K15 虽然在有效复制期大量表达，然而它们在潜伏感染细胞中（某些类型）也能被检测到，可能通过直接的自分泌方式参与病毒的致癌作用。裂解和潜伏活性之间的相互作用可能对 KS 非常重要，细胞因子失调被认为可导致该疾病。这种相互作用对 PEL 和 MCD 也很重要。这些问题和病毒宿主之间相互作用的详细分子生物学机制是本章的主题。

2　HHV-8 潜伏期产物与自分泌调节紊乱

2.1　潜伏相关核抗原（LANA）

LANA 由 HHV-8 病毒的 ORF73 编码，γ-2 疱疹病毒亚家族其他已确定序列的成员也编码同系产物。这些蛋白质的基本功能是作为潜伏起始结合蛋白，使病毒基因组结合到宿主染色体，从而在细胞分裂期间适当地分裂到姐妹细胞核中（Barbera et al. 2006；Verma et al. 2007）。这些活性等同于 γ-1 亚家族 EB 病毒的 EBNA1（Lindner and Sugden 2007）。然而，LANA 除了维持 HHV-8 病毒的潜伏感染外，还可能对病毒的致病性起作用。

已报道，LANA 的这种属性与抑制细胞周期关键蛋白和肿瘤抑制因子 p53 有关（Friborg et al. 1999）。然而，在大多数 PEL 细胞系中存在野生型的 p53，这表明 p53 的失活可能具有生物学相关性。PEL 细胞对 p53 激活的易感性表明，LANA 不能完全抑制肿瘤抑制因子（Chen et al. 2010；Petre et al. 2007）。LANA 也与视网膜母细胞瘤蛋白（Rb）相互作用介导 E2F 反应靶点的激活。LANA 还能联合

H-Ras 转导的转化大鼠胚胎成纤维细胞（Radkov et al. 2000）。此外，研究还发现 LANA 抑制周期蛋白依赖激酶抑制剂 p16INK4a 介导的细胞周期停滞和诱导 E2F 介导的淋巴类细胞进入 S 期（An et al. 2005）。然而，就像 p53 一样，这一实验结果与实际情况的相关性遭到了质疑，因为 Rb 在 PEL 细胞中表现出的功能是非常完整的（Platt et al. 2002）。

LANA 也与靶向参与调节细胞周期的各种蛋白质的 GSK3β 激酶之间相互作用。GSK3β 的靶点包括转录调节子 β-catenin 和原癌蛋白 c-Myc。GSK3β 通过磷酸化这些蛋白质，促进其降解（Karim et al. 2004；Sears et al. 2000）。β-caternin 与转录因子 TCF 共同诱导各种基因的表达，包括 c-myc、c-jun 和 cycinD1。这些基因主要参与促进细胞增值，它们在肿瘤发生过程中出现异常调节。LANA 结合到 GSK3β 后导致其核封存和蛋白激酶的失活，从而解除它对 β-catenin 的负调节作用，促进细胞扩增（Fujimuro and Hayward 2003；Fujimuro et al. 2003；Liu et al. 2007a，b）。c-Myc 的 T-58 残基为 GSK3b 的磷酸化靶点。研究发现，该位点在 PEL 细胞中处于低磷酸化状态。这种低磷酸化及其导致的 c-Myc 的稳定性依赖于 LANA 的表达（Bubman et al. 2007）。此外，LANA 直接与 c-Myc 相互作用，通过磷酸化 S-62 位点诱导 ERK 介导的 c-Myc 的激活（Liu et al. 2007b）。LANA 结合 c-Myc 并激活 ERK 活性，这些不依赖于 LANA 与 GSK3β 之间的相互作用。因此，通过这些不同的相互作用，LANA 能激活扩增途径，这可能对 HHV-8 病毒的潜伏和致病性都有意义。

近来报道 LANA 诱导血管生成素（angiongenin，ANG）的产生并与之相互作用。ANG 可上调 LANA 本身的表达，并且在建立潜伏感染和促进细胞活力方面起一定的作用（Paudel et al. 2012；Sadagopan et al. 2011）。而且，在 HHV-8 潜伏感染的、端粒酶永生化的内皮细胞（TIME）和 BCBL-1 的 PEL 细胞中，还发现 LANA 和 ANG 与膜联蛋白 A2（annexin A2）之间有相互作用。共聚焦分析结果也表明，除了 ANG-LANA 之间、ANG-膜联蛋白 A2 之间的相互作用外，这些蛋白质还通过共定位形成复合体（Paudel et al. 2012）。膜联蛋白 A2 也参与调节细胞扩增、凋亡和细胞骨架重建等（Shim et al. 2007；Thomas and Augustin 2009）。研究发现，抑制 PEL 细胞膜联蛋白 A2 或 ANG 的表达能增加细胞死亡，且删除膜联蛋白 A2 导致 ANG 和 LANA 的表达下降（Paudel et al. 2012；Sadagopan et al. 2011）。因此，LANA、ANG 和膜联蛋白 A2 之间在功能上存在整合的重要功能关系，增强被潜伏感染细胞的活性。此外，HHV-8 病毒感染的细胞中高水平的 ANG 可能通过诱导内皮细胞激活、迁移和血管生成作用来影响 KS 致病性（Sadagopan et al. 2009）。参与 LANA、ANG 和膜联蛋白 A2 相互调节、功能性的相互作用机制还不太清楚。然而，近来报道 ANG 通过与 p53 之间相互作用，使其去稳定，这可能对于 ANG 介导的促存活效应有一定的意义（Sadagopan et al.

2012）。

除了上面提到的 LANA 与各个细胞蛋白之间的相互作用外，LANA 还能通过一些常见的机制介导细胞基因的转录调控。其中的一个机制是参与转录调节抑制性 DNA 甲基化。LANA 与 DNA 甲基转移酶 DNMT3a 相互作用，导致其被招募并甲基化 LANA 靶向的启动子（Shamay et al. 2006）。LANA 也与组氨酸甲基转移酶 SUV39H1，以及转录组氨酸去乙酰酶相关的共抑制因子 mSin3、SAP30 和 CIR 相关。这些相互作用提示了 LANA 的另外一种直接的、启动子特异性的抑制机制（Krithivas et al. 2000；Sakakibara et al. 2004）。这种机制被认为对于抑制病毒的裂解和细胞的基因表达非常重要，最终促进潜伏和维持细胞长期的活力（Verma et al. 2007）。除了影响病毒潜伏期外，LANA 还通过靶向在各种癌症中遭到沉默的特定细胞基因，诱导发生表观遗传学抑制，从而参与 HHV-8 相关性肿瘤的发生（Shamay et al. 2006；Ziech et al. 2010）。

2.2 病毒 FLICE 抑制蛋白（vFLIP）

HHV-8 编码的 vFLIP 由 K13 开放阅读框编码，因此该蛋白质经常也被简称为 K13。vFLIP/K13 在结构上同其他病毒的含死亡效应结构域（DED）并与死亡受体相互作用的 vFLIP 相关，例如，来自传染性软疣病毒和马 2 型疱疹病毒 E8 的 MC159L。这些 vFLIP 对 Fas/CD95 和 TNF 受体介导的凋亡有保护作用（Bertin et al. 1997；Hu et al. 1997；Thome et al. 1997）。据报道，HHV-8 病毒的 vFLIP/K13 介导保护小鼠淋巴瘤和大鼠嗜铬细胞瘤细胞系的 Fas- 及 TNF-α 诱导的凋亡（Belanger et al. 2001；Djerbi et al. 1999）。然而，HHV-8 的 vFLIP/K13 能独特地诱导 NF-κB 信号，不能有效地抑制 Fas 诱导的凋亡，这表明 HHV-8 的 vFLIP/K13 主要是通过激活 NF-κB 起作用，而不是通过抑制死亡受体/级联酶发挥其功能（Chaudhary et al. 1999；Chugh et al. 2005；Matta and Chaudhary 2004）。HHV-8 的 vFLIP/K13 通过直接与抑制性的 κ 激酶（IKK）复合物相互作用来刺激其激酶活性，从而破坏 IκB 和 NF-κB 的 p50/p65 亚基之间的相互作用，以及导致蛋白酶介导的活性形式的 Rel/p52 从 RelB/p100 释放，最终激活 NF-κB 的经典和旁路途径（Field et al. 2003；Liu et al. 2002；Matta et al. 2007）。因此，vFLIP/K13 能通过不依赖信号接头和激酶（如 TRAF 和 RIP）等上游受体相关的机制激活 NF-κB。这样，vFLIP/K13 能避免激活 JNK 应急信号（Matta et al. 2007）。据报道，虽然 vFLIP/K13 与 TRAF2 相互作用对于 vFLIP/K13 结合到 BC-3 PEL 细胞的 IKKγ 是必需的，但 TRAF2 依赖的 vFLIP/K13 与 IKKγ 之间的相互作用和 vFLIP/K13 激活的 JNK/AP1 信号在随后的研究中不明显（Matta et al. 2007）。

vFLIP 激活的 NF-κB 具有重要的意义，因为 NF-κB 是被潜伏感染的 PEL 细胞裂解再激活的抑制因子，vFLIP 和 NF-κB 促进这些细胞存活（Brown et al. 2003；

Godfrey et al. 2005；Grossmann and Ganem 2008；Guasparri et al. 2004；Keller et al. 2000；Zhao et al. 2007）。这些效应提示潜伏期长期的维持和 vFLIP/K13 对 HHV-8 癌症的影响。除这些生物学特性外，NF-κB 信号还诱导促炎症细胞因子和血管生成因子，如 IL-6 和 IL-8。据预测，KS 病变区产生的这些细胞因子促进 KS 的致病性，并介导试验系统中 vFLIP/K13 诱导的细胞扩增和转化（An et al. 2003；Grossmann et al. 2006；Sun et al. 2006）。总之，这些研究表明，vFLIP/K13 通过对促存活和抗裂解 NF-κB 信号通路总体水平的激活，参与病毒潜伏的维持和 PEL、KS 致病作用。

2.3 kaposins

K12 转录单元组成 K12 开放阅读框，两套富含 GC 的重复单元（DR1、DR2）位于 K12 的上游（Sadler et al. 1999）。这个基因通过选择转录和翻译的起始产生卡波素（kaposin）A、B 和 C 三种蛋白质。kaposin A，对应于 K12 的翻译产物，起始于 K12 近端转录子的一个经典的密码子 AUG。kaposin B 和 C 起始于包含上游重复元素的转录子中不同读码框的 CUG。kaposin B 是从读码框 1 的 DR1 和 DR2 翻译来的，而读码框 2 翻译的 kaposin C 包含 DR1/2 翻译融合到 K12 的序列。此外，还发现了一个起始于 K12 上游较大的、5kb 的剪切转录子。这个序列有可能编码非 AUG 起始的蛋白质，该蛋白质有一个特异的、来自 DR2 上游密码子的 N 端序列（Li et al. 2002；Pearce et al. 2005）。研究还发现，尽管 K12 转录子在潜伏感染的细胞中有较高的表达，但在裂解复制期它也被诱导（Li et al. 2002；Sadler et al. 1999；Staskus et al. 1997；Sturzl et al. 1997；Zhong et al. 1996）。kaposin A、B 和 C 在不同类型细胞和组织中的相对表达水平不一样。例如，kaposin A 和 C 主要在原代 PEL 细胞中表达，而 kaposin B 主要存在于 BCBL-1 细胞系（Li et al. 2002）。尽管 kaposin A 和 B 的活性已经报道，但还没有 kaposin C 的功能研究。

因为 kaposin A 是开放阅读框 K12 的直接产物，所以它是第一个被鉴定和研究的蛋白质。转染试验研究表明，一个 6kDa 的蛋白质能转化永生化的 rat-3 细胞和 NIH3T3 细胞，转化后培养物中形成细胞克隆，且在无胸腺小鼠中形成肿瘤（Muralidhar et al. 1998）。这种转化依赖于结合到 kaposin A 上的鸟嘌呤核苷酸交换因子 cytohesin-1。这种相互作用促进膜对 cytohesin-1 的招募和激活，从而作用于膜相关的靶 GTPase，如 ARF1（Kliche et al. 2001）。在 kaposin A 转导的细胞中检测到一些激酶活性的升高，如 cdc2、PKC、ERK 和 CAM II，然而其潜在的机制还没有明确（Muralidhar et al. 2000）。基因芯片和信号通路研究表明，MEK/ERK、PI3K/AKT 和 STAT3 信号通路被 kaposin A 激活（Chen et al. 2009b）。初期的免疫荧光研究表明，kaposin A 可能定位于高尔基体（Muralidhar et al. 2000）。然而，后来的共聚焦荧光显微镜、细胞片段化和流式细胞分析发现大部分 kaposin

A 在核周围，有些在胞质膜（Tomkowicz et al. 2002，2005）。LXXLL 结构域是一个类似于核受体的配体相互作用区，是细胞永生化所必需的，它的突变导致核联合消失和 kaposin A 重新定位于细胞质（Tomkowicz et al. 2005）。然而，野生型和突变型 kaposin A 一样都能够激活 AP1 报告基因，这表明转化是通过一种完全不同于 AP1 激活的机制。最近发现，kaposin A 能与位于线粒体的 GTP 结合蛋白 septin-4 的一种变体相互作用，促进细胞凋亡（Lin et al. 2007；Mandel-Gutfreund et al. 2011）。在转染的细胞中共表达 kaposin A 和 septin-4 的变体抑制 septin-4 变体诱导的凋亡（Lin et al. 2007）。因此，抑制 septin-4 的功能可能是 kaposin A 通过促细胞生存从而影响癌症致病性的一种机制。通常，这种活性也被认为导致病毒潜伏感染。如果 septin-4 在 HHV-8 潜伏感染的细胞中表达，这种机制将具有一定的生物学意义。

Kaposin B，由 DR 重复序列和 K12 翻译而来，它通过 DR2 编码序列与 MK2 激酶相互作用，从而提高其活性（McCormick and Ganem 2005）。Kaposin B 结合到 MK2 的 C 端叶状区，这也是 p38 激酶靶向的区域。Kaposin B 结合到 C 端叶状区，就像被 p38 磷酸化一样，阻止 MK2 的 C 端叶状区和 C 端尾部序列之间的抑制性分子内相互作用，从而导致该激酶的激活。单个 DR1 联合单个 DR2 重复（但不是其中任何一个）就足够介导 MK2 激活（McCormick and Ganem 2006）。MK2 活性使含 ARE 的 mRNA 更加稳定。这些 mRNA 中许多都是编码细胞因子的，如促炎症和促血管生成的 IL-6。因此，kaposin B 有影响病毒致病性的潜能。根据预测，kaposin B 通过诱导细胞蛋白的促存活和有丝分裂活性，维持潜伏感染细胞群体和/或扩张潜伏细胞群。重要的是，kaposin B 能稳定编码淋巴内皮细胞分化关键调控子 PROX1 的 mRNA 的活性。ARE 结合蛋白 HuR 后靶向 PROX1，kaposin B 激活的 p38 蛋白激酶促进 HuR 从细胞核向细胞质的输出（Yoo et al. 2010）。HHV-8 感染对血管内皮细胞进行重新编程使之表达淋巴标志分子，这是 KS 发生和发展的关键步骤（Pyakurel et al. 2006；Wang et al. 2004）。Kaposin B 稳定 PROX1mRNA 的活性代表了 HHV-8 感染诱导从血管内皮到淋巴内皮转变的一种机制。因此，除了 kaposin A 外，kaposin B 也可能在 HHV-8 相关的疾病中起重要作用。

2.4　PEL 中的病毒白细胞介素-6（vIL-6）

病毒白细胞介素-6（vIL-6）与人类细胞的 IL-6（hIL-6）有大约 25%的序列同源性。这一病毒细胞因子分别由不同的研究组发现（Moore et al. 1996；Neipel et al. 1997a；Nicholas et al. 1997）。尽管病毒 IL-6 与人的序列同源性较低，但它们都采用同等的 4 个 α 螺旋束结构，有类似的受体相互作用和信号活性（Boulanger et al. 2003；Chow et al. 2001；Heinrich et al. 2003；Kishimoto et al. 1995）。hIL-6

的信号转导需要与信号传递者 gp130 和 gp80 受体亚基相互作用，导致 JAK 的激活、磷酸化、二聚化，以及 STAT1 和 STAT3 的重新定位（Heinrich et al. 1998）。几个研究组的研究表明，vIL-6 虽然利用与 hIL-6 同样的信号成分，但是它不需要 gp80 来形成活性复合物，而是能通过四聚体（$gp130_2$:$vIL-6_2$）或六聚体（$gp130_2$:$gp80_2$:$vIL-6_2$）复合物进行信号转导。最后，这两类细胞因子有一些共同的功能特征，如维持 IL-6 依赖性细胞系的生长（Burger et al. 1998；Nicholas et al. 1997）。然而，vIL-6 转导信号的能力很独特，不仅通过位于胞质膜上的 gp130 复合体，还在细胞内质网（ER）进行转导。vIL-6 与 hIL-6 不同，它的分泌型不多，大部分位于 ER。它们的这些独特属性可能参与维持病毒潜伏感染，对于 HHV-8 的致病性有重要作用。

几个研究表明，vIL-6 对于 PEL 细胞的生长起关键性作用。虽然在 PEL 细胞培养上清中都能检测到 vIL-6、IL-10 和血管内皮生长因子（VEGF），但只有 vIL-6 和 IL-10 诱导 PEL 细胞增殖（Aoki and Tosato 1999；Jones et al. 1999）。起初，因为 vIL-6 在有效复制时被诱导，所以在这些培养物中检测到 vIL-6 被认为是小部分细胞同步裂解导致重激活的结果。然而，现在 vIL-6 在潜伏感染的 PEL 细胞中也有低水平的表达（Chandriani and Ganem 2010；Chen et al. 2009a）。在这些细胞中删除 vIL-6 能诱导凋亡和减慢细胞生长率（Chen et al. 2009a）。细胞在用抗 vIL-6 单链抗体和靶向 vIL-6 转录物的多肽偶联磷酰吗啉寡聚体（PPMO）处理后，可以观察到类似的细胞生长效应（Kovaleva et al. 2006；Zhang et al. 2008）。完全滞留在 ER 中的 vIL-6（克隆有靶向 ER 性的 KDEL 结构域）能恢复 vIL-6 删除所介导的细胞生长效应（Chen et al. 2009a）。这些数据表明了 vIL-6 的细胞内自分泌信号在支持潜伏感染 PEL 细胞的生存和生长中的重要作用。

虽然高尔基体内 vIL-6 促进 PEL 细胞生长和活力的机制还不是很清楚，但是早期的研究表明，它与维生素 K 环氧还原酶复合体亚单位 1 的变体 2（vitamin K epoxide reductase complex subunit 1 variant 2，VKORC1v2）的新型相互作用是非常关键的。VKORC1v2 是高尔基体中的一种蛋白质，被认为是 vIL-6 的一种结合成分，对于 PEL 细胞生存是必需的（Chen et al. 2012）。删除 VKORC1v2 后能得到与删除 vIL-6 类似的细胞生长效应。此外，一种能破坏 VKORC1v2:vIL-6 之间相互作用的短肽抑制剂也模拟了 vIL-6 或 VKORC1v2 删除的细胞生长和凋亡效应，这些明确了 vIL-6:VKORC1v2 相互作用的生物学相关性（Chen et al. 2012）。这些研究同时表明，高尔基体内这种病毒细胞因子的活性，至少部分是通过 VKORC1v2 起作用的，对于维持潜伏感染 B 细胞内的病毒起重要作用；这些活性也参与病毒的致病作用。

在几个 PEL 细胞系中，检测到磷酸化（活性的）STAT3 的水平升高（Aoki et al. 2003）。当 vIL-6 通过 gp130 复合体信号转导通路时，STAT3 被激活。在 PEL

细胞中删除 STAT3 导致凋亡增加和存活素水平下降（Aoki et al. 2003）。存活素是凋亡抑制剂（IAP）家族成员，研究表明其在几个癌症细胞系中能抑制凋亡（Ambrosini et al. 1997）。这些结果具有重要意义，因为它们把存活素的抗凋亡活性与 STAT3 信号和可能的 vIL-6 信号联系到了一起。在这方面值得一提的是，PEL 细胞 gp130 的删除导致细胞生长抑制和凋亡增加（E. Cousins and J. Nicholas，未发表）。除了 vIL-6:gp130 信号外，STAT3 也能被 VEGF 激活（Bartoli et al. 2000）。重要的是，研究发现 vIL-6 在实验性转导的细胞系中诱导 VEGF，并且对 PEL 细胞生长和异种移植肿瘤的迁移起重要作用（Aoki et al. 1999; Aoki and Tosato 1999）。因此，vIL-6 在 PEL 细胞参与一系列的活动，不仅能启动促生长和通过 ER 的生存信号（图 15-1），还能通过激活 STAT3/生存素和 VEGF 信号影响 PEL 的致病性。

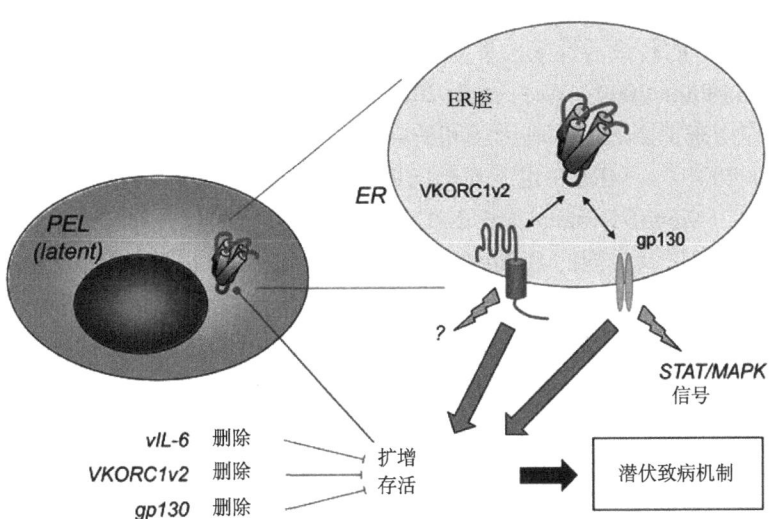

图 15-1 潜伏感染的 PEL 细胞内 vIL-6 的活性和 ER 内的相互作用。在 PEL 的潜伏感染期，vIL-6 虽然表达较低，且主要隔离在 ER 内，但仍能发挥其功能。潜伏表达的 vIL-6 支持 PEL 细胞生长和活性。在 vIL-6 删除的 PEL 细胞，这些活性能被限制在 ER 内转导的（带 KDEL 标签的）vIL-6 补偿。vIL-6 的信号转导者 gp130 和一个新的剪切变体蛋白 VKORC1v2，每一个都能结合 ER 内的 vIL-6，删除任何一个都能抑制 PEL 细胞生长和活性。已有的证据表明，vIL-6 通过每一个这些 ER 受体的活性是独立的。虽然 PEL 细胞中检测到 gp130 介导的 STAT 和 MAPK 信号的激活，但 gp130 信号（与其对生长和存活的效应相反）不受 VKORC1v2 的删除，以及多肽介导的破坏 vIL-6 和 VKORC1v2 之间相互作用的影响。在潜伏感染的 PEL 细胞中，vIL-6 的表达、促生长和促存活的活性表明，病毒细胞因子可能参与 B 细胞潜伏感染的维持和 PEL 疾病。

2.5 PEL 中病毒干扰素调节因子 3（vIRF-3）

HHV-8 有 4 种病毒干扰素因子（vIRF 1~4），其作用是抵抗细胞 IRF，以及抑制细胞对病毒感染和有效复制（见下文）的天然免疫反应（Cunningham et al. 2003；Lee et al. 2009a）。所有 vIRF 都在裂解复制期表达，这与其逃逸宿主抗病毒防御的主要作用一致，然而，vIRF-3 实际上作为一种潜伏期产物在 PEL 细胞中表达（Jenner et al. 2001；Paulose-Murphy et al. 2001；Rivas et al. 2001）。正因为如此，有些研究者把 vIRF-3 称为潜伏相关核抗原-2（LANA2），尽管它部分定位于细胞质（Munoz-Fontela et al. 2005），并且在其他任何检查的细胞中缺少可论证的潜伏表达，但是，在 PEL/B 细胞，vIRF-3 有可能影响病毒潜伏细胞途径和病毒相关的致病性。与其他 vIRF 的共同之处是，vIRF-3 能抑制细胞 IRF 的功能。vIRF-3 除了抑制促凋亡激酶 PKR（被干扰素和 dsRNA 激活）外，还通过干扰 IRF-3、IRF-5 和 IRF-7 的转录活性来发挥其功能（Esteban et al. 2003；Joo et al. 2007；Lubyova and Pitha 2000；Wies et al. 2009）。重要的是，研究发现 vIRF-3 直接与 p53 相互作用来抑制肿瘤抑制因子和诱导 Myc 指导的转录（Lubyova et al. 2007；Rivas et al. 2001）。vIRF-3 也能与靶向促凋亡基因的转录因子 FOXO3a 作用，并抑制其功能（Munoz-Fontela et al. 2007）。这些活性表明，vIRF-3 在促进 PEL 细胞存活和扩增，以及常规的 B 细胞潜伏方面起重要作用。实际上，研究表明 vIRF-3 的删除触发了细胞凋亡，因此其对培养物中 PEL 细胞活力起至关重要的作用（Wies et al. 2008）。vIRF-3 的促存活作用部分是由于其抑制 PML 介导的对生物素的抑制（Marcos-Villar et al. 2009）。而且，近来还报道，在 PEL 细胞中，vIRF-3 抑制 CIITA 转录因子介导的、对干扰素 γ 和 II 型主要组织相容性复合体的抑制（Schmidt et al. 2011）。vIRF-3 的这种免疫逃逸活性可能对于体内这些细胞的长期存活是至关重要的。因此，vIRF-3 的活性至少在有些细胞（vIRF-3 潜伏表达）对于其潜伏持续性起非常重要的作用，也可能显著参与 PEL 的恶性化。

2.6 MicroRNA（miRNA）

微小 RNA（miRNA）是长度约 22 个核苷酸的非编码 RNA，其作用是通过裂解作用或通过抑制翻译来调节 mRNA 的表达。miRNA 是由初级 miRNA（pri-miRNA）编码，通过 RNA 聚合酶 II 合成，在由 exportin 5 进行核输出之前，被 DROSHA 的 RNase III 结构域处理成为 pre-miRNA（杆环结构）。在胞质中，pre-miRNA 被 DICER 的 RNAse III 结构域裂解为 21~24 个核苷酸的双链 RNA。整合的 miRNA 指导装载的 RISC 靶向 mRNA（Schwarz et al. 2003）。一般来说，如果 miRNA 与它的靶向序列能很好地互补，那么靶 mRNA 就会被降解。另外，miRNA 的结合即使在不完全互补的情况下也能抑制 mRNA 的翻译（Zeng et al.

2003)。

虽然 miRNA 已经在所有的多细胞动物中都能检测到，但病毒编码的 miRNA 是最近才被发现的（Pfeffer et al. 2004）。迄今为止，已经有 12 个 HHV-8 病毒编码的 miRNA 被鉴定，命名为 miR-K12-1 至 miR-K12-12。这 12 个 miRNA 中有 10 个位于 HHV-8 基因组中潜伏表达的开放阅读框 71 和 K12 之间。Mi-k12-10 位于 ORF K12 内，而 miR-K12-12 位于 K12 的 3′-UTR（Pfeffer et al. 2005；Samols et al. 2005）。所有 HHV-8 的 12 个 miRNA 都是朝着从 ORF 71 到 K12 的方向，它们在潜伏期表达（Cai et al. 2005）。许多的 miRNA 都能在裂解感染期被检测到（有些甚至是被诱导的）（Cai et al. 2005；Umbach and Cullen 2010）。生物信息学方法是利用 miRNA 种子序列（miRNA 的 2~7/8 个核苷酸）去寻找 miRNA 的靶基因，但这些方法能产生大量的潜在候选者（Gottwein and Cullen 2010；Lu et al. 2010b；Nachmani et al. 2009；Qin et al. 2010）。然而，那些不是完全互补的种子序列的靶标可能被忽视，因此，有必要通过验证试验对鉴定的候选者进行真伪评价。常用的功能性方法包括：转导含单个或组合 HHV-8 的 miRNA 重组病毒；通过微芯片检测 mRNA 水平可能发生的变化（Ziegelbauer et al. 2009）。最近，还进行了 RISC 和/或相关的 Argonaute 蛋白的免疫共沉淀，以及共沉淀 mRNA 的微芯片分析（RIP-CHIP）（Dolken et al. 2010）。通过这些方法，在宿主细胞中已经鉴定了多个 miRNA 靶点。从这些实验数据，已经推导出一些病毒编码的 miRNA：①限制 NK 细胞对病毒感染细胞的识别（Nachmani et al. 2009）；②抑制 RTA 蛋白表达，从而抑制潜伏-裂解之间的转变（Bellare and Ganem 2009；Lin et al. 2011；Lu et al.2010a）；③干扰 TGF-β 信号（Liu et al. 2012）；④改变 NF-κB 信号途径（Lei et al. 2010）；⑤调控细胞因子产生（Abend et al. 2010）；⑥修饰细胞周期进程（Gottwein and Cullen 2010）。这些 miRNA 的靶点和信号途径总结于表 15-1，下面将进一步讨论。

表 15-1　HHV-8 编码的 microRNA 及其功能

功能类别	病毒 microRNA	靶基因	活性/功能	参考文献
细胞周期调节	miR-K12-1	p21	抑制细胞周期停滞	Gottwein and Cullen（2010）
凋亡	miR-K12-10a	TWEAKR	减少的 caspase 活性	Abend et al.（2010）
	miR-K12-5，9，10	BCLAF1	抑制凋亡	Ziegelbauer et al.（2009）
	miR-K12-1，3，4-3p	Caspase 3	抑制凋亡	Suffert et al.（2011）
	miR-K12-11	BACH1	促存活	Gottwein et al.（2007），Skalsky et al.（2007），Qin et al.（2010）

续表

功能类别	病毒 microRNA	靶基因	活性/功能	参考文献
潜伏维持	miR-K12-3	NFIB	抑制 RTA，稳定潜伏	Lu et al.（2010a，b）
	miR-K12-5，7-5p，9	RTA	稳定潜伏	Bellare and Ganem（2009），Lin et al.（2011），Lu et al.（2010a，b）
生长信号	miR-K12-11	SMAD5	抑制 TGF-信号	Liu et al.（2012）
	miR-K12-6，11	MAF	细胞命运重新编程	Hansen et al.（2010）
免疫逃逸	miR-K12-7	MICB	逃逸 NK 细胞监视	Nachmani et al.（2009）
血管生成作用	miR-K12-1，3，6，11	THBS1	增强血管生成作用	Samols et al.（2007）
病毒复制	miR-K12-1	IkBalpha	限制病毒复制	Lei et al.（2010）
染色质修饰	miR-K12-4-5p	Rb12	全面表观遗传修饰	Lu et al.（2010a，b）
没有验证的靶点	miR-K12-3	NHP2L1	剪切子组装？	Dolken et al.（2010）
	miR-K12 簇	LRRC8D	不明确	Dolken et al.（2010）
	miR-K12 簇	SEC15L	囊泡运载？	Dolken et al.（2010）
	miR-K12-4-3	GEMIN8	mRNA 剪切？	Dolken et al.（2010）
	miR-K12 簇	ZNF684	转录调节？	Dolken et al.（2010）
	miR-K12 簇	CDK5RAP1	CDK5 抑制剂？	Dolken et al.（2010）

HHV-8 通过多种策略来保持其不被宿主免疫反应识别，而病毒 miRNA 被认为起关键性作用。HHV-8 编码的 miR-K12-7 靶向一个病毒干扰诱导的细胞表面标记分子 MICB。MICB 能通过 NK 细胞表达的 NKG2D 受体诱导 NK 细胞的识别和杀伤活性（Glas et al. 2000；Nachmani et al. 2009）。病毒编码的 miRNA 靶向的 MICB 在人类巨细胞病毒（Stern-Ginossar et al. 2007；Stern-Ginossar et al.2008）和 EB 病毒感染（Nachmani et al. 2009）中都比较保守。几个 HHV-8 miRNA 除了起免疫逃逸作用外，还靶向 RTA，抑制病毒复制和维持病毒潜伏感染。几个研究组已经鉴定了 miR-K12-3、miR-12-5、miR-K12-9 和 miR-K12-11，它们直接或间接地靶向 RTA 的表达（Bellare and Ganem 2009；Lin et al. 2011；Lu et al. 2010b）。miR-K12-1 通过下调 NF-κB 的抑制蛋白 IκB-α、上调 NF-κB 信号，从而限制病毒复制和终止 HHV-8 病毒的裂解性复制（Lei et al. 2010）。病毒通过降低其病毒子的产生来避免宿主的免疫反应。

除了免疫逃逸外，病毒还能抵抗宿主细胞感染后诱导的促凋亡途径。Caspase 3 是多个病毒 miRNA（miR-K12-1、miR-K12-3 和 miR-K12-4-3p）的靶基因，它被抑制就会降低 HHV-8 感染细胞对 caspase 诱导凋亡的敏感性（Suffert et al. 2011）。类似地，miR-K12-10a 抑制 TWEAK 受体（TWEAKR）表达，从而限制 TWEAK 诱导的 caspase 激活和凋亡（Abend et al. 2010）。TWEAKR 的失活降低了促炎症细胞因子 IL8/CXCL8 和 MCP-1/CCL2 的产生（Abend et al. 2010）。几个 HHV-8 的 microRNA（miR-K12-5、miR-K12-9 和 miR-K12-10a/b）都能靶向转录抑制因子 BCLAF1，导致泊苷诱导的 PEL 细胞凋亡减少（Ziegelbauer et al. 2009）。最后，细胞 miR-155 的同源物 miR-K12-11 能改变 BACH1 的表达，从而导致多种表型变化，包括：HMOX1 上调（细胞存活率增加）；xCT 上调（巨噬细胞和内皮细胞对病毒感染的易感性增加）；对活性氮诱导的细胞凋亡产生保护（Gottwein et al. 2007；Qin et al. 2010；Skalsky et al. 2007）。

HHV-8 编码的 microRNA 也在细胞生长和血管生成中起显著性的作用。miR-K12-11 可以直接靶向 SMAD5，下调 TGF-β 信号（Liu et al. 2012），从而诱导细胞扩增。研究者们已经注意到，HHV-8$^+$B 细胞系的 miR-155（miR-K12-11 的细胞类似物）的水平下降，而 miR-K12-11 可能弥补这些细胞中被下调的 miR-155 水平（Skalsky et al. 2007）。抑制 miR-K12-11 能激活 HHV-8$^+$B 细胞的 TGF-β 信号（Liu et al. 2012）。TGF-β 信号受 HHV-8 miRNA（miR-K12-1miR-K12-3、miR-K12-6 和 miR-K12-11）的靶点凝血栓蛋白（thrombospondin 1，THBS1）调控。THBS1 是一种抗血管生成因子，它的下调导致 TGF-β 信号的抑制（Samols et al. 2005）。因此，病毒的多个 microRNA 能改变细胞的生长信号和增强血管生成作用，从而支撑 HHV-8 相关肿瘤发生。在 KS 中，血管内皮细胞（BEC）和淋巴内皮细胞（LEC）的标志分子表达均能找到。在适当的刺激下，KS 可发生命运重编程，转向 LEC 或 BEC。此外，病毒的 miRNA 还能改变内皮细胞的转录组，帮助细胞重编程。尤其是，miR-12-6 和 miR-K12-11 靶向细胞的转录因子 MAF（肌肉腱膜纤维肉瘤癌基因类似物）（Hansen et al. 2010），这一现象通常发生在 LEC，而不是 BEC。在 KS 组织中，通过 microRNA 沉默 MAF，会增加 BEC 标记基因的表达（Rodriguez et al. 2007）。

几个其他的研究虽然发现了病毒 microRNA 的潜在靶基因，但这些靶基因仍在验证中。例如，视网膜母细胞瘤样蛋白 2（retinoblastoma-like protein 2，Rbl2）被鉴定为 miR-K12-4-5p 的靶点（Lu et al. 2010b）。Rbl2 是一个特异性 DNA 甲基转移酶（DNMT3a 和 3b）的抑制剂，抑制 Rbl2 之后发现有表观遗传学的变化，但是这些变化的后果还不清楚（Lu et al. 2010b）。最后，用荧光素酶检测方法的大规模研究鉴定了一些 HHV-8 的 miRNA 潜在靶点，包括参与囊泡运输、剪切体组装、转录调控和细胞周期进展的一些蛋白质（Dolken et al. 2010）。这些靶蛋白还有待验证，其结果将有助于理解miRNA在HHV-8病毒生物学和致病性中的作用。

3 通过裂解活性的新型病毒-宿主相互作用

3.1 病毒白细胞介素-6（vIL-6）

vIL-6在PEL致病性方面主要通过直接自分泌作用，而在KS和MCD主要通过旁分泌信号起作用。新感染的细胞和那些正在进行裂解复制的细胞表达vIL-6作为早期基因产物，在RTA表达之后，vIL-6很快就被诱导表达（Sun et al. 1999）。在KS病变中，大部分HHV-8感染的细胞仍然保持潜伏感染状态，但小部分细胞处于裂解活性状态。这小部分细胞表达裂解蛋白，包括vIL-6、vGPCR和K1。这些蛋白质最后增强细胞炎症因子和血管生成因子的表达（Mesri et al. 2010）。例如，vIL-6能诱导VEGF的表达（Aoki and Tosato 1999），被认为是KS发展的关键因素。VEGF和其他细胞因子（IL6、CXCL8和bFGF）从裂解活性的细胞中分泌后，可以进一步以旁分泌形式激活周围潜伏感染的和未感染的细胞。分泌的蛋白质调节HHV-8感染细胞的存活，主要通过VEGF的血管生成和招募未感染的细胞到病变位置。炎症细胞因子（包括IL-6）和血管生成因子被认为在KS发展的起始阶段起作用（Ensoli and Sturzl 1998）。

在同一MCD患者，感染的淋巴结IL-6水平比未感染的淋巴结高很多（Yoshizaki et al. 1989）。此外，疾病的严重程度与IL-6水平相关。当感染的淋巴结被切除后，IL-6水平就下降（Yoshizaki et al. 1989）。同样，来自HIV阳性KS患者的细胞系表达IL-6，KS组织产生的IL-6的量比正常组织也高（Miles et al. 1990）。研究发现，IL-6的反义寡核苷酸抑制HIV阳性患者KS细胞生长和IL-6产生，而外源性重组IL-6能恢复细胞生长和扩增（Miles et al. 1990）。另外一个研究还发现，MCD患者的癌变浆细胞产生的IL-6水平大大升高，但是其他B细胞瘤的IL-6没有明显变化（Burger et al. 1994）。当发现这些现象时，疾病相关的IL-6失调机制还不清楚。近来越来越多的报道表明，vIL-6在一些细胞中能诱导IL-6和VEGF的表达（Aoki et al. 1999; Mori et al. 2000）。vIL-6也可能直接影响MCD。此外，vIL-6在B细胞急性感染过程中下调CCL2和抑制中性粒细胞浸润（Fielding et al. 2005）。

3.2 病毒CC趋化因子配体（vCCL）

HHV-8的三个趋化因子vCCL-1、vCCL-2和vCCL-3分别由K6、K4和K4.1阅读框编码（Moore et al. 1996; Neipel et al. 1997b; Nicholas et al. 1997; Russo et al.1996），都是在裂解周期的早期表达（Jenner et al. 2001; Paulose-Murphy et al.

2001）。vCCL-1 和 vCCL-2 在结构上分别与细胞趋化因子 CCL3 和 CCL4 很类似，而 vCCL-3 与一些 CC 趋化因子有明显的一级序列相似性。然而，病毒趋化因子的属性与细胞来源的趋化因子显著不同。从受体的使用来看，vCCL-1 是 CCR8 类似物；vCCL-2 通过 CCR3、CCR8 转导信号，也可能通过 CCR5 转导信号；vCCL-3 功能性地靶向 CCR4 和 XCR1（Boshoff et al. 1997；Dairaghi et al. 1999；Luttichau 2008；Luttichau et al. 2007；Nakano et al. 2003；Stine et al. 2000）。此外，vCCL-2 还结合几个 CCR 型和 CXCR 型趋化因子受体，作为中性配体（不产生信号）结合 CX3XR1，它通过这些受体有效地抑制细胞趋化因子活性（Chen et al. 1998；Crump et al. 2001；Dairaghi et al. 1999；Kledal et al. 1997；Luttichau et al. 2001）。病毒趋化因子所靶向的受体的特性表明，它们可能通过 Th2 极化和阻断白细胞迁移来介导免疫逃逸，这些通过 vCCL-2 的体内实验已得到了证实（Chen et al. 1998；Weber et al. 2001）。

除了这些免疫逃逸的特性外，每一种病毒趋化因子还能通过诱导 VEGF 促进血管生成（Boshoff et al. 1997；Liu et al. 2001；Stine et al. 2000）。像 vIL-6 一样，HHV-8 的 vCCL 可能通过旁分泌信号促进 KS 的致病作用，它们也可能在 PEL 中起作用。小鼠研究数据表明，VEGF 是 PEL 的一个重要因素（Aoki and Tosato 1999；Ensoli and Sturzl 1998；Haddad et al. 2008）。vCCL-1 和 vCCL-2 的其他致病作用可能还包括：通过 CCR8 产生促生存信号，这在 HHV-8 感染的和未感染的内皮细胞中得到了证实（Choi and Nicholas 2008）。研究还发现，vCCL-1 和 vCCL-2 能促进 PEL 和小鼠细胞系的存活（Liu et al. 2001；Louahed et al. 2003）。不像大多数（非分泌型的）病毒蛋白，病毒趋化因子具有通过旁分泌途径发挥其功能的潜力。因此，这些趋化因子可能促进潜伏感染和未感染细胞的存活，而这些细胞包围了那些支持裂解复制的细胞，这些都与病毒致病性相关。然而，vCCL-1 和 vCCL-2 的促生存活性的一个重要方面是，它们通过自分泌信号对有效复制起正调节作用。内源性产生的病毒趋化因子抑制裂解周期诱导的细胞凋亡，提高病毒在 HHV-8 感染的内皮细胞中的产量（Choi and Nicholas 2008）。这一活性涉及 CCR8 信号依赖性抑制裂解周期应激诱导的促凋亡蛋白 Bim，它是一个强有力的病毒有效复制的抑制剂。

3.3 病毒 G 蛋白偶联受体（vGPCR）

vGPCR 虽然不是 HHV-8 所特有的，但 HHV-8 编码的 vGPCR 在结构和功能上都与其他 γ-2 疱疹病毒的 vGPCR 不一样，它通过旁分泌方式作用于 KS 的发展（Cannon 2007；Nicholas 2005；Rosenkilde et al. 2001；Verzijl et al. 2004）。HHV-8 的 vGPCR 除了通过直接关联并激活信号蛋白 SHP2 外，还不寻常地与 3 个类型的 Gα 蛋白有功能上的联系（Couty et al. 2001；Liu et al. 2004；Philpott et al. 2011；

Shepard et al. 2001）。早期报道，在 vGPCR 转导的细胞系的体外和体内实验系统中，vGPCR 能作为一类经典的自分泌癌基因发挥其功能，这暗示 vGPCR 可能是作为一种潜伏蛋白表达的（使其直接参与 HHV-8 的肿瘤形成）。然而，目前还没有发现 vGPCR 潜伏表达的证据。尽管如此，vGPCR 能在受体转导的小鼠中诱导 KS 样的肿瘤。尽管只有少量的细胞表达 vGPCR，但这种表型能持续存在（Montaner et al. 2003；Yang et al. 2000）。vGPCR 信号诱导产生血管生成因子、有丝分裂原和炎症细胞因子，最终导致局部内皮细胞激活、扩增和肿瘤形成（Montaner et al. 2004），这些能解释以上现象。像前面提到的一样，细胞因子失调被认为是 KS 疾病的主要驱动力。已知 vGPCR 能激活一些关键因子，如 VEGF、bFGF、CXCL8 和 IL-6，这些在 KS 病变中都能观察到，被认为是促进 KS 发展和进程所必需的（Bais et al. 1998；Cannon et al. 2003；Pati et al. 2001；Schwarz and Murphy 2001）。因此，小量同步再激活的内皮细胞产生的 vGPCR，可能诱导了足够的细胞因子水平来促进 KS 发展。应当指出的是，在动物模型中，表达 vGPCR 的细胞能够与表达潜伏基因 v-cyclin 和/或 vFLIP 的细胞合作，提高单独接种 vGPCR 阳性细胞的 KS 发生率（Montaner et al. 2003）。这支持了在 HHV-8 相关的肿瘤中自分泌潜伏和旁分泌裂解活性能一起起作用的观点。

3.4 病毒干扰素调节因子（vIRF）

HHV-8 的 vIRF 1~4 由基因组区域包含的 ORF K9 至 K11 所编码。一个同等位点（编码 8 个 vIRF）只发现于关系很近的恒河猴猴病毒属（Alexander et al. 2000；Cunningham et al. 2003；Moore et al. 1996；Searles et al. 1999）。所有 4 个 vIRF 都在裂解复制期间表达，但 vIRF-1 和 vIRF-3 也在 PEL 潜伏期表达（Pozharskaya et al. 2004；Rivas et al. 2001）。此外，通过 RT-PCR 能在 KS 细胞检测到 vIRF-1 转录子（Dittmer 2003）。因此，vIRF-3 被认为是 PEL 细胞活力所必需的（Wies et al. 2008）。然而，没有检测到缺失 vIRF-1 对培养中的 PEL 细胞生长或存活的影响（Choi and Nicholas，未发表数据）。vIRF 好像主要起逃避宿主细胞对从头（de novo）感染和病毒有效复制的防御作用，这些能驱使细胞 IRF 和干扰素信号级联反应，导致细胞周期停止和诱导凋亡信号（Lee et al. 2009a；Offermann 2007）。vIRF-3 通过直接结合到 IRF5 和 IRF7 的功能性二聚体、启动子相关的部位，从而拮抗其相应的功能。vIRF-3 也能抑制 IRF3 的活性（Joo et al. 2007；Wies et al. 2009）。vIRF-1 通过竞争性地结合到转录共激活因子来阻断 IRF 指导的启动子招募 p300/CBP，从而介导转录抑制 IRF 靶向的基因（Burysek et al. 1999a；Li et al. 2000；Lin et al. 2001；Seo et al. 2000；Zimring et al. 1998）。vIRF-2 介导的转录抑制 IRF-1、IRF-3 和 ISGF3 靶向基因，部分是通过激活 caspase 3 介导的 IRF3 去稳定性而实现的（Areste et al. 2009；Burysek et al. 1999b；Fuld et al. 2006）。此外，vIRF-2

和 vIRF-3 直接靶向和/或抑制 dsRNA 激活的 PKR 激酶活性，从而抑制 PKR 诱导的蛋白质翻译和干扰素信号（Burysek and Pitha 2001；Esteban et al. 2003）。有趣的是，vIRF-3 和促血管生成转录因子 HIF-1α 有关联，且能使其呈稳定状态（Shin et al. 2008），这不仅能促进内皮细胞存活，还能通过诱导细胞因子（如 VEGF）来影响 KS 和 PEL 的致病性。研究表明，vIRF-1、3 和 4 通过以下方式抑制 p53 活性：①直接结合到肿瘤抑制因子（vIRF-1 和 vIRF-3）；②通过与 p53 磷酸化的和 p53 激活的 ATM 激酶相互作用（vIRF-1）；③通过稳定 MDM2（vIRF-4），从而促进 p53 的泛素化和蛋白酶体降解（Lee et al. 2009b；Nakamura et al. 2001；Rivas et al. 2001；Seo et al. 2001；Shin et al. 2006）。据报道，vIRF-4 与去泛素化酶 HAUSP 抑制性的相互作用参与了 p53 的去稳定（Lee et al. 2011）。因此，p53 代表一个 vIRF 的主要靶点，对于控制病毒有效复制很重要。vIRF-4 也结合到 Notch 通路的靶点 CSL，然而这种相互作用的意义还不是很清楚（Heinzelmann et al. 2010）。

vIRF-1 还和其他一些细胞蛋白有关联并抑制其活性，这些蛋白质主要参与细胞对感染的天然免疫反应和促进凋亡。它们的作用靶点包括维甲酸、干扰素诱导蛋白 GRIM19，以及 TGF-β 受体激活的转录因子 Smad3（肿瘤抑制）和 Smad4（co-Smad）（Angell et al. 2000；Ma et al. 2007；Seo et al. 2002，2005）。最近，研究还发现 vIRF-1 直接结合到所谓的 BOP（BH3-only protein）蛋白家族的成员（Choi and Nicholas 2010；Choi et al. 2012）。BOP 是 Bcl-2 相关蛋白，通过抑制 Bcl-2 家族促存活成员或直接激活凋亡执行者 Bax 和 Bak，发挥其促凋亡作用（Kuwana et al. 2005；Willis and Adams 2005）。vIRF-1 中由 170~184 位氨基酸组成的区域（BOP 结合域，BBD）与 BOP 的 BH3 结构域相互作用，从而介导抑制 BOP，这是其促凋亡活性所必需的（Choi and Nicholas 2010；Choi et al. 2012）。据预测，vIRF-1 的 BBD 是一个两亲性 α 螺旋结构，类似于 Bid 的 BH3 抑制性 BH3-B 结构域，代表的仅仅是 BH3 的 B 型 BH3 抑制性结构域的第二个例子，因此是一个新的病毒凋亡抑制机制。BBD 介导的、与 BOP 之间的相互作用具有重要的功能，证据如下：①BBD 突变的 vIRF-1 促有效复制，其抑制裂解感染内皮细胞凋亡的活性比野生型 vIRF-1 的弱；②vIRF-1:BOP 的 BBD 多肽破坏后，被感染细胞中病毒的产生明显受到抑制；③vIRF-1 靶向的 BOP 成员 Bim 或 Bid 的表达受到干扰后，病毒复制滴度显著上升（Choi and Nicholas 2010；Choi et al. 2012）。

总之，大量发表的数据表明，HHV-8 的 vIRF 代表一组有效的抗凋亡蛋白，它们通过与一组重要的、参与宿主抗感染防御的细胞蛋白相互作用，促进病毒的有效复制（总结于图 15-2）。

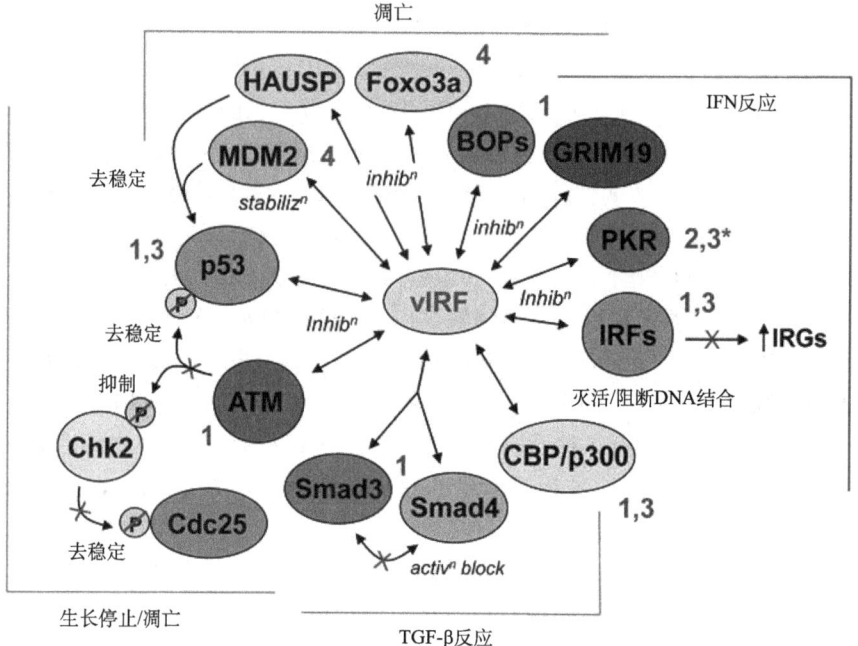

图 15-2　vIRF 与细胞蛋白之间的抑制性相互作用总结。相邻的数字表明了特定的 vIRF 与每一个靶点相互作用，这种作用的效应用斜体字表示。vIRF 相互作用的活性分为 4 个一般性、有相互重叠的生物学类别，分别用不同颜色的线框标记。vIRF 和蛋白质之间的相互作用及其意义在文中进行了充分的讨论（*功能抑制；没有检测到物理性相互作用）。

3.5　K7 编码的病毒凋亡抑制蛋白（vIAP）

与其他疱疹病毒一样，HHV-8 编码与细胞 Bcl-2 蛋白同源的蛋白质。然而，HHV-8 额外还编码一个含 BH 样结构域的抗凋亡蛋白，是细胞存活素的同系物。HHV-8 的这种蛋白质称为 K7（对应于该编码的 ORF）或病毒凋亡抑制蛋白（vIAP）。K7/vIAP 是一种膜相关蛋白，含一个假定的线粒体靶向信号，定位于线粒体和内质网（ER），也可能定位于其他的膜结构（Feng et al. 2002；Wang et al. 2002）。据报道，K7/vIAP 通过 C 端 BH2 样结构结合到细胞的 Bcl-2，也可结合到由蛋白酶裂解作用激活的 caspase 3，通过这种桥梁作用发挥其抑制 caspase 3 的蛋白裂解活性（Wang et al. 2002）。这种在凋亡级联反应中与末端的 caspase 3 的相互作用导致的抑制作用类似于细胞中 IAP（生存素、XIAP 和 cIAP1、cIAP2）的活性。然而，关于具有 K7/vIAP 与 Bcl-2 之间的相互作用的类似特性，在细胞中还没有报道有同类蛋白。这种相互作用的功能和生物学意义还有待进一步研究。然而，K7/vIAP 能够抑制 Fas 抗体和 TNF-α 处理细胞的促凋亡信号，这表明在裂解周期诱导的应急期，它可能通过促存活活性而作为一个裂解复制启动子（Wang et al. 2002）。K7/vIAP 也与钙调节的亲环素配体（CAML）相互作用，调节细胞内钙离子浓度（Bram and Crabtree 1994；Feng et al. 2002）。野生型（但不是 CAML 结合抵抗的）K7/vIAP 能抑制转染细胞中化学诱导线粒体去极化，证实了这种相互作用在功能上的意义（Feng et al. 2002）。因此，K7/vIAP 除了抑制性地结合到 caspase 3 外，它似乎还通过与 CAML 相互作用介导凋亡抑制。K7/vIAP 也与细胞蛋白 PLIC1（蛋白连接整合素相关蛋白和细胞骨架蛋白 1，又叫泛素）相互作用，这与泛素偶联蛋白抑制蛋白酶体降解有关（Feng et al. 2004；Kleijnen et al. 2000；Wu et al. 1999）。K7/vIAP 可以拮抗 PLIC1 活性，从而使泛素化蛋白去稳定，如同 p53 和抑制 NF-κB 的 IκB（Feng et al. 2004）。综上所述，K7/vIAP 与细胞蛋白 PLIC1、caspase 3/Bcl-2 和 CAML 之间的抑制性相互作用在裂解复制期可能促进细胞生存，并进一步提高病毒产生的效率。

4 末端膜蛋白

4.1 K1/可变包含 ITAM 的蛋白（VIP）

HHV-8 的 K1 开放阅读框（ORF）位于基因组的左侧末端，与编码信号膜蛋白的其他 γ 疱疹病毒基因共线性，包括塞米日肉瘤病毒（HVS）的塞米日转化相关蛋白（STP）、EBV 的潜伏膜蛋白-1（LMP-1）和恒河猴病毒 K1 同源 R1 受体（Albrecht et al. 1992；Damania et al. 1999；Kaye et al. 1993；Lagunoff and Ganem 1997；Murthy et al. 1989）。K1 蛋白是一种 I 型跨膜信号蛋白，其胞质 C 端包含一个功能性的免疫受体酪氨酸激活结构模式（immunoreceptortyrosine-based activation motif，ITAM）（Lagunoff et al. 2001；Lee et al. 1998a）。不同 HHV-8 分离株的 K1 测序结果发现，在编码蛋白的细胞外区域，有一个不寻常的氨基酸序列可变区（Nicholas et al. 1998；Zong et al.1999），因此称之为 K1/可变包含 ITAM 的蛋白（variable ITAM-containing protein，VIP）。这种可变区的功能意义还不清楚，而 K1 基因是用作 HHV-8 株病毒分布和感染性流行病毒研究的基础（Hayward and Zong 2007；Mbulaiteye et al. 2006；Whitby et al. 2004）。早期的研究主要集中在 K1 的基因组位置，后来趋向于 K1/VIP 的基本信号通路和转化特性。K1/VIP 对于 HHV-8 的致病性有潜在的作用。K1/VIP 类似于 RRV 的 R1，在体内致瘤实验中能够从功能上代替 HVS 上位置相当的 ORF1/STP，独立地促进细胞生长和转化（Lee et al. 1998b；Prakash et al. 2002）。K1/VIP 可能是通过激活 AKT 途径参与这些活性，并进一步激活细胞生长相关的 mTOR，促使凋亡蛋白 GSK3、Bad 和 forkhead 转录因子失活（Tomlinson and Damania 2004；Wang et al. 2006）。然而，K1 好像主要在裂解复制期表达（Jenner et al. 2001；Lagunoff and Ganem 1997；Nakamura et al. 2003；Paulose-Murphy et al.2001），因此，其在 KS、PEL 和 MCD 中的潜在作用可能只限于 K1/VIP 诱导细胞因子的旁分泌效应（见下文），而不是早期功能分析所表明的直接效应。虽然有报道在 KS 和 MCD 组织中通过免疫学方法能检测到 K1/VIP，但是这不与潜伏感染的细胞相关（Lee et al. 2003a；Wang et al. 2006）。然而，应该注意的是，原位检测 K1 转录物研究表明，在一些缺少可检测的裂解标记物（主要囊膜蛋白）mRNA 表达的 KS 细胞中，K1/VIP 可能至少在一些潜伏感染的 KS 细胞中表达（Wang et al. 2006）。

K1/VIP 招募并激活 Src 家族激酶 PI3K 和 PLCγ 后，通过几条基本的配体非依赖性的信号通路介导信号转导（Lagunoff et al. 2001；Lee et al. 2005，1998a；Samaniego et al. 2001；Tomlinson and Damania 2004）。研究还表明，K1/VIP 可能还通过诱导细胞因子引起 HHV-8 相关性疾病，特别是 KS。这些 K1/VIP 诱导的细胞因子包括促炎症因子 IL-1β、IL-6 和 GM-CSF，以及血管生成因子 VEGF、CXCL8 和 bFGF（Lee et al. 2005；Prakash et al. 2002；Samaniego et al. 2001；Wang et al. 2006）。HHV-8 受体通过诱导细胞因子参与的致病作用，理论上在裂解复制期或潜伏期都可能发生。在 KS、PEL 和 MCD 中，少部分细胞支持裂解再激活，使与 K1 一样的裂解期表达蛋白通过旁分泌途径影响周围未感染和潜伏感染的细胞（Aoki et al. 2003；Aoki and Tosato 2003；Ensoli et al. 2001）。

4.2 K15 编码的膜蛋白

K15 编码的全长蛋白是一个含 12 个跨膜结构域的信号受体。与 K1 一样，K15 在致病性方面可能通过诱导细胞因子表达失调发挥作用。在潜伏期，K15 可能通过促生存信号引起癌症疾病。尽管 K15 转录物主要在裂解期表达，但是在静止期（潜伏期）PEL 培养物也检测到一些 K15 产物（Choi et al. 2000；Glenn et al. 1999；Sharp et al. 2002）。因为 K15 初级转录物含 8 个外显子，能剪切为不同的产物，从而使问题变得很复杂。剪切导致 mRNA 和编码蛋白的表达差异，取决于细胞类型和病毒所处的阶段。虽然所有形式的 K15 都包含 C 端含功能信号结构模式的蛋白质序列（见下文），但不同蛋白异型在它们的跨膜结构域的互补部分是不一样的。在 PEL 细胞的潜伏期，检测到了 K15 转录子和 23kDa 的蛋白质，然而一旦裂解复制重新激活，K15 的 mRNA 水平就被诱导（Choi et al. 2000；Glenn et al. 1999；Sharp et al. 2002；Tsai et al. 2009）。只有在用丁酸诱导裂解后，K15 全长蛋白才能在含 HHV-8 杆粒（bacmid）的 HEK293 细胞中检测到（Brinkmann et al. 2007）。在自然感染 HHV-8 的细胞中观察不到全长蛋白，即早期裂解触发蛋白 RTA 激活 K15 启动子转录的能力与 K15 优势裂解表达一致（Wong and Damania 2006）。然而，对于 K15 转录物和蛋白表达的特征，以及 K15 受体信号是否与自分泌方式下的潜伏特性和 HHV-8 肿瘤有关,这些仍然不确定。

　　所有 K15 亚型的细胞质尾部,以及 M、P 等位基因的蛋白质类型的信号结构都包括两个 SH2、一个 SH3 和一个 TRAF 结合位点(Brinkmann et al. 2003;Choi et al. 2000;Glenn et al. 1999)。SH2 结合介导的与 Src 家族激酶之间的相互作用是通过 K15 一级磷酸化位点 Y48EEV 结构来实现的(Brinkmann et al. 2003;Choi et al. 2000)。这样,在 SH3 结合序列 PPLP 的参与下,共同抑制 B 细胞受体(BCR)信号。PPLP 结构与交叉素 2(细胞内接头蛋白)和 Src 激酶之间的相互作用对于这种抑制活性很重要(Lim et al. 2007;Pietrek et al. 2010)。K15 受体对 BCR 的抑制与 EBV 的共线性编码的 LMP-2 是平行的,每一个都可能通过抑制 BCR 信号促使的裂解周期重新活化来促进潜伏感染。研究表明,Y481EEV 结构参与 NF-κB 和 MAPK 蛋白激酶 ERK、JNK 的激活,这些都发生在 Y481 磷酸化之后(Brinkmann and Schulz 2006;Choi et al. 2000;Pietrek et al. 2010)。K15 受体与 TRAF1、2、3 之间的相互作用可能与 NF-κB 和 MAPK 信号有关(Brinkmann and Schulz 2006;Glenn et al. 1999)。第二个含酪氨酸的结构 Y432ASI 的磷酸化不可检测,其意义还不确定。然而,它与凋亡调节蛋白 HAX-1、ER 之间的相互作用,以及 HAX-1 与 K15 在线粒体中的共定位表明,病毒受体可能通过这一结构促进细胞存活(Sharp et al. 2002)。

　　通过研究 K15 信号下游的效应发现,受体可能在 HHV-8 的生物学和潜在的病毒致病机制中发挥一定的功能。K15 除了可能通过与 HAX-1 相互作用具有抗凋亡活性外,还能诱导几个抗凋亡基因的表达,包括 A20、Bcl-2A1、Birc2 和 Birc3(Brinkmann et al. 2007)。这些基因的诱导可能有助于促进裂解复制周期中细胞的存活,从而进一步增强病毒的有效复制。如果 K15 在潜伏期表达,那么它的促存活信号可能使潜伏细胞活性延长并有利于体内潜伏池(latency pool)的维持和病毒致病作用。另一方面,在 K15 转导的细胞内观察到诱导的细胞因子,这表明 K15 通过来自裂解感染细胞的旁分泌信号影响周围(潜伏感染和未感染)细胞。潜伏感染表达 K15 的细胞对微环境表现出类似的效应。K15 受体信号诱导的细胞因子包括 IL-6、CCL2、CXCL3 和 CXCL8,每一个都具有血管生成活性,参与 KS 的致病作用(Brinkmann et al. 2007;Caselli et al. 2007;Ensoli and Sturzl 1998)。令人惊奇的是,K15 也诱导血管生成 VEGF 信号下游靶基因的表达。这清楚地表明,如果受体在潜伏期表达,那么 K15 通过自分泌方式在致病机制中发挥作用,然而 K15 的这种活性可能也导致病毒有效的复制。K15 血管生成作用的靶点包括 *Dscr-1* 和 *Cox-2*(Brinkmann et al. 2007)。值得注意的是,据报道,Cox-2 在 HHV-8 开始感染和随后潜伏感染的内皮细胞中都被诱导表达,而 Cox-2 对于几个炎性因子和血管生成因子的产生起重要作用(Sharma-Walia et al. 2010)。因此,K15 在 HHV-8 裂解复制和致病性中的促生存作用,以及旁分泌介导的促血管生成作用是可能的。如果受体潜伏表达，通过促存活信号的自分泌活性有可能导致潜伏感染和肿瘤发生。

5 小结

HHV-8 的发现和研究为鉴定以前不清楚的病毒蛋白或者那些以前没有涉足过或没有深入研究过的蛋白质的独特活性提供了机会。HHV-8 也为鉴定和了解病毒 miRNA 特征提供了模型。病毒的 miRNA 是一个新的研究领域，为认识病毒操纵宿主细胞过程提供了独到而重要的视角。这种作用过程实际上是正常病毒生物学和潜在病毒致病性的一部分。这些过程中蛋白质的特征和 miRNA 的特性已经得到了详细的描述，形成了几个重要的观点。首先，认为"只有自分泌、潜伏的病毒活性与病毒相关性肿瘤发生有关"的观点需要修改，特别是对于 KS，也可能是 PEL 和 MCD。裂解性复制过程中产生的（病毒的和/或细胞的）旁分泌因素可能促进扩增、促进生存和引起致病相关的其他功能。与 HHV-8 致病性相关的潜伏和裂解病毒蛋白，以及它们可能的自分泌和旁分泌对疾病的作用总结见图 15-3。其次，病毒产物的裂解和潜伏的分类与以前的想法没有明显的区别。例如，病毒在有效复制过程中，vIL-6、vIRF-1、vIRF-3、K1 和 K15 明显得到最大限度的表达，然而，在一些细胞类型中，病毒潜伏期也有这些蛋白质的表达。而且，值得注意的是，潜伏表达的 vIL-6 和 vIRF-3 对于 PEL 细胞的生长和存活很重要。第三个重要的观点是病毒编码的趋化因子 vCCL-1 和 vCCL-2，当在病毒有效复制过程中分泌时，以及被认为通过旁分泌作用于微环境从而促使病毒产生时（最值得注意的是逃避宿主的免疫反应），也能直接作用于产生感染的细胞，通过抗凋亡信号来提高病毒的产生。vGPCR 也表现了这种直接的促病毒复制活性。对于病毒趋化因子和 vGPCR，诱导的细胞因子可能通过类似的和/或其他活性，以一种自分泌方式促进病毒复制，同时也对宿主微环境产生广泛的效应。最后，几个 HHV-8 蛋白与广泛的宿主因子之间有多重相互作用（这一观点总结于表 15-2），并以 LANA 和 vIRF-1 进行了例证。因此，病毒蛋白通常通过蛋白质之间的相互作用发挥其多重活性。这些相互作用的详细特征和它们的功能效应对于理解各自和联合参与病毒生物学及致病机制很重要。这种特征性研究为研发新的抗病毒和治疗药物提供了基础，主要通过干扰特异性病毒与宿主之间的相互作用来抑制病毒复制或致病作用。本章概述了 HHV-8 与宿主之间的各种新型相互作用，以及参与这些过程的相关活动，它们都可能成为靶点。描述的这些相互作用也表明了病毒与宿主之间相互作用的广度和复杂度，提示了在其他病毒系统中可能存在类似的活性和机制。

第 15 章 人疱疹病毒 8 型分子生物学：病毒致病性和复制相关的新功能及病毒-宿主相互作用 · 277 ·

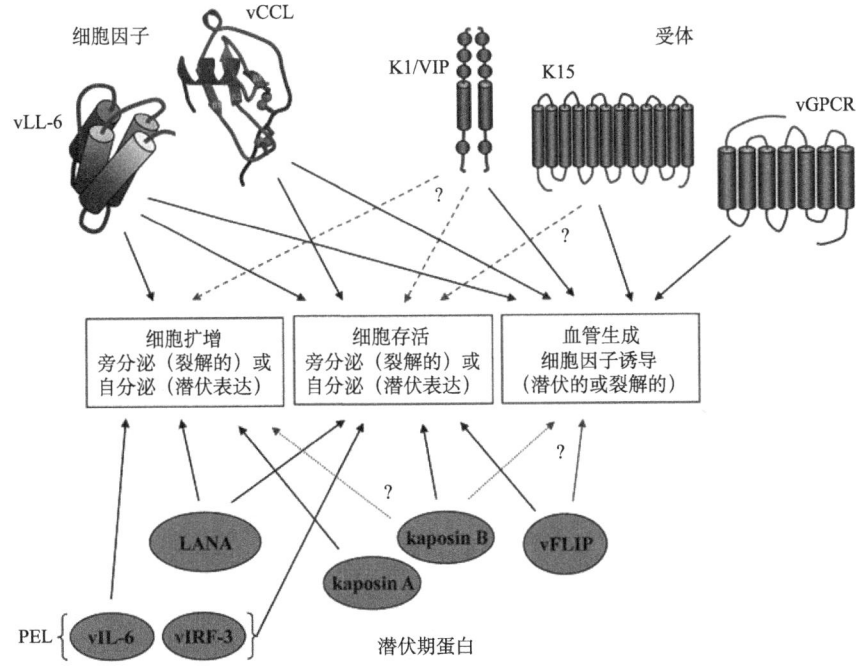

图 15-3 HHV-8 蛋白对病毒相关肿瘤的潜在作用。图中显示了与 HHV-8 肿瘤致病作用相关的一般活性。潜伏蛋白和裂解蛋白都通过自分泌和旁分泌活性在疾病中发挥潜在作用。ORF K1 和 K15 编码的信号受体的潜伏表达至今还没有明确的结论。因此，这种实验检测到的自分泌活性（虚线）是否反映了受体在 HHV-8 致病性中的直接作用仍然不确定。然而，K1 和 K15 通过诱导有丝分裂、促存活和血管生成分泌细胞因子作用于肿瘤。趋化因子受体 vGPCR 也起同样的作用。裂解期的病毒细胞因子被分泌后，通过自分泌和旁分泌机制影响细胞生长及存活。这些活性除了影响病毒致病性外（通过旁分泌效应），还能促进病毒复制（通过自分泌信号）。PEL 细胞中 vIL-6 的潜伏表达可能主要通过内分泌信号影响致病性。vIRF-3 也在 PEL 细胞的潜伏期表达，像 vIL-6 一样促进 PEL 细胞活性。潜伏期蛋白可能通过两个方面影响 HHV-8 相关肿瘤：一方面，通过直接自分泌效应影响细胞增殖；另一方面，通过典型的癌基因和肿瘤抑制因子的机制影响存活。Kaposin B 和 vFLIP 可能作为细胞扩增和/或血管生成作用的启动子而发挥作用，然而这些功能还没有得到直接的证实。

表 15-2 病毒和宿主蛋白之间的相互作用及它们的活性

蛋白	类别	靶点	活性/功能	参考文献
LANA	潜伏复制	p53	促存活	Friborg et al.（1999）
		血管生成素/膜黏蛋白 A2	促存活	Paudel et al.（2012）
		pRb	促有丝分裂	Radkov et al.（2000）
		GSK3b	促有丝分裂	Fujimuro et al.（2003）

续表

蛋白	类别	靶点	活性/功能	参考文献
		c-Myc	促有丝分裂	Liu et al.（2007b）
		组蛋白 H2A/B	病毒基因组和染色体束缚	Barbera et al.（2006）
		DNMT3a	转录抑制	Shamay et al.（2006）
		SUV39H1	转录抑制	Sakakibara et al.（2004）
		mSin3/SAP30/CIR	转录抑制	Krithivas et al.（2000）
K13/vFLIP	潜伏信号	IKKa/b	NF-κB 激活/生存	Matta et al.（2007）
		TRAF2/IKKg?	NF-κB/Jnk 激活	Guasparri et al.（2006）
		Procaspase-8	抑制 caspase 活性/存活	Belanger et al.（2001）
Kaposin A	潜伏信号	Cytohesin-1，Septin 4 变体	几个信号激酶的 GTP 酶介导的信号转导和激活；存活/扩增中的作用？	Kliche et al.（2001），Lin et al.（2007）
Kaposin B	潜伏，mRNA 调节	MK2 激酶	激活 MK2，稳定包含 mRNA 的 ARE（如 IL-6、PROX1）；潜在的促存活和/或有丝分裂活性；内皮重新编程	McCormick and Ganem（2005）
vIL-6	配体，细胞因子	gp130/gp80	激活 STAT/MAKPK；扩增/存活；促炎症/血管生成	Chow et al.（2001），Boulanger et al.（2004）
		VKORC1v2	扩增/存活（PEL），机制不明	Chen et al.（2012）
vCCL-1	配体，趋化因子	CCR8	类似物，Th2 极化；促生存；促进病毒复制；促血管生成	Dairaghi et al.（1999），Choi and Nicholas（2008）
vCCL-2	配体，趋化因子	CCR3，CCR8，CCR5?	类似物，Th2 极化；促生存；促进病毒复制；促血管生成	Choi and Nicholas（2008），Boshoff et al.（1997），Nakano et al.（2003）
		CCR5，CCR2，CCR10，CXCR4，CX3CR1，XCR1	趋化因子拮抗剂；促生存；促进病毒复制	Chen et al.（1998），Boshoff et al.（1997），Kledal et al.（1997），Luttichau et al.（2001），（2007）
vCCL-3	配体，趋化因子	CCR4，XCR1	类似物，Th2 极化；促血管生成	Stine et al.（2000），Luttichau et al.（2007）
vGPCR	信号受体	Ga（i，q，12/13），SHP2	激活各种促生存和有丝分裂信号途径；促进病毒复制；促血管生成	Couty et al.（2001），Liu et al.（2004），Philpott et al.（2011），Shepard et al.（2001），Sandford et al.（2009）

续表

蛋白	类别	靶点	活性/功能	参考文献
vIRF-1	天然免疫调节	p53，ATM，p300/CBP，GRIM19，Smads3/4，BOP，（包括：Bim 和 Bid），IRF1，IRF3	促存活；抑制 IFN 信号	Burysek et al.（1999a），Choi et al.（2012）Li et al.（2000），Lin et al.（2001），Nakamura et al.（2001），Seo et al.（2001），（2002），（2005），Shin et al.（2006）
vIRF-2	天然免疫调节	PKR，IRF1，IRF2，p65，p300	抑制 IFN 信号	Burysek and Pitha（2001），Burysek et al.（1999b）
vIRF-3	天然免疫调节	p53，IRF3，IRF5，IRF7，14-3-3，HIF-1a，Foxo3a	促存活；抑制 IFN 信号；血管生成信号	Joo et al.（2007），Munoz-Fontela et al.（2007），Rivas et al.（2001），Shin et al.（2008），Weis et al.（2008）
vIRF-4	天然免疫调节	MDM2	促存活（通过 p53 的去稳定）	Lee et al.（2009b）
		HAUSP	促存活（通过 p53 的去稳定）	Lee et al.（2011）
		CSL	未知	Heinzelmann et al.(2010)
K7/vIAP	凋亡调节	Bcl-2/caspase 3	促存活	Wang et al.（2002）
		CAML	促存活	Feng et al.（2002）
		PLIC	促存活	Feng et al.（2004）
K1/VIP	凋亡调节	Src kinases，PI3K，SHP2，PLCc	促存活/有丝分裂原；促血管生成/炎症	Lee et al.（1998a），（2005）
K15	受体信号传导	Src kinases，TRAFs，intersectin 2，HAX-1	促存活/有丝分裂原；促血管生成	Brinkmann et al.（2003），Lim et al.（2007），Pietrek et al.（2010），Sharp et al.（2002）

（刘红旗，陶玉芬 译）

参 考 文 献

Abend JR, Uldrick T, Ziegelbauer JM (2010) Regulation of tumor necrosis factor-like weak inducer of apoptosis receptor protein (TWEAKR) expression by Kaposi's sarcoma-associated herpesvirus microRNA prevents TWEAK-induced apoptosis and inflammatory cytokine expression. J Virol

84:12139–12151

Albrecht JC, Nicholas J, Cameron KR, Newman C, Fleckenstein B, Honess RW (1992) Herpesvirus saimiri has a gene specifying a homologue of the cellular membrane glycoprotein CD59. Virology 190:527–530

Alexander L, Denekamp L, Knapp A, Auerbach MR, Damania B, Desrosiers RC (2000) The primary sequence of rhesus monkey rhadinovirus isolate 26–95: sequence similarities to Kaposi's sarcoma-associated herpesvirus and rhesus monkey rhadinovirus isolate 17577. J Virol 74:3388–3398

Ambrosini G, Adida C, Altieri DC (1997) A novel anti-apoptosis gene, survivin, expressed in cancer and lymphoma. Nat Med 3:917–921

An FQ, Compitello N, Horwitz E, Sramkoski M, Knudsen ES, Renne R (2005) The latency-associated nuclear antigen of Kaposi's sarcoma-associated herpesvirus modulates cellular gene expression and protects lymphoid cells from p16 INK4A-induced cell cycle arrest. J Biol Chem 280:3862–3874

An J, Sun Y, Sun R, Rettig MB (2003) Kaposi's sarcoma-associated herpesvirus encoded vFLIP induces cellular IL-6 expression: the role of the NF-kappaB and JNK/AP1 pathways. Oncogene 22:3371–3385

Angell JE, Lindner DJ, Shapiro PS, Hofmann ER, Kalvakolanu DV (2000) Identification of GRIM-19, a novel cell death-regulatory gene induced by the interferon-beta and retinoic acid combination, using a genetic approach. J Biol Chem 275:33416–33426

Aoki Y, Feldman GM, Tosato G (2003) Inhibition of STAT3 signaling induces apoptosis and decreases survivin expression in primary effusion lymphoma. Blood 101:1535–1542

Aoki Y, Jaffe ES, Chang Y, Jones K, Teruya-Feldstein J, Moore PS, Tosato G (1999) Angiogenesis and hematopoiesis induced by Kaposi's sarcoma-associated herpesvirus- encoded interleukin-6. Blood 93:4034–4043

Aoki Y, Narazaki M, Kishimoto T, Tosato G (2001) Receptor engagement by viral interleukin-6 encoded by Kaposi sarcoma-associated herpesvirus. Blood 98:3042–3049

Aoki Y, Tosato G (1999) Role of vascular endothelial growth factor/vascular permeability factor in the pathogenesis of Kaposi's sarcoma-associated herpesvirus-infected primary effusion lymphomas. Blood 94:4247–4254

Aoki Y, Tosato G (2003) Targeted inhibition of angiogenic factors in AIDS-related disorders. Curr Drug Targets Infect Disord 3:115–128

Areste C, Mutocheluh M, Blackbourn DJ (2009) Identification of caspase-mediated decay of interferon regulatory factor-3, exploited by a Kaposi sarcoma-associated herpesvirus immunoregulatory protein. J Biol Chem 284:23272–23285

Arvanitakis L, Mesri EA, Nador RG, Said JW, Asch AS, Knowles DM, Cesarman E (1996)

Establishment and characterization of a primary effusion (body cavity-based) lymphoma cell line (BC-3) harboring kaposi's sarcoma-associated herpesvirus (KSHV/HHV-8) in the absence of Epstein-Barr virus. Blood 88:2648–2654

Bais C, Santomasso B, Coso O, Arvanitakis L, Raaka EG, Gutkind JS, Asch AS, Cesarman E, Gershengorn MC, Mesri EA (1998) G-protein-coupled receptor of Kaposi's sarcoma-associated herpesvirus is a viral oncogene and angiogenesis activator. Nature 391:86–89

Barbera AJ, Chodaparambil JV, Kelley-Clarke B, Joukov V, Walter JC, Luger K, Kaye KM (2006) The nucleosomal surface as a docking station for Kaposi's sarcoma herpesvirus LANA. Science 311:856–861

Bartel DP (2004) MicroRNAs: genomics, biogenesis, mechanism, and function. Cell 116:281–297

Bartoli M, Gu X, Tsai NT, Venema RC, Brooks SE, Marrero MB, Caldwell RB (2000) Vascular endothelial growth factor activates STAT proteins in aortic endothelial cells. J Biol Chem 275:33189–33192

Belanger C, Gravel A, Tomoiu A, Janelle ME, Gosselin J, Tremblay MJ, Flamand L (2001) Human herpesvirus 8 viral FLICE-inhibitory protein inhibits Fas-mediated apoptosis through binding and prevention of procaspase-8 maturation. J Hum Virol 4:62–73

Bellare P, Ganem D (2009) Regulation of KSHV lytic switch protein expression by a virus- encoded microRNA: an evolutionary adaptation that fine-tunes lytic reactivation. Cell Host Microbe 6:570–575

Bertin J, Armstrong RC, Ottilie S, Martin DA, Wang Y, Banks S, Wang GH, Senkevich TG, Alnemri ES, Moss B, Lenardo MJ, Tomaselli KJ, Cohen JI (1997) Death effector domain-containing herpesvirus and poxvirus proteins inhibit both Fas- and TNFR1-induced apoptosis. Proc Natl Acad Sci U S A 94:1172–1176

Boshoff C, Endo Y, Collins PD, Takeuchi Y, Reeves JD, Schweickart VL, Siani MA, Sasaki T, Williams TJ, Gray PW, Moore PS, Chang Y, Weiss RA (1997) Angiogenic and HIV- inhibitory functions of KSHV-encoded chemokines. Science 278:290–294

Boulanger MJ, Chow DC, Brevnova EE, Garcia KC (2003) Hexameric structure and assembly of the interleukin-6/IL-6 alpha-receptor/gp130 complex. Science 300:2101–2104

Boulanger MJ, Cow DC, Brevnova, EE, Martick M. Sandford G, Nicholas J, Garcia KC (2004) Molecular mechanisms for viral mimicry of a human cytokine: activation of gp130 by HHV-8 interleukin 6. J Mol Biol 335:641–654

Bram RJ, Crabtree GR (1994) Calcium signalling in T cells stimulated by a cyclophilin B-binding protein. Nature 371:355–358

Brinkmann MM, Glenn M, Rainbow L, Kieser A, Henke-Gendo C, Schulz TF (2003) Activation of mitogen-activated protein kinase and NF-kappaB pathways by a Kaposi's sarcoma- associated herpesvirus K15 membrane protein. J Virol 77:9346–9358

Brinkmann MM, Pietrek M, Dittrich-Breiholz O, Kracht M, Schulz TF (2007) Modulation of host gene expression by the K15 protein of Kaposi's sarcoma-associated herpesvirus. J Virol 81:42–58

Brinkmann MM, Schulz TF (2006) Regulation of intracellular signalling by the terminal membrane proteins of members of the Gammaherpesvirinae. J Gen Virol 87:1047–1074

Brown HJ, Song MJ, Deng H, Wu TT, Cheng G, Sun R (2003) NF-kappaB inhibits gammaherpesvirus lytic replication. J Virol 77:8532–8540

Bubman D, Guasparri I, Cesarman E (2007) Deregulation of c-Myc in primary effusion lymphoma by Kaposi's sarcoma herpesvirus latency-associated nuclear antigen. Oncogene 26:4979–4986

Burger R, Neipel F, Fleckenstein B, Savino R, Ciliberto G, Kalden JR, Gramatzki M (1998) Human herpesvirus type 8 interleukin-6 homologue is functionally active on human myeloma cells. Blood 91:1858–1863

Burger R, Wendler J, Antoni K, Helm G, Kalden JR, Gramatzki M (1994) Interleukin-6 production in B-cell neoplasias and Castleman's disease: evidence for an additional paracrine loop. Ann Hematol 69:25–31

Burysek L, Pitha PM (2001) Latently expressed human herpesvirus 8-encoded interferon regulatory factor 2 inhibits double-stranded RNA-activated protein kinase. J Virol 75:2345–2352

Burysek L, Yeow WS, Lubyova B, Kellum M, Schafer SL, Huang YQ, Pitha PM (1999a) Functional analysis of human herpesvirus 8-encoded viral interferon regulatory factor 1 and its association with cellular interferon regulatory factors and p300. J Virol 73:7334–7342

Burysek L, Yeow WS, Pitha PM (1999b) Unique properties of a second human herpesvirus 8-encoded interferon regulatory factor (vIRF-2). J Hum Virol 2:19–32

Cai X, Lu S, Zhang Z, Gonzalez CM, Damania B, Cullen BR (2005) Kaposi's sarcoma-associated herpesvirus expresses an array of viral microRNAs in latently infected cells. Proc Natl Acad Sci U S A 102:5570–5575

Cannon M (2007) The KSHV and other human herpesviral G protein-coupled receptors. Curr Top Microbiol Immunol 312:137–156

Cannon M, Philpott NJ, Cesarman E (2003) The Kaposi's sarcoma-associated herpesvirus G protein-coupled receptor has broad signaling effects in primary effusion lymphoma cells. J Virol 77:57–67

Carbone A, Cilia AM, Gloghini A, Capello D, Perin T, Bontempo D, Canzonieri V, Tirelli U, Volpe R, Gaidano G (2000) Primary effusion lymphoma cell lines harbouring human herpesvirus type-8. Leuk Lymphoma 36:447–456

Caselli E, Fiorentini S, Amici C, Di Luca D, Caruso A, Santoro MG (2007) Human herpesvirus 8 acute infection of endothelial cells induces monocyte chemoattractant protein 1-dependent capillary-like structure formation: role of the IKK/NF-kappaB pathway. Blood 109:2718–2726

Chandriani S, Ganem D (2010) Array-based transcript profiling and limiting-dilution reverse transcription-PCR analysis identify additional latent genes in Kaposi's sarcoma-associated herpesvirus. J Virol 84:5565–5573

Chang Y, Moore PS (1996) Kaposi's Sarcoma (KS)-associated herpesvirus and its role in KS. Infect Agents Dis 5:215–222

Chaudhary PM, Jasmin A, Eby MT, Hood L (1999) Modulation of the NF-kappa B pathway by virally encoded death effector domains-containing proteins. Oncogene 18:5738–5746

Chen D, Cousins E, Sandford G, Nicholas J (2012) Human herpesvirus 8 viral interleukin-6 interacts with splice variant 2 of vitamin K epoxide reductase complex subunit 1. J Virol 86:1577–1588

Chen D, Nicholas J (2006) Structural requirements for gp80 independence of human herpesvirus 8 interleukin-6 (vIL-6) and evidence for gp80 stabilization of gp130 signaling complexes induced by vIL-6. J Virol 80:9811–9821

Chen D, Sandford G, Nicholas J (2009a) Intracellular signaling mechanisms and activities of human herpesvirus 8 interleukin-6. J Virol 83:722–733

Chen S, Bacon KB, Li L, Garcia GE, Xia Y, Lo D, Thompson DA, Siani MA, Yamamoto T, Harrison JK, Feng L (1998) In vivo inhibition of CC and CX3C chemokine-induced leukocyte infiltration and attenuation of glomerulonephritis in Wistar-Kyoto (WKY) rats by vMIP-II. J Exp Med 188:193–198

Chen W, Hilton IB, Staudt MR, Burd CE, Dittmer DP (2010) Distinct p53, p53:LANA, and LANA complexes in Kaposi's Sarcoma–associated Herpesvirus Lymphomas. J Virol 84:3898–3908

Chen X, Cheng L, Jia X, Zeng Y, Yao S, Lv Z, Qin D, Fang X, Lei Y, Lu C (2009b) Human immunodeficiency virus type 1 Tat accelerates Kaposi sarcoma-associated herpesvirus Kaposin A-mediated tumorigenesis of transformed fibroblasts in vitro as well as in nude and immunocompetent mice. Neoplasia 11:1272–1284

Choi JK, Lee BS, Shim SN, Li M, Jung JU (2000) Identification of the novel K15 gene at the rightmost end of the Kaposi's sarcoma-associated herpesvirus genome. J Virol 74:436–446

Choi YB, Nicholas J (2008) Autocrine and paracrine promotion of cell survival and virus replication by human herpesvirus 8 chemokines. J Virol 82:6501–6513

Choi YB, Nicholas J (2010) Bim nuclear translocation and inactivation by viral interferon regulatory factor. PLoS Pathog 6:e1001031

Choi YB, Sandford G, Nicholas J (2012) Human herpesvirus 8 interferon regulatory factor- mediated BH3-only protein Inhibition via Bid BH3-B mimicry. PLoS Pathog 8(6):e1002748 Chow D, He X, Snow AL, Rose-John S, Garcia KC (2001) Structure of an extracellular gp130 cytokine receptor signaling complex. Science 291:2150–2155

Chugh P, Matta H, Schamus S, Zachariah S, Kumar A, Richardson JA, Smith AL, Chaudhary PM (2005) Constitutive NF-kappaB activation, normal Fas-induced apoptosis, and increased incidence of lymphoma in human herpes virus 8 K13 transgenic mice. Proc Natl Acad Sci U S A 102:12885–

12890

Couty JP, Geras-Raaka E, Weksler BB, Gershengorn MC (2001) Kaposi's sarcoma-associated herpesvirus G protein-coupled receptor signals through multiple pathways in endothelial cells. J Biol Chem 276:33805–33811

Crump MP, Elisseeva E, Gong J, Clark-Lewis I, Sykes BD (2001) Structure/function of human herpesvirus-8 MIP-II (1–71) and the antagonist N-terminal segment (1–10). FEBS Lett 489:171–175

Cunningham C, Barnard S, Blackbourn DJ, Davison AJ (2003) Transcription mapping of human herpesvirus 8 genes encoding viral interferon regulatory factors. J Gen Virol 84:1471–1483
Dairaghi DJ, Fan RA, McMaster BE, Hanley MR, Schall TJ (1999) HHV8-encoded vMIP-I selectively engages chemokine receptor CCR8. Agonist and antagonist profiles of viral chemokines. J Biol Chem 274:21569–21574

Damania B, Li M, Choi JK, Alexander L, Jung JU, Desrosiers RC (1999) Identification of the R1 oncogene and its protein product from the rhadinovirus of rhesus monkeys. J Virol 73:5123–5131

Dittmer DP (2003) Transcription profile of Kaposi's sarcoma-associated herpesvirus in primary Kaposi's sarcoma lesions as determined by real-time PCR arrays. Cancer Res 63:2010–2015
Djerbi M, Screpanti V, Catrina AI, Bogen B, Biberfeld P, Grandien A (1999) The inhibitor of death receptor signaling, FLICE-inhibitory protein defines a new class of tumor progression factors. J Exp Med 190:1025–1032

Dolken L, Malterer G, Erhard F, Kothe S, Friedel CC, Suffert G, Marcinowski L, Motsch N, Barth S, Beitzinger M, Lieber D, Bailer SM, Hoffmann R, Ruzsics Z, Kremmer E, Pfeffer S, Zimmer R, Koszinowski UH, Grasser F, Meister G, Haas J (2010) Systematic analysis of viral and cellular microRNA targets in cells latently infected with human gamma-herpesviruses by RISC immunoprecipitation assay. Cell Host Microbe 7:324–334

Ensoli B, Sgadari C, Barillari G, Sirianni MC, Sturzl M, Monini P (2001) Biology of Kaposi's sarcoma. Eur J Cancer 37:1251–1269

Ensoli B, Sturzl M (1998) Kaposi's sarcoma: a result of the interplay among inflammatory cytokines, angiogenic factors and viral agents. Cytokine Growth Factor Rev 9:63–83

Esteban M, Garcia MA, Domingo-Gil E, Arroyo J, Nombela C, Rivas C (2003) The latency protein LANA2 from Kaposi's sarcoma-associated herpesvirus inhibits apoptosis induced by dsRNA-activated protein kinase but not RNase L activation. J Gen Virol 84:1463–1470

Feng P, Park J, Lee BS, Lee SH, Bram RJ, Jung JU (2002) Kaposi's sarcoma-associated herpesvirus mitochondrial K7 protein targets a cellular calcium-modulating cyclophilin ligand to modulate intracellular calcium concentration and inhibit apoptosis. J Virol 76:11491–11504

Feng P, Scott CW, Cho NH, Nakamura H, Chung YH, Monteiro MJ, Jung JU (2004) Kaposi's sarcoma-associated herpesvirus K7 protein targets a ubiquitin-like/ubiquitin-associated domain-containing protein to promote protein degradation. Mol Cell Biol 24:3938–3948

Field N, Low W, Daniels M, Howell S, Daviet L, Boshoff C, Collins M (2003) KSHV vFLIP binds to IKK-gamma to activate IKK. J Cell Sci 116:3721–3728

Fielding CA, McLoughlin RM, Colmont CS, Kovaleva M, Harris DA, Rose-John S, Topley N, Jones SA (2005) Viral IL-6 blocks neutrophil infiltration during acute inflammation. J Immunol 175:4024–4029

Friborg J Jr, Kong W, Hottiger MO, Nabel GJ (1999) p53 inhibition by the LANA protein of KSHV protects against cell death. Nature 402:889–894

Fujimuro M, Hayward SD (2003) The latency-associated nuclear antigen of Kaposi's sarcoma-associated herpesvirus manipulates the activity of glycogen synthase kinase-3beta. J Virol 77:8019–8030

Fujimuro M, Wu FY, ApRhys C, Kajumbula H, Young DB, Hayward GS, Hayward SD (2003) A novel viral mechanism for dysregulation of beta-catenin in Kaposi's sarcoma-associated herpesvirus latency. Nat Med 9:300–306

Fuld S, Cunningham C, Klucher K, Davison AJ, Blackbourn DJ (2006) Inhibition of interferon signaling by the Kaposi's sarcoma-associated herpesvirus full-length viral interferon regulatory factor 2 protein. J Virol 80:3092–3097

Gaidano G, Pastore C, Gloghini A, Volpe G, Capello D, Polito P, Vaccher E, Tirelli U, Saglio G, Carbone A (1997) Human herpesvirus type-8 (HHV-8) in haematopoietic neoplasia. Leuk Lymphoma 24:257–266

Glas R, Franksson L, Une C, Eloranta ML, Ohlen C, Orn A, Karre K (2000) Recruitment and activation of natural killer (NK) cells in vivo determined by the target cell phenotype. An adaptive component of NK cell-mediated responses. J Exp Med 191:129–138

Glenn M, Rainbow L, Aurade F, Davison A, Schulz TF (1999) Identification of a spliced gene from Kaposi's sarcoma-associated herpesvirus encoding a protein with similarities to latent membrane proteins 1 and 2A of Epstein-Barr virus. J Virol 73:6953–6963

Godfrey A, Anderson J, Papanastasiou A, Takeuchi Y, Boshoff C (2005) Inhibiting primary effusion lymphoma by lentiviral vectors encoding short hairpin RNA. Blood 105:2510–2518 Gottwein E, Corcoran DL, Mukherjee N, Skalsky RL, Hafner M, Nusbaum JD, Shamulailatpam P, Love CL, Dave SS, Tuschl T, Ohler U, Cullen BR (2011) Viral microRNA targetome of KSHV-infected primary effusion lymphoma cell lines. Cell Host Microbe 10:515–526

Gottwein E, Cullen BR (2010) A human herpesvirus microRNA inhibits p21 expression and attenuates p21-mediated cell cycle arrest. J Virol 84:5229–5237

Gottwein E, Mukherjee N, Sachse C, Frenzel C, Majoros WH, Chi JT, Braich R, Manoharan M, Soutschek J, Ohler U, Cullen BR (2007) A viral microRNA functions as an orthologue of cellular miR-155. Nature 450:1096–1099

Grossmann C, Ganem D (2008) Effects of NFkappaB activation on KSHV latency and lytic reactivation are complex and context-dependent. Virology 375:94–102

Grossmann C, Podgrabinska S, Skobe M, Ganem D (2006) Activation of NF-kappaB by the latent vFLIP gene of Kaposi's sarcoma-associated herpesvirus is required for the spindle shape of virus-infected endothelial cells and contributes to their proinflammatory phenotype. J Virol 80:7179–7185

Guasparri I, Keller SA, Cesarman E (2004) KSHV vFLIP is essential for the survival of infected lymphoma cells. J Exp Med 199:993–1003

Guasparri I, Wu H, Cesarman E (2006) The KSHV oncoprotein vFLIP contains a TRAF- interacting motif and requires TRAF2 and TRAF3 for signalling. EMBO Rep 7:114–119

Haddad L, El Hajj H, Abou-Merhi R, Kfoury Y, Mahieux R, El-Sabban M, Bazarbachi A (2008) KSHV-transformed primary effusion lymphoma cells induce a VEGF-dependent angiogenesis and establish functional gap junctions with endothelial cells. Leukemia 22:826–834

Hansen A, Henderson S, Lagos D, Nikitenko L, Coulter E, Roberts S, Gratrix F, Plaisance K, Renne R, Bower M, Kellam P, Boshoff C (2010) KSHV-encoded miRNAs target MAF to induce endothelial cell reprogramming. Genes Dev 24:195–205

Hayward GS, Zong JC (2007) Modern evolutionary history of the human KSHV genome. Curr Top Microbiol Immunol 312:1–42

Heinrich PC, Behrmann I, Haan S, Hermanns HM, Muller-Newen G, Schaper F (2003) Principles of interleukin (IL)-6-type cytokine signalling and its regulation. Biochem J 374:1–20

Heinrich PC, Behrmann I, Muller-Newen G, Schaper F, Graeve L (1998) Interleukin-6-type cytokine signalling through the gp130/Jak/STAT pathway. Biochem J 334(Pt 2):297–314 Heinzelmann K, Scholz BA, Nowak A, Fossum E, Kremmer E, Haas J, Frank R, Kempkes B (2010) Kaposi's sarcoma-associated herpesvirus viral interferon regulatory factor 4 (vIRF4/ K10) is a novel interaction partner of CSL/CBF1, the major downstream effector of Notch signaling. J Virol 84:12255–12264

Hu S, Vincenz C, Buller M, Dixit VM (1997) A novel family of viral death effector domain-containing molecules that inhibit both CD-95- and tumor necrosis factor receptor-1-induced apoptosis. J Biol Chem 272:9621–9624

Ishiyama T, Nakamura S, Akimoto Y, Koike M, Tomoyasu S, Tsuruoka N, Murata Y, Sato T, Wakabayashi Y, Chiba S (1994) Immunodeficiency and IL-6 production by peripheral blood monocytes in multicentric Castleman's disease. Br J Haematol 86:483–489

Jenner RG, Alba MM, Boshoff C, Kellam P (2001) Kaposi's sarcoma-associated herpesvirus latent and lytic gene expression as revealed by DNA arrays. J Virol 75:891–902

Jones KD, Aoki Y, Chang Y, Moore PS, Yarchoan R, Tosato G (1999) Involvement of interleukin-10 (IL-10) and viral IL-6 in the spontaneous growth of Kaposi's sarcoma herpesvirus-associated infected primary effusion lymphoma cells. Blood 94:2871–2879

Joo CH, Shin YC, Gack M, Wu L, Levy D, Jung JU (2007) Inhibition of interferon regulatory factor 7 (IRF7)-mediated interferon signal transduction by the Kaposi's sarcoma-associated herpesvirus viral IRF homolog vIRF3. J Virol 81:8282–8292

Karim R, Tse G, Putti T, Scolyer R, Lee S (2004) The significance of the Wnt pathway in the pathology of human cancers. Pathology 36:120–128

Kawa K (2000) Epstein-Barr virus–associated diseases in humans. Int J Hematol 71:108–117

Kaye KM, Izumi KM, Kieff E (1993) Epstein-Barr virus latent membrane protein 1 is essential for B-lymphocyte growth transformation. Proc Natl Acad Sci U S A 90:9150–9154

Keller SA, Schattner EJ, Cesarman E (2000) Inhibition of NF-kappaB induces apoptosis of KSHV-infected primary effusion lymphoma cells. Blood 96:2537–2542

Kishimoto T, Akira S, Narazaki M, Taga T (1995) Interleukin-6 family of cytokines and gp130. Blood 86:1243–1254

Kledal TN, Rosenkilde MM, Coulin F, Simmons G, Johnsen AH, Alouani S, Power CA, Luttichau HR, Gerstoft J, Clapham PR, Clark-Lewis I, Wells TN, Schwartz TW (1997) A broad-spectrum chemokine antagonist encoded by Kaposi's sarcoma-associated herpesvirus. Science 277:1656–1659

Kleijnen MF, Shih AH, Zhou P, Kumar S, Soccio RE, Kedersha NL, Gill G, Howley PM (2000) The hPLIC proteins may provide a link between the ubiquitination machinery and the proteasome. Mol Cell 6:409–419

Kliche S, Nagel W, Kremmer E, Atzler C, Ege A, Knorr T, Koszinowski U, Kolanus W, Haas J (2001) Signaling by human herpesvirus 8 kaposin A through direct membrane recruitment of cytohesin-1. Mol Cell 7:833–843

Kovaleva M, Bussmeyer I, Rabe B, Grotzinger J, Sudarman E, Eichler J, Conrad U, Rose-John S, Scheller J (2006) Abrogation of viral interleukin-6 (vIL-6)-induced signaling by intracellular retention and neutralization of vIL-6 with an anti-vIL-6 single-chain antibody selected by phage display. J Virol 80:8510–8520

Krithivas A, Young DB, Liao G, Greene D, Hayward SD (2000) Human herpesvirus 8 LANA interacts with proteins of the mSin3 corepressor complex and negatively regulates Epstein-Barr virus gene expression in dually infected PEL cells. J Virol 74:9637–9645

Kuwana T, Bouchier-Hayes L, Chipuk JE, Bonzon C, Sullivan BA, Green DR, Newmeyer DD (2005) BH3 domains of BH3-only proteins differentially regulate Bax-mediated mitochon- drial membrane permeabilization both directly and indirectly. Mol Cell 17:525–535

Lagunoff M, Ganem D (1997) The structure and coding organization of the genomic termini of Kaposi's sarcoma-associated herpesvirus. Virology 236:147–154

Lagunoff M, Lukac DM, Ganem D (2001) Immunoreceptor tyrosine-based activation motif- dependent signaling by Kaposi's sarcoma-associated herpesvirus K1 protein: effects on lytic viral replication. J Virol 75:5891–5898

Lee BS, Connole M, Tang Z, Harris NL, Jung JU (2003a) Structural analysis of the Kaposi's sarcoma-associated herpesvirus K1 protein. J Virol 77:8072–8086

Lee BS, Lee SH, Feng P, Chang H, Cho NH, Jung JU (2005) Characterization of the Kaposi's sarcoma-associated herpesvirus K1 signalosome. J Virol 79:12173–12184

Lee H, Guo J, Li M, Choi JK, DeMaria M, Rosenzweig M, Jung JU (1998a) Identification of an immunoreceptor tyrosine-based activation motif of K1 transforming protein of Kaposi's sarcoma-associated herpesvirus. Mol Cell Biol 18:5219–5228

Lee H, Veazey R, Williams K, Li M, Guo J, Neipel F, Fleckenstein B, Lackner A, Desrosiers RC, Jung JU (1998b) Deregulation of cell growth by the K1 gene of Kaposi's sarcoma-associated herpesvirus. Nat Med 4:435–440

Lee HR, Choi WC, Lee S, Hwang J, Hwang E, Guchhait K, Haas J, Toth Z, Jeon YH, Oh TK, Kim MH, Jung JU (2011) Bilateral inhibition of HAUSP deubiquitinase by a viral interferon regulatory factor protein. Nat Struct Mol Biol 18:1336–1344

Lee HR, Kim MH, Lee JS, Liang C, Jung JU (2009a) Viral interferon regulatory factors. J Interferon Cytokine Res 29:621–627

Lee HR, Toth Z, Shin YC, Lee JS, Chang H, Gu W, Oh TK, Kim MH, Jung JU (2009b) Kaposi's sarcoma-associated herpesvirus viral interferon regulatory factor 4 targets MDM2 to deregulate the p53 tumor suppressor pathway. J Virol 83:6739–6747

Lee Y, Ahn C, Han J, Choi H, Kim J, Yim J, Lee J, Provost P, Radmark O, Kim S, Kim VN (2003b) The nuclear RNase III Drosha initiates microRNA processing. Nature 425:415–419 Lei X, Bai Z, Ye F, Xie J, Kim CG, Huang Y, Gao SJ (2010) Regulation of NF-kappaB inhibitor IkappaB alpha and viral replication by a KSHV microRNA. Nat Cell Biol 12:193–199

Li H, Komatsu T, Dezube BJ, Kaye KM (2002) The Kaposi's sarcoma-associated herpesvirus K12 transcript from a primary effusion lymphoma contains complex repeat elements, is spliced, and initiates from a novel promoter. J Virol 76:11880–11888

Li M, Damania B, Alvarez X, Ogryzko V, Ozato K, Jung JU (2000) Inhibition of p300 histone acetyltransferase by viral interferon regulatory factor. Mol Cell Biol 20:8254–8263

Liang D, Lin X, Lan K (2012) Looking at Kaposi's Sarcoma-Associated Herpesvirus-Host Interactions from a microRNA Viewpoint. Front Microbiol 2:271

Lim CS, Seet BT, Ingham RJ, Gish G, Matskova L, Winberg G, Ernberg I, Pawson T (2007) The K15 protein of Kaposi's sarcoma-associated herpesvirus recruits the endocytic regulator intersectin 2 through a selective SH3 domain interaction. Biochemistry 46:9874–9885

Lin CW, Tu PF, Hsiao NW, Chang CY, Wan L, Lin YT, Chang HW (2007) Identification of a novel septin 4 protein binding to human herpesvirus 8 kaposin A protein using a phage display cDNA library. J Virol Methods 143:65–72

Lin R, Genin P, Mamane Y, Sgarbanti M, Battistini A, Harrington WJ Jr, Barber GN, Hiscott J (2001) HHV-8 encoded vIRF-1 represses the interferon antiviral response by blocking IRF-3 recruitment of the CBP/p300 coactivators. Oncogene 20:800–811

Lin X, Liang D, He Z, Deng Q, Robertson ES, Lan K (2011) miR-K12-7-5p encoded by Kaposi's sarcoma-associated herpesvirus stabilizes the latent state by targeting viral ORF50/RTA. PLoS One 6:e16224

Lindner SE, Sugden B (2007) The plasmid replicon of Epstein-Barr virus: mechanistic insights into efficient, licensed, extrachromosomal replication in human cells. Plasmid 58:1–12

Liu C, Okruzhnov Y, Li H, Nicholas J (2001) Human herpesvirus 8 (HHV-8)-encoded cytokines induce expression of and autocrine signaling by vascular endothelial growth factor (VEGF) in HHV-8-infected primary-effusion lymphoma cell lines and mediate VEGF-independent antiapoptotic effects. J Virol 75:10933–10940

Liu C, Sandford G, Fei G, Nicholas J (2004) Galpha protein selectivity determinant specified by a viral chemokine receptor-conserved region in the C tail of the human herpesvirus 8 g protein- coupled receptor. J Virol 78:2460–2471

Liu J, Martin H, Shamay M, Woodard C, Tang QQ, Hayward SD (2007a) Kaposi's sarcoma- associated herpesvirus LANA protein downregulates nuclear glycogen synthase kinase 3 activity and consequently blocks differentiation. J Virol 81:4722–4731

Liu J, Martin HJ, Liao G, Hayward SD (2007b) The Kaposi's sarcoma-associated herpesvirus LANA protein stabilizes and activates c-Myc. J Virol 81:10451–10459

Liu L, Eby MT, Rathore N, Sinha SK, Kumar A, Chaudhary PM (2002) The human herpes virus 8-encoded viral FLICE inhibitory protein physically associates with and persistently activates the Ikappa B kinase complex. J Biol Chem 277:13745–13751

Liu Y, Sun R, Lin X, Liang D, Deng Q, Lan K (2012) Kaposi's sarcoma-associated herpesvirus-encoded microRNA miR-K12-11 attenuates transforming growth factor beta signaling through suppression of SMAD5. J Virol 86:1372–1381

Louahed J, Struyf S, Demoulin JB, Parmentier M, Van Snick J, Van Damme J, Renauld JC (2003) CCR8-dependent activation of the RAS/MAPK pathway mediates anti-apoptotic activity of I-309/CCL1 and vMIP-I. Eur J Immunol 33:494–501

Lu CC, Li Z, Chu CY, Feng J, Sun R, Rana TM (2010a) MicroRNAs encoded by Kaposi's sarcoma-associated herpesvirus regulate viral life cycle. EMBO Rep 11:784–790

Lu F, Stedman W, Yousef M, Renne R, Lieberman PM (2010b) Epigenetic regulation of Kaposi's sarcoma-associated herpesvirus latency by virus-encoded microRNAs that target Rta and the cellular Rbl2-DNMT pathway. J Virol 84:2697–2706

Lubyova B, Kellum MJ, Frisancho JA, Pitha PM (2007) Stimulation of c-Myc transcriptional activity by vIRF-3 of Kaposi sarcoma-associated herpesvirus. J Biol Chem 282:31944–31953 Lubyova B, Pitha PM (2000) Characterization of a novel human herpesvirus 8-encoded protein, vIRF-3, that shows homology to viral and cellular interferon regulatory factors. J Virol 74:8194–8201

Lund E, Guttinger S, Calado A, Dahlberg JE, Kutay U (2004) Nuclear export of microRNA precursors. Science 303:95–98

Luttichau HR (2008) The herpesvirus 8 encoded chemokines vCCL2 (vMIP-II) and vCCL3 (vMIP-III) target the human but not the murine lymphotactin receptor. Virol J 5:50

Luttichau HR, Johnsen AH, Jurlander J, Rosenkilde MM, Schwartz TW (2007) Kaposi sarcoma-associated herpes virus targets the lymphotactin receptor with both a broad spectrum antagonist vCCL2 and a highly selective and potent agonist vCCL3. J Biol Chem 282:17794–17805

Luttichau HR, Lewis IC, Gerstoft J, Schwartz TW (2001) The herpesvirus 8-encoded chemokine vMIP-II, but not the poxvirus-encoded chemokine MC148, inhibits the CCR10 receptor. Eur J Immunol 31:1217–1220

Ma X, Kalakonda S, Srinivasula SM, Reddy SP, Platanias LC, Kalvakolanu DV (2007) GRIM-19 associates with the serine protease HtrA2 for promoting cell death. Oncogene 26:4842–4849 Mandel-Gutfreund Y, Kosti I, Larisch S (2011) ARTS, the unusual septin: structural and functional aspects. Biol Chem 392:783–790

Marcos-Villar L, Lopitz-Otsoa F, Gallego P, Munoz-Fontela C, Gonzalez-Santamaria J, Campagna M, Shou-Jiang G, Rodriguez MS, Rivas C (2009) Kaposi's sarcoma-associated herpesvirus protein LANA2 disrupts PML oncogenic domains and inhibits PML-mediated transcriptional repression of the survivin gene. J Virol 83:8849–8858

Matta H, Chaudhary PM (2004) Activation of alternative NF-kappa B pathway by human herpes virus 8-encoded Fas-associated death domain-like IL-1 beta-converting enzyme inhibitory protein (vFLIP). Proc Natl Acad Sci U S A 101:9399–9404

Matta H, Mazzacurati L, Schamus S, Yang T, Sun Q, Chaudhary PM (2007) Kaposi's sarcoma-associated herpesvirus (KSHV) oncoprotein K13 bypasses TRAFs and directly interacts with the IkappaB kinase complex to selectively activate NF-kappaB without JNK activation. J Biol Chem 282:24858–24865

Mbulaiteye S, Marshall V, Bagni RK, Wang CD, Mbisa G, Bakaki PM, Owor AM, Ndugwa CM, Engels EA, Katongole-Mbidde E, Biggar RJ, Whitby D (2006) Molecular evidence for mother-to-child transmission of Kaposi sarcoma-associated herpesvirus in Uganda and K1 gene evolution within the host. J Infect Dis 193:1250–1257

McCormick C, Ganem D (2005) The kaposin B protein of KSHV activates the p38/MK2 pathway and stabilizes cytokine mRNAs. Science 307:739–741

McCormick C, Ganem D (2006) Phosphorylation and function of the kaposin B direct repeats of

Kaposi's sarcoma-associated herpesvirus. J Virol 80:6165–6170

Mesri EA, Cesarman E, Boshoff C (2010) Kaposi's sarcoma and its associated herpesvirus. Nat Rev Cancer 10:707–719

Miles SA, Rezai AR, Salazar-Gonzalez JF, Vander Meyden M, Stevens RH, Logan DM, Mitsuyasu RT, Taga T, Hirano T, Kishimoto T et al (1990) AIDS Kaposi sarcoma-derived cells produce and respond to interleukin 6. Proc Natl Acad Sci U S A 87:4068–4072

Montaner S, Sodhi A, Molinolo A, Bugge TH, Sawai ET, He Y, Li Y, Ray PE, Gutkind JS (2003) Endothelial infection with KSHV genes in vivo reveals that vGPCR initiates Kaposi's sarcomagenesis and can promote the tumorigenic potential of viral latent genes. Cancer Cell 3:23–36

Montaner S, Sodhi A, Servitja JM, Ramsdell AK, Barac A, Sawai ET, Gutkind JS (2004) The small GTPase Rac1 links the Kaposi sarcoma-associated herpesvirus vGPCR to cytokine secretion and paracrine neoplasia. Blood 104:2903–2911

Moore PS, Boshoff C, Weiss RA, Chang Y (1996) Molecular mimicry of human cytokine and cytokine response pathway genes by KSHV. Science 274:1739–1744

Mori Y, Nishimoto N, Ohno M, Inagi R, Dhepakson P, Amou K, Yoshizaki K, Yamanishi K (2000) Human herpesvirus 8-encoded interleukin-6 homologue (viral IL-6) induces endog- enous human IL-6 secretion. J Med Virol 61:332–335

Munoz-Fontela C, Collado M, Rodriguez E, Garcia MA, Alvarez-Barrientos A, Arroyo J, Nombela C, Rivas C (2005) Identification of a nuclear export signal in the KSHV latent protein LANA2 mediating its export from the nucleus. Exp Cell Res 311:96–105

Munoz-Fontela C, Marcos-Villar L, Gallego P, Arroyo J, Da Costa M, Pomeranz KM, Lam EW, Rivas C (2007) Latent protein LANA2 from Kaposi's sarcoma-associated herpesvirus interacts with 14-3-3 proteins and inhibits FOXO3a transcription factor. J Virol 81:1511–1516

Muralidhar S, Pumfery AM, Hassani M, Sadaie MR, Kishishita M, Brady JN, Doniger J, Medveczky P, Rosenthal LJ (1998) Identification of kaposin (open reading frame K12) as a human herpesvirus 8 (Kaposi's sarcoma-associated herpesvirus) transforming gene. J Virol 72:4980–4988

Muralidhar S, Veytsmann G, Chandran B, Ablashi D, Doniger J, Rosenthal LJ (2000) Characterization of the human herpesvirus 8 (Kaposi's sarcoma-associated herpesvirus) oncogene, kaposin (ORF K12). J Clin Virol 16:203–213

Murthy SC, Trimble JJ, Desrosiers RC (1989) Deletion mutants of herpesvirus saimiri define an open reading frame necessary for transformation. J Virol 63:3307–3314

Nachmani D, Stern-Ginossar N, Sarid R, Mandelboim O (2009) Diverse herpesvirus microRNAs target the stress-induced immune ligand MICB to escape recognition by natural killer cells. Cell Host Microbe 5:376–385

Nakamura H, Li M, Zarycki J, Jung JU (2001) Inhibition of p53 tumor suppressor by viral interferon regulatory factor. J Virol 75:7572–7582

Nakamura H, Lu M, Gwack Y, Souvlis J, Zeichner SL, Jung JU (2003) Global changes in Kaposi's sarcoma-associated virus gene expression patterns following expression of a tetracycline-inducible Rta transactivator. J Virol 77:4205–4220

Nakano K, Isegawa Y, Zou P, Tadagaki K, Inagi R, Yamanishi K (2003) Kaposi's sarcoma- associated herpesvirus (KSHV)-encoded vMIP-I and vMIP-II induce signal transduction and chemotaxis in monocytic cells. Arch Virol 148:871–890

Neipel F, Albrecht JC, Ensser A, Huang YQ, Li JJ, Friedman-Kien AE, Fleckenstein B (1997a) Human herpesvirus 8 encodes a homolog of interleukin-6. J Virol 71:839–842

Neipel F, Albrecht JC, Fleckenstein B (1997b) Cell-homologous genes in the Kaposi's sarcoma-associated rhadinovirus human herpesvirus 8: determinants of its pathogenicity? J Virol 71:4187–4192

Nicholas J (2005) Human gammaherpesvirus cytokines and chemokine receptors. J Interferon Cytokine Res 25:373–383

Nicholas J, Ruvolo VR, Burns WH, Sandford G, Wan X, Ciufo D, Hendrickson SB, Guo HG, Hayward GS, Reitz MS (1997) Kaposi's sarcoma-associated human herpesvirus-8 encodes homologues of macrophage inflammatory protein-1 and interleukin-6. Nat Med 3:287–292

Nicholas J, Zong JC, Alcendor DJ, Ciufo DM, Poole LJ, Sarisky RT, Chiou CJ, Zhang X, Wan X, Guo HG, Reitz MS, Hayward GS (1998) Novel organizational features, captured cellular genes, and strain variability within the genome of KSHV/HHV8. J Natl Cancer Inst Monogr 23:79–88

Offermann MK (2007) Kaposi sarcoma herpesvirus-encoded interferon regulator factors. Curr Top Microbiol Immunol 312:185–209

Okano M (2000) Haematological associations of Epstein-Barr virus infection. Baillieres Best Pract Res Clin Haematol 13:199–214

Pati S, Cavrois M, Guo HG, Foulke JS Jr, Kim J, Feldman RA, Reitz M (2001) Activation of NF- kappaB by the human herpesvirus 8 chemokine receptor ORF74: evidence for a paracrine model of Kaposi's sarcoma pathogenesis. J Virol 75:8660–8673

Paudel N, Sadagopan S, Balasubramanian S, Chandran B (2012) Kaposi's Sarcoma-Associated Herpesvirus Latency-Associated Nuclear Antigen and Angiogenin Interact with Common Host Proteins, Including Annexin A2, Which Is Essential for Survival of Latently Infected Cells. J Virol 86:1589–1607

Paulose-Murphy M, Ha NK, Xiang C, Chen Y, Gillim L, Yarchoan R, Meltzer P, Bittner M, Trent J, Zeichner S (2001) Transcription program of human herpesvirus 8 (kaposi's sarcoma- associated herpesvirus). J Virol 75:4843–4853

Pearce M, Matsumura S, Wilson AC (2005) Transcripts encoding K12, v-FLIP, v-cyclin, and the microRNA cluster of Kaposi's sarcoma-associated herpesvirus originate from a common promoter. J Virol 79:14457–14464

Petre CE, Sin SH, Dittmer DP (2007) Functional p53 signaling in Kaposi's sarcoma-associated herpesvirus lymphomas: implications for therapy. J Virol 81:1912–1922

Pfeffer S, Sewer A, Lagos-Quintana M, Sheridan R, Sander C, Grasser FA, van Dyk LF, Ho CK, Shuman S, Chien M, Russo JJ, Ju J, Randall G, Lindenbach BD, Rice CM, Simon V, Ho DD, Zavolan M, Tuschl T (2005) Identification of microRNAs of the herpesvirus family. Nat Methods 2:269–276

Pfeffer S, Zavolan M, Grasser FA, Chien M, Russo JJ, Ju J, John B, Enright AJ, Marks D, Sander C, Tuschl T (2004) Identification of virus-encoded microRNAs. Science 304:734–736

Philpott N, Bakken T, Pennell C, Chen L, Wu J, Cannon M (2011) The Kaposi's sarcoma- associated herpesvirus G protein-coupled receptor contains an immunoreceptor tyrosine-based inhibitory motif that activates Shp2. J Virol 85:1140–1144

Pietrek M, Brinkmann MM, Glowacka I, Enlund A, Havemeier A, Dittrich-Breiholz O, Kracht M, Lewitzky M, Saksela K, Feller SM, Schulz TF (2010) Role of the Kaposi's sarcoma- associated herpesvirus K15 SH3 binding site in inflammatory signaling and B-cell activation. J Virol 84:8231–8240

Platt G, Carbone A, Mittnacht S (2002) p16INK4a loss and sensitivity in KSHV associated primary effusion lymphoma. Oncogene 21:1823–1831

Poole LJ, Zong JC, Ciufo DM, Alcendor DJ, Cannon JS, Ambinder R, Orenstein JM, Reitz MS, Hayward GS (1999) Comparison of genetic variability at multiple loci across the genomes of the major subtypes of Kaposi's sarcoma-associated herpesvirus reveals evidence for recombination and for two distinct types of open reading frame K15 alleles at the right- hand end. J Virol 73:6646–6660

Pozharskaya VP, Weakland LL, Zimring JC, Krug LT, Unger ER, Neisch A, Joshi H, Inoue N, Offermann MK (2004) Short duration of elevated vIRF-1 expression during lytic replication of human herpesvirus 8 limits its ability to block antiviral responses induced by alpha interferon in BCBL-1 cells. J Virol 78:6621–6635

Prakash O, Tang ZY, Peng X, Coleman R, Gill J, Farr G, Samaniego F (2002) Tumorigenesis and aberrant signaling in transgenic mice expressing the human herpesvirus-8 K1 gene. J Natl Cancer Inst 94:926–935

Pyakurel P, Pak F, Mwakigonja AR, Kaaya E, Heiden T, Biberfeld P (2006) Lymphatic and vascular origin of Kaposi's sarcoma spindle cells during tumor development. Int J Cancer 119:1262–1267

Qin Z, Freitas E, Sullivan R, Mohan S, Bacelieri R, Branch D, Romano M, Kearney P, Oates J, Plaisance K, Renne R, Kaleeba J, Parsons C (2010) Upregulation of xCT by KSHV-encoded microRNAs facilitates KSHV dissemination and persistence in an environment of oxidative stress. PLoS

Pathog 6:e1000742

Radkov SA, Kellam P, Boshoff C (2000) The latent nuclear antigen of Kaposi sarcoma-associated herpesvirus targets the retinoblastoma-E2F pathway and with the oncogene Hras transforms primary rat cells. Nat Med 6:1121–1127

Rivas C, Thlick AE, Parravicini C, Moore PS, Chang Y (2001) Kaposi's sarcoma-associated herpesvirus LANA2 is a B-cell-specific latent viral protein that inhibits p53. J Virol 75:429–438

Rodriguez A, Vigorito E, Clare S, Warren MV, Couttet P, Soond DR, van Dongen S, Grocock RJ, Das PP, Miska EA, Vetrie D, Okkenhaug K, Enright AJ, Dougan G, Turner M, Bradley A (2007) Requirement of bic/microRNA-155 for normal immune function. Science 316:608–611

Rosenkilde MM, Waldhoer M, Luttichau HR, Schwartz TW (2001) Virally encoded 7TM receptors. Oncogene 20:1582–1593

Roth WK (1991) HIV-associated Kaposi's sarcoma: new developments in epidemiology and molecular pathology. J Cancer Res Clin Oncol 117:186–191

Russo JJ, Bohenzky RA, Chien MC, Chen J, Yan M, Maddalena D, Parry JP, Peruzzi D, Edelman IS, Chang Y, Moore PS (1996) Nucleotide sequence of the Kaposi sarcoma-associated herpesvirus (HHV8). Proc Natl Acad Sci U S A 93:14862–14867

Sadagopan S, Sharma-Walia N, Veettil MV, Bottero V, Levine R, Vart RJ, Chandran B (2009) Kaposi's sarcoma-associated herpesvirus upregulates angiogenin during infection of human dermal microvascular endothelial cells, which induces 45S rRNA synthesis, antiapoptosis, cell proliferation, migration, and angiogenesis. J Virol 83:3342–3364

Sadagopan S, Valiya Veettil M, Paudel N, Bottero V, Chandran B (2011) Kaposi's sarcoma- associated herpesvirus-induced angiogenin plays roles in latency via the phospholipase C gamma pathway: blocking angiogenin inhibits latent gene expression and induces the lytic cycle. J Virol 85:2666–2685

Sadagopan S, Veettil MV, Chakraborty S, Sharma-Walia N, Paudel N, Bottero V, Chandran B (2012) Angiogenin functionally interacts with p53 and regulates p53-mediated apoptosis and cell survival. Oncogene 31:4835–4847

Sadler R, Wu L, Forghani B, Renne R, Zhong W, Herndier B, Ganem D (1999) A complex translational program generates multiple novel proteins from the latently expressed kaposin (K12) locus of Kaposi's sarcoma-associated herpesvirus. J Virol 73:5722–5730

Sakakibara S, Ueda K, Nishimura K, Do E, Ohsaki E, Okuno T, Yamanishi K (2004) Accumulation of heterochromatin components on the terminal repeat sequence of Kaposi's sarcoma-associated herpesvirus mediated by the latency-associated nuclear antigen. J Virol 78:7299–7310

Samaniego F, Pati S, Karp JE, Prakash O, Bose D (2001) Human herpesvirus 8 K1-associated nuclear factor-kappa B-dependent promoter activity: role in Kaposi's sarcoma inflammation? J Natl

Cancer Inst Monogr 28:15–23

Samols MA, Hu J, Skalsky RL, Renne R (2005) Cloning and identification of a microRNA cluster within the latency-associated region of Kaposi's sarcoma-associated herpesvirus. J Virol 79:9301–9305

Samols MA, Skalsky RL, Maldonado AM, Riva A, Lopez MC, Baker HV, Renne R (2007) Identification of cellular genes targeted by KSHV-encoded microRNAs. PLoS Pathogens 3:e65

Sandford G, Choi YB, Nicholas J (2009) Role of ORF74-encoded viral G protein-coupled receptor in human herpesvirus 8 lytic replication. J Virol 83:13009–13014

Schmidt K, Wies E, Neipel F (2011) Kaposi's sarcoma-associated herpesvirus viral interferon regulatory factor 3 inhibits gamma interferon and major histocompatibility complex class II expression. J Virol 85:4530–4537

Schwarz DS, Hutvagner G, Du T, Xu Z, Aronin N, Zamore PD (2003) Asymmetry in the assembly of the RNAi enzyme complex. Cell 115:199–208

Schwarz M, Murphy PM (2001) Kaposi's sarcoma-associated herpesvirus G protein-coupled receptor constitutively activates NF-kappa B and induces proinflammatory cytokine and chemokine production via a C-terminal signaling determinant. J Immunol 167:505–513

Searles RP, Bergquam EP, Axthelm MK, Wong SW (1999) Sequence and genomic analysis of a Rhesus macaque rhadinovirus with similarity to Kaposi's sarcoma-associated herpesvirus/ human herpesvirus 8. J Virol 73:3040–3053

Sears R, Nuckolls F, Haura E, Taya Y, Tamai K, Nevins JR (2000) Multiple Ras-dependent phosphorylation pathways regulate Myc protein stability. Genes Dev 14:2501–2514

Seo T, Lee D, Lee B, Chung JH, Choe J (2000) Viral interferon regulatory factor 1 of Kaposi's sarcoma-associated herpesvirus (human herpesvirus 8) binds to, and inhibits transactivation of, CREB-binding protein. Biochem Biophys Res Commun 270:23–27

Seo T, Lee D, Shim YS, Angell JE, Chidambaram NV, Kalvakolanu DV, Choe J (2002) Viral interferon regulatory factor 1 of Kaposi's sarcoma-associated herpesvirus interacts with a cell death regulator, GRIM19, and inhibits interferon/retinoic acid-induced cell death. J Virol 76:8797–8807

Seo T, Park J, Choe J (2005) Kaposi's sarcoma-associated herpesvirus viral IFN regulatory factor 1 inhibits transforming growth factor-beta signaling. Cancer Res 65:1738–1747

Seo T, Park J, Lee D, Hwang SG, Choe J (2001) Viral interferon regulatory factor 1 of Kaposi's sarcoma-associated herpesvirus binds to p53 and represses p53-dependent transcription and apoptosis. J Virol 75:6193–6198

Shamay M, Krithivas A, Zhang J, Hayward SD (2006) Recruitment of the de novo DNA methyltransferase Dnmt3a by Kaposi's sarcoma-associated herpesvirus LANA. Proc Natl Acad Sci U S A 103:14554–14559

Sharma-Walia N, Paul AG, Bottero V, Sadagopan S, Veettil MV, Kerur N, Chandran B (2010) Kaposi's sarcoma associated herpes virus (KSHV) induced COX-2: a key factor in latency, inflammation, angiogenesis, cell survival and invasion. PLoS Pathog 6:e1000777

Sharp TV, Wang HW, Koumi A, Hollyman D, Endo Y, Ye H, Du MQ, Boshoff C (2002) K15 protein of Kaposi's sarcoma-associated herpesvirus is latently expressed and binds to HAX-1, a protein with antiapoptotic function. J Virol 76:802–816

Shepard LW, Yang M, Xie P, Browning DD, Voyno-Yasenetskaya T, Kozasa T, Ye RD (2001) Constitutive activation of NF-kappa B and secretion of interleukin-8 induced by the G protein-coupled receptor of Kaposi's sarcoma-associated herpesvirus involve G alpha(13) and RhoA. J Biol Chem 276:45979–45987

Shim WS, Ho IA, Wong PE (2007) Angiopoietin: a TIE(d) balance in tumor angiogenesis. Mol Cancer Res 5:655–665

Shin YC, Joo CH, Gack MU, Lee HR, Jung JU (2008) Kaposi's sarcoma-associated herpesvirus viral IFN regulatory factor 3 stabilizes hypoxia-inducible factor-1 alpha to induce vascular endothelial growth factor expression. Cancer Res 68:1751–1759

Shin YC, Nakamura H, Liang X, Feng P, Chang H, Kowalik TF, Jung JU (2006) Inhibition of the ATM/p53 signal transduction pathway by Kaposi's sarcoma-associated herpesvirus interferon regulatory factor 1. J Virol 80:2257–2266

Skalsky RL, Samols MA, Plaisance KB, Boss IW, Riva A, Lopez MC, Baker HV, Renne R (2007) Kaposi's sarcoma-associated herpesvirus encodes an ortholog of miR-155. J Virol 81:12836–12845

Staskus KA, Zhong W, Gebhard K, Herndier B, Wang H, Renne R, Beneke J, Pudney J, Anderson DJ, Ganem D, Haase AT (1997) Kaposi's sarcoma-associated herpesvirus gene expression in endothelial (spindle) tumor cells. J Virol 71:715–719

Stern-Ginossar N, Elefant N, Zimmermann A, Wolf DG, Saleh N, Biton M, Horwitz E, Prokocimer Z, Prichard M, Hahn G, Goldman-Wohl D, Greenfield C, Yagel S, Hengel H, Altuvia Y, Margalit H, Mandelboim O (2007) Host immune system gene targeting by a viral miRNA. Science 317:376–381

Stern-Ginossar N, Gur C, Biton M, Horwitz E, Elboim M, Stanietsky N, Mandelboim M, Mandelboim O (2008) Human microRNAs regulate stress-induced immune responses mediated by the receptor NKG2D. Nat Immunol 9:1065–1073

Stine JT, Wood C, Hill M, Epp A, Raport CJ, Schweickart VL, Endo Y, Sasaki T, Simmons G, Boshoff C, Clapham P, Chang Y, Moore P, Gray PW, Chantry D (2000) KSHV-encoded CC chemokine vMIP-III is a CCR4 agonist, stimulates angiogenesis, and selectively chemoat- tracts TH2 cells. Blood 95:1151–1157

Sturzl M, Blasig C, Schreier A, Neipel F, Hohenadl C, Cornali E, Ascherl G, Esser S, Brockmeyer NH, Ekman M, Kaaya EE, Tschachler E, Biberfeld P (1997) Expression of HHV- 8 latency-associated T0.7 RNA in spindle cells and endothelial cells of AIDS-associated, classical and African Kaposi's sarcoma. Int J Cancer 72:68–71

Suffert G, Malterer G, Hausser J, Viiliainen J, Fender A, Contrant M, Ivacevic T, Benes V, Gros F, Voinnet O, Zavolan M, Ojala PM, Haas JG, Pfeffer S (2011) Kaposi's sarcoma herpesvirus microRNAs target caspase 3 and regulate apoptosis. PLoS Pathog 7:e1002405

Sun Q, Matta H, Lu G, Chaudhary PM (2006) Induction of IL-8 expression by human herpesvirus 8 encoded vFLIP K13 via NF-kappaB activation. Oncogene 25:2717–2726

Sun R, Lin SF, Staskus K, Gradoville L, Grogan E, Haase A, Miller G (1999) Kinetics of Kaposi's sarcoma-associated herpesvirus gene expression. J Virol 73:2232–2242

Thomas M, Augustin HG (2009) The role of the Angiopoietins in vascular morphogenesis. Angiogenesis 12:125–137

Thome M, Schneider P, Hofmann K, Fickenscher H, Meinl E, Neipel F, Mattmann C, Burns K, Bodmer JL, Schroter M, Scaffidi C, Krammer PH, Peter ME, Tschopp J (1997) Viral FLICE- inhibitory proteins (FLIPs) prevent apoptosis induced by death receptors. Nature 386:517–521

Tomkowicz B, Singh SP, Cartas M, Srinivasan A (2002) Human herpesvirus-8 encoded Kaposin: subcellular localization using immunofluorescence and biochemical approaches. DNA Cell Biol 21:151–162

Tomkowicz B, Singh SP, Lai D, Singh A, Mahalingham S, Joseph J, Srivastava S, Srinivasan A (2005) Mutational analysis reveals an essential role for the LXXLL motif in the transformation function of the human herpesvirus-8 oncoprotein, kaposin. DNA Cell Biol 24:10–20

Tomlinson CC, Damania B (2004) The K1 protein of Kaposi's sarcoma-associated herpesvirus activates the Akt signaling pathway. J Virol 78:1918–1927

Tsai YH, Wu MF, Wu YH, Chang SJ, Lin SF, Sharp TV, Wang HW (2009) The M type K15 protein of Kaposi's sarcoma-associated herpesvirus regulates microRNA expression via its SH2-binding motif to induce cell migration and invasion. J Virol 83:622–632

Umbach JL, Cullen BR (2010) In-depth analysis of Kaposi's sarcoma-associated herpesvirus microRNA expression provides insights into the mammalian microRNA-processing machin- ery. J Virol 84:695–703

Verma SC, Lan K, Robertson E (2007) Structure and function of latency-associated nuclear antigen. Curr Top Microbiol Immunol 312:101–136

Verschuren EW, Jones N, Evan GI (2004) The cell cycle and how it is steered by Kaposi's sarcoma-associated herpesvirus cyclin. J Gen Virol 85:1347–1361

Verzijl D, Fitzsimons CP, Van Dijk M, Stewart JP, Timmerman H, Smit MJ, Leurs R (2004) Differential activation of murine herpesvirus 68- and Kaposi's sarcoma-associated herpes- virus-encoded ORF74 G protein-coupled receptors by human and murine chemokines. J Virol 78:3343–3351

Wang HW, Sharp TV, Koumi A, Koentges G, Boshoff C (2002) Characterization of an anti- apoptotic glycoprotein encoded by Kaposi's sarcoma-associated herpesvirus which resembles a spliced variant of human survivin. EMBO J 21:2602–2615

Wang HW, Trotter MW, Lagos D, Bourboulia D, Henderson S, Makinen T, Elliman S, Flanagan AM, Alitalo K, Boshoff C (2004) Kaposi sarcoma herpesvirus-induced cellular reprogram- ming contributes to the lymphatic endothelial gene expression in Kaposi sarcoma. Nat Genet 36:687–693

Wang L, Dittmer DP, Tomlinson CC, Fakhari FD, Damania B (2006) Immortalization of primary endothelial cells by the K1 protein of Kaposi's sarcoma-associated herpesvirus. Cancer Res 66:3658–3666

Weber KS, Grone HJ, Rocken M, Klier C, Gu S, Wank R, Proudfoot AE, Nelson PJ, Weber C (2001) Selective recruitment of Th2-type cells and evasion from a cytotoxic immune response mediated by viral macrophage inhibitory protein-II. Eur J Immunol 31:2458–2466

Whitby D, Marshall VA, Bagni RK, Wang CD, Gamache CJ, Guzman JR, Kron M, Ebbesen P, Biggar RJ (2004) Genotypic characterization of Kaposi's sarcoma-associated herpesvirus in asymptomatic infected subjects from isolated populations. J Gen Virol 85:155–163

Wies E, Hahn AS, Schmidt K, Viebahn C, Rohland N, Lux A, Schellhorn T, Holzer A, Jung JU, Neipel F (2009) The Kaposi's Sarcoma-associated Herpesvirus-encoded vIRF-3 Inhibits Cellular IRF-5. J Biol Chem 284:8525–8538

Wies E, Mori Y, Hahn A, Kremmer E, Sturzl M, Fleckenstein B, Neipel F (2008) The viral interferon-regulatory factor-3 is required for the survival of KSHV-infected primary effusion lymphoma cells. Blood 111:320–327

Willis SN, Adams JM (2005) Life in the balance: how BH3-only proteins induce apoptosis. Curr Opin Cell Biol 17:617–625

Wong EL, Damania B (2006) Transcriptional regulation of the Kaposi's sarcoma-associated herpesvirus K15 gene. J Virol 80:1385–1392

Wu AL, Wang J, Zheleznyak A, Brown EJ (1999) Ubiquitin-related proteins regulate interaction of vimentin intermediate filaments with the plasma membrane. Mol Cell 4:619–625

Yang TY, Chen SC, Leach MW, Manfra D, Homey B, Wiekowski M, Sullivan L, Jenh CH, Narula SK, Chensue SW, Lira SA (2000) Transgenic expression of the chemokine receptor encoded by human herpesvirus 8 induces an angioproliferative disease resembling Kaposi's sarcoma. J Exp Med 191:445–454

Yoo J, Kang J, Lee HN, Aguilar B, Kafka D, Lee S, Choi I, Lee J, Ramu S, Haas J, Koh CJ, Hong YK (2010) Kaposin-B enhances the PROX1 mRNA stability during lymphatic reprogram- ming of vascular endothelial cells by Kaposi's sarcoma herpes virus. PLoS Pathog 6:e1001046

Yoshizaki K, Matsuda T, Nishimoto N, Kuritani T, Taeho L, Aozasa K, Nakahata T, Kawai H, Tagoh H,

Komori T et al (1989) Pathogenic significance of interleukin-6 (IL-6/BSF-2) in Castleman's disease. Blood 74:1360–1367

Young LS, Murray PG (2003) Epstein-Barr virus and oncogenesis: from latent genes to tumours. Oncogene 22:5108–5121

Zeng Y, Yi R, Cullen BR (2003) MicroRNAs and small interfering RNAs can inhibit mRNA expression by similar mechanisms. Proc Natl Acad Sci U S A 100:9779–9784

Zhang YJ, Bonaparte RS, Patel D, Stein DA, Iversen PL (2008) Blockade of viral interleukin-6 expression of Kaposi's sarcoma-associated herpesvirus. Mol Cancer Ther 7:712–720

Zhao J, Punj V, Matta H, Mazzacurati L, Schamus S, Yang Y, Yang T, Hong Y, Chaudhary PM (2007) K13 blocks KSHV lytic replication and deregulates vIL6 and hIL6 expression: a model of lytic replication induced clonal selection in viral oncogenesis. PLoS One 2:e1067

Zhong W, Wang H, Herndier B, Ganem D (1996) Restricted expression of Kaposi sarcoma- associated herpesvirus (human herpesvirus 8) genes in Kaposi sarcoma. Proc Natl Acad Sci U S A 93:6641–6646

Ziech D, Franco R, Pappa A, Malamou-Mitsi V, Georgakila S, Georgakilas AG, Panayiotidis MI (2010) The role of epigenetics in environmental and occupational carcinogenesis. Chem Biol Interact 188:340–349

Ziegelbauer JM, Sullivan CS, Ganem D (2009) Tandem array-based expression screens identify host mRNA targets of virus-encoded microRNAs. Nat Genet 41:130–134

Zimring JC, Goodbourn S, Offermann MK (1998) Human herpesvirus 8 encodes an interferon regulatory factor (IRF) homolog that represses IRF-1-mediated transcription. J Virol 72:701–707

Zong JC, Ciufo DM, Alcendor DJ, Wan X, Nicholas J, Browning PJ, Rady PL, Tyring SK, Orenstein JM, Rabkin CS, Su IJ, Powell KF, Croxson M, Foreman KE, Nickoloff BJ, Alkan S, Hayward GS (1999) High-level variability in the ORF-K1 membrane protein gene at the left end of the Kaposi's sarcoma-associated herpesvirus genome defines four major virus subtypes and multiple variants or clades in different human populations. J Virol 73:4156–4170

第 16 章　抗病毒治疗与癌症控制

Wei-Liang Shih, Chi-Tai Fang 和 Pei-Jer Chen

摘　要　乙肝病毒（HBV）、丙肝病毒（HCV）、人乳头瘤病毒（HPV）和 EB 病毒（EBV）引起的肿瘤占全球人类肿瘤病的 10%~15%。传统化疗或分子靶向治疗常常用于治疗病毒相关的肿瘤。然而，更加积极的方法首先应该是通过抗病毒治疗来抑制或减少病毒感染，从而预防肿瘤的发生。针对慢性 HBV 和 HCV 感染的抗病毒治疗达到了一定的目标，能明显减少受治患者肝细胞癌症的发生。然而，对于某些病毒相关的癌症，抗病毒治疗的效果并不明显，如治疗抵抗性 EBV 相关淋巴瘤和移植后淋巴增殖紊乱、艾滋病（AIDS）患者中 KSHV 相关的卡波西肉瘤，以及 HTLV-1 相关的急性、慢性和成人慢性生长型 T 细胞淋巴瘤。对于 HPV 相关的宫颈癌，治疗性 HPV 疫苗和基于 RNA 干扰的治疗也显示了一定可喜的结果。总之，抗病毒治疗对于癌症的预防和治疗已经取得了令人满意的成果。然而，我们还需要通过更大规模的研究来证实抗病毒治疗的效果，并且需要注重深层次研究更加有效和便利的抗病毒方案。

1　引言

乙肝病毒（HBV）、丙肝病毒（HCV）、人乳头瘤病毒（HPV）、EB 病毒（EBV）、人 T 淋巴细胞病毒 1 型（HTLV-1）、卡波西肉瘤相关疱疹病毒（KSHV）和梅克尔细胞多瘤病毒（MCV）是目前已知引起慢性感染、与人类特定肿瘤相关的 7 类病毒（Moore and Chang 2010）。总的来说，全世界人类肿瘤中 10%~15% 是由病毒感染引起的。尽管只有少部分感染个体真正发展为癌症，但临床预后通常很不好。

病毒因子在癌变过程中的重要作用很早就被提出来。目前分子技术的进步允

P.-J. Chen (✉)
Institute of Clinical Medicine, National Taiwan University, Taipei, Taiwan
e-mail: peijerchen@ntu.edu.tw

W.-L. Shih _ C.-T. Fang
Institute of Epidemiology and Preventive Medicine, National Taiwan University,
Taipei, Taiwan

许对病毒载量（即人体病毒复制活力的标志）进行快速、精确的定量。越来越多的数据表明,对于病毒相关的肿瘤,病毒的载量与发生肿瘤的风险成正比,如 HBV 和 HCV 引起的肝细胞癌（HCC）、EB 病毒引起的鼻咽癌（NPC）。鉴于病毒复制活力在病毒相关癌症中的重要性,抑制或减少病毒的抗病毒治疗可能是一个预防癌症的重要策略。目前,抗病毒治疗已经应用到了 7 种病毒相关的癌症治疗中（表 16-1）,而且临床资料证实 HBV 和 HCV 的抗病毒治疗是有疗效的。

本章我们对目前已证明了病毒载量和临床结果（如癌症风险和存活率）相关性的一些证据进行了评估,并阐述目前抗病毒治疗对癌症相关病毒的影响。

表 16-1　人类肿瘤病毒、相关肿瘤以及特异的抗病毒治疗

病毒[a]	肿瘤类型[b]	抗病毒治疗[c]	
HBV	HCC	干扰素	(α-干扰素和 PEG 化α2a 干扰素)
		核苷酸类似物	(拉米夫定、阿德福韦、恩替卡韦、替比夫定和替诺福韦)
HCV	HCC	PEG 化的干扰素和利巴韦林	
		直接的抗病毒试剂（蛋白酶抑制剂）	(波西普韦和特拉匹韦)
KSHV	AIDS-KS	抗疱疹病毒药物	(更昔洛韦和缬更昔洛韦)
		HAART（基于 PI）；HAART（基于 NNRTI）	
	HIV 阴性 KS	HIV 蛋白酶抑制剂	(茚地那韦)
HTLV-1	ALT（急性、慢性和闷烧型）	干扰素加齐多夫定/扎西他滨或联合化疗	
EBV	PTLD, NPC, HL	免疫治疗	(EBV 特异性的细胞毒 T 细胞)
	EBV 相关的淋巴瘤	针对病毒	(裂解复制诱导剂加阿昔洛韦/更昔洛韦)
HPV	宫颈癌	治疗性 HPV 疫苗（集中在 HPV-16 和 HPV-18）	
		基于 RNA 干扰的治疗	(反义寡核苷酸,核酶和 siRNA)
MCV	MCC	干扰素	干扰素和　干扰素

a.HBV, 乙肝病毒；HCV, 丙肝病毒；EBV, EB 病毒；HPV, 人肉瘤病毒；HTLV-1, 人 T 细胞嗜淋巴病毒 1 型；KSHV, 卡波西肉瘤相关疱疹病毒；MCV, 梅克尔细胞多瘤病毒。

b.HCC, 肝细胞肿瘤；AIDS-KS, AIDS-卡波西肉瘤；ATL, 成人 T 细胞淋巴瘤；PTLD, 移植后淋巴扩增紊乱；NPC, 鼻咽癌；HL, 霍奇金淋巴瘤；MCC, 梅克尔细胞癌。

c.HAART, 高度活性抗逆转录病毒治疗；PI, 蛋白酶抑制剂；NNRTI, 非核苷酸逆转录酶抑制剂

2　乙肝病毒（HBV）和丙肝病毒（HCV）

慢性 HBV 和 HCV 感染是 HCC 的主要病因,占全球 HCC 病例的 75%~80%。

在中国台湾，自 1985 年以来，针对新生儿的 HBV 通用免疫计划已经使青少年 HBV 相关性 HCC 降低了 70%（Chang et al. 2009）。然而，大量 HBV 慢性感染的人群仍然有发展成为 HCC 的危险。不幸的是，目前还没有能有效预防 HCV 感染的疫苗。HCV 相关的 HCC 的比例在不断增长，尤其是在发达国家（El-Serag 2012）。对于这些 HBV 或 HCV 持续性感染的患者，靶向 HBV 和 HCV 的抗病毒治疗可能是一种有效降低 HCC 风险的策略。

2.1 抗乙肝病毒治疗

乙肝病毒复制是驱动乙肝病毒相关疾病的关键因素（Liaw 2006）。乙肝病毒表面抗原（HBeAg）是一个已知的 HBV 复制的标记（Chen et al. 2009；Fang et al. 2003）。流行病学研究也一致表明，HBV 病毒载量的增加，代表了 HBV 复制活性的升高，与 HCC 的高风险、病情恶化和低存活率相关（Chen et al. 2009）。HBV 抗病毒治疗的目标是将 HBV 的 DNA 降低到不可检测的水平，或诱导血清表面抗原逆转（Feld et al. 2009）。

目前已获批准的用于治疗慢性 HBV 感染的方法有：传统的α干扰素、PGE 化的干扰素α2a 和核苷酸类似物，包括拉米夫定、阿德福韦、恩替卡韦、替比夫定和替诺福韦。较新的核酸类似物（恩替卡韦、替比夫定和替诺福韦）治疗能分别抑制 HBeAg 阳性患者（Chang et al. 2006；Lai et al. 2007；Marcellin et al. 2008）和 HBeAg 阴性患者（Lai et al. 2006，2007；Marcellin et al. 2008）中 HBV 的 DNA 至 $6.2\sim6.9\ \log_{10}$ IU/mL 和 $4.6\sim5.2\ \log_{10}$ IU/mL。通过药物治疗，60%~80%的 HBeAg 表面抗原阳性患者（Chang et al. 2006；Dienstag 2009；Lai et al. 2007；Marcellin et al. 2008）和 88%~95%的 HBeAg 表面抗原阴性患者中 HBV 的 DNA 可以控制在不可检测的水平（Dienstag 2009；Lai et al. 2006，2007；Marcellin et al. 2008）。然而，用拉米夫定和阿德福韦治疗只能轻微地减少 HBeAg 阳性和阴性患者中 HBV 的 DNA 量，不可检出的 HBV 的 DNA 的比例也较低。此外，核苷酸类似物（NUC）治疗的患者 HBeAg 血清阴转率为 12%~23%（Chang et al. 2006；Dienstag 2009；Lai et al. 2007；Marcellin et al. 2008）。经过 1 年的 NUC 治疗后，相对较小比例的初始反应者中存在病毒学反应（Dienstag 2009）。因此，NUC 通常作为一种长程治疗药物。尽管目前还没有最佳的 NUC 治疗疗程，但是为了进一步巩固反应，在 HBeAg 血清阴转后再延长 6 个月以上的治疗是一种目前可以接受的方法。

尽管 NUC 是高效和安全的，但在长时间使用后，其抗药性的出现是一个备受关注的问题。据报道，与不受 NUC 影响的患者相比，产生了拉米夫定药物抗药性的患者发生 HCC 的风险较高（Papatheodoridis et al. 2010）。拉米夫定在使用 12 个月后，药物抗药性很快就累计达 15%~25%，使用 4 年后高达 60%~65%（Papatheo-doridis et al. 2008）。阿德福韦和替诺福韦在长期使用后也能产生

25%~30%的抗药性。只有恩替卡韦和替诺福韦的治疗还没有表现出抗药性。因此，恩替卡韦和替诺福韦具有较好的抗药性谱、高效性和安全性，是目前建议的首选治疗药物（Dienstag 2009）。

与使用核苷类似物（NUC）相比，基于干扰素的治疗因其副作用和较差的耐受性而较少用于 HBV 感染的治疗。尽管如此，近来的一些研究为干扰素抗 HBV 的治疗提供了一些支持性的证据。HBeAg 阳性患者在用聚乙二醇（PEG）化干扰素治疗 48~56 周后，10%~25%患者 HBV 的 DNA 降低到不可检测水平，平均下降至低于 2~4.5$\log_{10}$拷贝/mL（Janssen et al. 2005；Lau et al. 2005）。药物治疗后 3 年的平均跟踪研究表明，拉米夫定共治疗和单独干扰素治疗后，分别有 81%和 70%初始反应者的 HBeAg 减少和阴转能持续一段时间（Buster et al. 2008）。PEG 化干扰素治疗 48 周后，HBeAg 患者 HBV 的 DNA 低于检测水平的比例为 63%，平均病毒载量降低至 4.1$\log_{10}$拷贝/mL（Marcellin et al. 2004）。跟踪 24 周后（第 72 周），HBV 的 DNA 不可检测率下降至 19%，平均病毒载量降低至 2.3$\log_{10}$拷贝/mL（Marcellin et al. 2004）。治疗结束后 3 年的跟踪研究表明，46%的 HBeAg 阴性初始反应者表现为 HBV 的 DNA 持续性被抑制在不可检测水平（Marcellin et al. 2009）。尽管 PEG 化干扰素只在少部分患者中引起病毒学反应，但大多数在撤销治疗后仍具有持久性反应。由于这一优点和固有的治疗持久性，PEG 化干扰素对于特定患者仍然具有治疗作用。

对于用 NUC 和干扰素进行抗 HBV 治疗后，降低 HCC 发生和患者存活的长期疗效也有一定的研究。基于干扰素的治疗有两个研究报道，持续的病毒学反应者明显表现出较好的存活状态和较低 HCC 的风险（Niederau et al. 1996；van Zonneveld et al. 2004）。与未治疗组相比，干扰素治疗的患者有较低的 HCC 发生率（RR 为 0.23~0.66）（表 16-2）。对于 NUC，早期两个大的随机对照治疗试验针对有严重肝病患者的 HBV 慢性感染进行了研究，结果表明，拉米夫定能降低治疗过的患者和有持续性病毒抑制患者的疾病进一步发展（包括发展为 HCC）的风险（Di Marco et al. 2004；Liaw et al. 2004）。几个 Meta 分析一致表明，NUC 治疗与较低的 HCC 发生率相关（表 16-2）。

表 16-2　Meta 分析基于核苷酸类似物和干扰素治疗 HBV 和 HCV 的感染

研究	设计	受试者的数目	治疗	终端	主要发现
HBV					
Mommeja-Marin et al.（2003）	26 项前瞻性研究	N=3428（2524 个是乙肝表面抗原阳性）	IFN vs. CN 和 NUC vs. CN	组织学反应 生物化学反应 血清学反应	治疗诱导的 HBV DNA 减少与组织学、生物化学及血清学反应相关

续表

研究	设计	受试者的数目	治疗	终端	主要发现
Sung et al.（2008）	12 项研究	N=2742，治疗者1292人，未治疗者1450人	IFN vs. CN	HBV 相关的 HCC	RR=0.66（0.48~0.89）
	5 项研究	N=2289，治疗者1267人，未治疗者1022人	NUCs vs. CN	HBV 相关的 HCC	RR=0.22（0.10~0.50）
Yang et al.（2009）	11 项临床试验	N=2082，治疗者1006人，未治疗者1076人	IFN vs. CN	HBV 相关的 HCC 发生	RR=0.59（0.43~0.81）
	5 项临床试验	N=935，治疗者516人，为治疗者419人	IFN vs. CN	HBV 相关的硬化	RR=0.65（0.41~0.91）
Wong et al.（2010）	11 项研究	N=2122，治疗者975人，未治疗者1147人	IFN vs. CN	整个肝脏的反应	RR=0.55（0.43~0.70）
				肝脏相关的死亡	RR=0.63（0.42~0.96）
Papatheodoridis et al.（2010）	21 项研究	N=4415，治疗者3381人，未治疗者534人	IFN vs. CN	发生 HCC	HCC 发生率：治疗组2.8%；为治疗组：6.4%
Zhang et al.（2011）	2 项随机对照研究	N=158，治疗者95人，未治疗者63人	非维持性 IFN vs. CN	HBV 相关的 HCC 发生	RR=0.23（0.05~1.04）
HCV					
Camma et al.（2001）	14 项研究	HCV 相关的硬化，N=3109人	IFN 治疗和非治疗	HCC 发生	OR=0.28（0.22~0.36）
Papatheodoridis et al.（2001）	11 项研究	HCV 相关的硬化，N=2178	CN vs. IFN	HCC 发生	OR=3.02（2.35-3.89）
	5 项研究	HCV 相关的硬化	Non-SVR vs. SVR	HCC 发生	OR=3.65（1.71~7.78）
Zhang et al.（2011）	4 个随机控制实验	HCV 患者，N=378	非维持性 IFN 治疗和非治疗	HCV 相关的 HCC 发生	RR=0.39（0.26~0.59）
	2 个随机控制实验	HCV 患者，N=223	非维持性 IFN 治疗和非治疗	HCV-SVR	RR=0.30（0.04~2.15）
	2 个随机控制实验	起初对干扰素治疗无反应，N=1101	非维持性 IFN 治疗和非治疗	HCV 相关的 HCC 发生	RR=0.96（0.59~1.56）

续表

研究	设计	受试者的数目	治疗	终端	主要发现
Singal et al.（2010）	20 项研究	HCV 相关的硬化，$N=4700$	治疗和未治疗组	HCC 发生	RR=0.43（0.33~0.56）
	14 项研究		SVR vs. non-SVR	HCC 发生	RR=0.35（0.26~0.46）
Qu et al.（2012）	8 个随机控制实验	HCV 相关的硬化，$N=1505$	治疗和未治疗组	HCC 发生	Or=0.29（0.10~0.80）
	3 个随机控制实验	HCV 相关的硬化，$N=1155$	维持干扰素治疗和未治疗	HCC 发生	OR=0.54（0.32~0.90）

CN，对照组（安慰剂或无处理）；RR，相关性风险；OR，优势比；SVR，持续病毒学应答；IFN，干扰素；NUC，核苷酸类似物；RCT，随机对照实验

2.2 抗 HCV 治疗

对于 HCV，目前仍然没有疫苗。幸运的是，对于 HCV 患者来说，有效的抗 HCV 治疗在临床上已经取得了好的疗效。基于干扰素通过联合 PEG 化干扰素和利巴韦林的治疗是目前治疗 HCV 的标准方法。这种治疗在 50%基因 1 型 HCV 患者中导致持续病毒反应（SVR），在基因 2 和 3 型 HCV 患者中引起的 SVR 高达 80%（Munir et al. 2010）。这种 SVR 具有持久性（Hofmann and Zeuzem 2011），而且与良好的临床结果高度相关，包括降低 HCC（表 16-2）和肝脏相关死亡的风险（Masuzaki et al. 2010）。尽管如此，非 SVR 患者在疾病进程方面的风险没有减少，持续的抗 HCV 治疗对这些患者的临床结果并没有帮助（表 16-2）。

高病毒载量和基因 1 型通常预测慢性丙肝患者对于抗 HCV 治疗的反应率较低。然而，近年来由于治疗手段越来越先进，无反应者的百分比减少了。PEG 化干扰素和利巴韦林联合治疗使高病毒载量的 HCV 基因 1b 型患者中的 SVR 上升至大约 40%（Masuzaki et al. 2010）。此外，当我们在治疗前对治疗方法进行优化时，可以通过许多临床标志（如肥胖、IL-28 的多态性）来鉴定这些非反应者。而且，即将推出的新药（两个 HCV 非结构 3/4A 蛋白酶抑制剂波普瑞韦和替拉瑞韦）能较好地抑制基因 1 型病毒感染患者（对干扰素的治疗不反应）的 HCV RNA（Hofmann and Zeuzem 2011）。以上研究表明，我们离找到高效和低副作用的抗 HCV 治疗方案应该为期不远了。

3 HBV-HCV 共感染

由于 HBV 和 HCV 有共同的传播途径及增加肝病（包括 HCC）的风险，因此，HBV-HCV 共感染的治疗在流行地区非常重要。尽管还没有建立起特异性的治疗

方案，但是根据肝炎病毒学、抗病毒治疗史、肝病的发展阶段和等级，已经有了一些建议性的个性化治疗（Potthoff et al. 2010）。

在起始治疗前，有必要确定引起感染的优势病毒。干扰素/PGE化干扰素和利巴韦林联合治疗是目前治疗 HCV 优势感染患者的选择。干扰素和利巴韦林治疗的 24 周末，43%~69%的患者表现为 HCV-SVR（Potthoff et al. 2010）。HCV 基因 2/3 型和 1 型患者在联合治疗 24 周或 48 周以后，HCV-SVR 率分别高达 83%和 72%（Liu et al. 2009）。在跟踪 24~48 周末期，干扰素和利巴韦林联合治疗组的 HBV DNA 不可检测率为 11%~18%，而 PGE 化干扰素和利巴韦林联合治疗组的高达 56%（Liu et al. 2009；Potthoff et al. 2010）。有趣的是，联合治疗好像有较高的 HBsAg 清除率，这也是优化治疗的目标。对于这两种治疗方案，HBsAg 清除的比例为 11%~19%（Liu et al. 2009；Yeh et al. 2011）。然而，有报道称治疗后出现严重的肝耀斑和 HBV 复发，因此，在一些共感染的患者中需谨慎使用联合治疗，并且应该长期进行病毒学检测。对于 HBV 感染或 HBV-HCV 共感染的患者，还没有建立起最佳的治疗方案。

4 HBV-HIV 共感染和 HCV-HIV 共感染

HBV-HIV 共感染和 HCV-HIV 共感染通常加速肝脏疾病（包括纤维化和 HCC）的发展。一般来说，单一的药物治疗（干扰素、PEG 化干扰素、拉米夫定、阿德福韦、恩替卡韦和替比夫定）在 HBV-HIV 共感染患者中不能取得满意的疗效（Lacombe and Rockstroh 2012）。尽管如此，单一的替诺福韦治疗会有一些帮助，如有效的病毒学抑制作用、较好的耐药性谱和组织学的改善。然而，必须避免中断使用，否则病毒的突破会带来不良后果。

根据欧洲 AIDS 临床协会提议的指南（Lacombe and Rockstroh 2012；Soriano et al. 2010），对于不需要 HIV 治疗的 HBV-HIV 共感染患者（>500 CD4$^+$细胞/uL），建议早期接受替诺福韦和拉米夫定/恩曲他滨联合治疗，或当患者的 HBV DNA 水平在 2000IU/mL 以上时，采取早期追加 NUC（阿德福韦或替比夫定）的治疗策略。对于那些对干扰素治疗有反应的患者，建议采用 48 周的干扰素治疗。当需要同时进行 HBV 和 HIV 治疗时，要根据以前拉米夫定的使用情况来选择治疗方法。对于初次使用拉米夫定的患者，应选择替诺福韦加拉米夫定/恩曲他滨的联合治疗。对于已经用拉米夫定治疗过的患者，建议再使用替诺福韦、恩替卡韦或其他 HIV 核苷酸逆转录酶抑制剂治疗。此外，研究表明，含拉米夫定的 HAART 在 HBeAg 阴性 HBV-HIV 共感染的患者中能抑制 HBV 的复制（Fang et al. 2003）。尽管上面已经提出了一些治疗指南，我们还需要更加有力的证据，以便作出基于证据的治疗决策。

关于HCV-HIV共感染患者的治疗，目前标准的治疗方法是联合PEG化干扰素和利巴韦林，这种治疗的SVR率能达到27%~50%。而对于基因2型和3型患者，该种治疗表现出更高的SVR（44%~73%）。相比之下，基因1和4型患者的SVR只有17%~35%（Lacombe and Rockstroh 2012）。

HCV-HIV共感染患者的治疗应根据HCV的基因型和病毒反应的不同进行选择。对于非HCV基因1型、具有快速病毒学反应的基因2/3和4型的患者（在第4周时的病毒载量为不可检测水平），建议分别采用24周和48周的PEG化干扰素联合利巴韦林治疗。如果在治疗的第12周还没有病毒学反应，应该停止治疗。在12周有病毒学反应和在24周不能检测到HCV RNA的患者，对于基因2/3型和4型建议分别接受48周和72周的治疗（Lacombe and Rockstroh 2012；Soriano et al. 2010）。对于HCV基因1型患者，在12周出现早期病毒学反应和在24周不可检测到病毒的情况下，长时间的治疗可能有好处。然而，患者处于高度肝纤维化阶段时，建议接受干扰素/利巴韦林和HCV蛋白酶抑制剂联合治疗。近来的前期试验表明，在共感染的患者中实施三重治疗，与二重治疗相比，能提高SVR率（Ingiliz and Rockstroh 2012）。此外，基于临床研究结果，HAART可能对控制HCV-HIV共感染患者的肝损伤预后有积极影响，而且大多数患者第一次使用HAART就产生了好的疗效。

5 卡波西肉瘤相关疱疹病毒

卡波西肉瘤相关疱疹病毒（KSHV），也叫人疱疹病毒8（HHV-8），是卡波西肉瘤（KS，免疫缺陷的HIV患者最为常见的恶性肿瘤）的必需病原因子。KS患者与感染了KSHV但没有症状的患者相比，升高的KSHV病毒载量更为常见，这也与高风险的AIDS-KS有关（Gantt and Casper 2011；Sunil et al. 2010）。尽管如此，仍有多项研究表明抗疱疹病毒药物，如更昔洛韦和缬更昔洛韦，不仅能降低KSHV的病毒载量，还能防止AIDS-KS（Gantt and Casper 2011）。虽然这些小规模研究还需要进一步确认（Gantt and Casper 2011），但在将来的临床试验中，研究这些有前景的药物与DNA合成阻断剂或裂解复制诱导剂联合运用的效果，应该很有意思。

KSHV的复制主要依赖于HIV诱导的免疫缺陷（Mesri et al. 2010）。早期使用高活性抗逆转录病毒治疗（HAART）能恢复宿主的免疫力，降低HAART治疗患者AIDS-KS的发生率和死亡率（Bower et al. 2006；Mesri et al. 2010）。与前HAART时代相比，HAART时代KS的发生率下降了6倍（Sunil et al. 2010）。即使在资源有限的地区，早期使用HAART也能降低KS的发生率（Casper 2011）。从单个患者的水平上看，HAART也与KSHV的病毒血症的控制有高度的相关性

（Bourboulia et al. 2004）。然而，对于初始诊断时已经是 KS 晚期的患者，HAART 单一治疗只能使一半的患者完全康复（Nguyen et al. 2008）。对于那些单一 HAART 治疗后没有完全康复的 AIDS-KS 患者，再用 HAART 和化疗联合治疗能将反应率提高到 81.5%（Bower et al. 2006）。HAART 可分为基于蛋白酶抑制剂（PI）的治疗和基于非核苷酸逆转录酶抑制剂（NNRTI）的治疗。对于这两种治疗，在小规模的观察研究中发现 KS 的发生率没有区别（Gantt and Casper 2011），但基于 PI 的 HAART 治疗好像有更好的效果，因为当从基于 PI 的治疗转变为基于 NNRTI 的 HAART 治疗时，报道有更加彻底的复发和缓解（Gantt and Casper 2011）。尽管如此，基于 PI 的 HAART 治疗对于 KSHV 是否有治疗效果，还需要更多的、令人信服的证据来支持，并迫切需要大规模的、严格控制的试验和优化了的 HAART 治疗方法。

一个针对 28 人的临床研究表明，单一的 ART（indinavir）治疗可以诱导一些 HIV 阴性患者中 KS 肿瘤的抑制和病情的稳定（Monini et al. 2009）。除了引起 KS 外，KSHV 还与预后很差的罕见癌症如原发性扩散淋巴瘤（PEL）和多中心 Castleman 疾病（MCD）有关（Chang et al. 2006）。近来，很少有研究证明单独的 HAART 治疗或与其他方法的联合治疗，可以长期地缓解 PEL 和 MCD 的症状（Sunil et al. 2010）。

6 人类嗜 T 淋巴细胞病毒 1 型（HTLV-1）

人类嗜 T 淋巴细胞病毒 1 型是成人 T 细胞淋巴瘤（ATL）的致病因子（Poiesz et al. 1980）。尽管经过 10~40 年的潜伏期后（Proietti et al. 2005），全球 1500 万~2000 万感染人群中只有小部分（<6%）发展成为 ATL，但 ATL 患者的预后很差。急性和淋巴性 ATL 的平均存活时间不到一年（Goncalves et al. 2010）。

与没有症状的携带者相比，ATL 患者有显著高水平的 HTLV-1 原病毒 DNA 和抗体滴度（Manns et al. 1999）。HTLV-1 原病毒 DNA 的量是 ATL 发展的一个预测因素，与临床结果相关（Etoh et al. 1999；Iwanaga et al. 2010；Okayama et al. 2004）。大量的研究数据表明，抗病毒治疗是目前 ATL 治疗中的一个选择（Tsukasaki et al. 2009）。20 世纪 80 年代早期，ATL 的抗病毒药物治疗在日本就有研究，然而真正鼓舞人心的是 1995 年报道的 α 干扰素和 AZT（zidovudine）联合治疗 ATL 患者的两个临床研究（Gill et al. 1995；Hermine et al. 1995）。这种联合治疗表现出很高的反应率（在 50%以上）和中等毒副作用，且存活时间在 1 年以上。从那以后，许多关于使用 α 干扰素和叠氮胸腺（zidovudine，AZT）联合治疗 30 人以下的小规模研究分别在法国（Hermine et al. 2002）、英国（Matutes et al. 2001）、马提尼克（法属西印度群岛）（Besson et al. 2002）和美国进行（Ratner et al. 2009）。总体看来，这些研究都表明了一致的抗病毒治疗效果。近来，一个世界范围内元分析[包含了 254 个 α 干扰素和 AZT（zidovudine）联合治疗或化疗的 ATL 患者]进一步证明，α 干扰素和 AZT 的联合治疗引起高的反应率和使存活时间显著延长（Bazarbachi et al. 2010）。然而，这种存活时间的优势只限于急性、慢性和慢性生长亚型。对于淋巴性 ATL，化疗似乎比抗病毒治疗更有效。此外，联合 α 干扰素/AZT 和 As_2O_3 治疗在 7 个反复发作的急性或淋巴性 ATL 患者中表现出较好的效果（Hermine et al. 2004）。另外，对 10 个慢性 ATL 患者的研究表明，治疗的反应率为 100%（Kchour et al. 2009）。尽管这些都是初步的观察，但这一方法的可能性值得考虑。

改善抗病毒治疗的反应性和存活时间是治疗 ATL 的一个非常重要的进展。研究也表明，ATL 患者在抗病毒治疗后，HTLV-1 原病毒 DNA 减少，且与对治疗的反应性相关（Kchour et al. 2007，2009）。然而，所有这些结果都来自于小量样本的研究。

7 EB 病毒（EBV）

EBV 作为第一个被鉴定的致瘤病毒，与多种癌症有关，包括伯基特淋巴瘤、霍奇金淋巴瘤、免疫抑制 B 细胞淋巴瘤、移植后淋巴增生性疾病（PTLD）、胃癌和鼻咽癌（Kutok and Wang 2006）。尽管目前还没有标准的检测方法，EBV 病毒载量的定量分析已经用于 PTLD 和鼻咽癌（NPC）患者。因为 EBV 相关的癌症的病理致病和临床特征都不一样，而且情况复杂，所以 EBV 的病毒载量的临床意义在所有类型中也不一样（Kimura et al. 2008）。

EBV 相关疾病的抗病毒治疗包括药物治疗、免疫治疗和直接针对病毒的治疗。对于 EBV 相关的肿瘤，由于病毒维持潜伏复制，使得核苷酸类似物的药物治疗不能产生效果。通过转移 EBV 特异性细胞毒 T 细胞（EBV-CTL）的免疫治疗，能杀死感染细胞，已经用于治疗 PTLD（Rooney et al. 1995）、NPC（Chua et al. 2001）和 HL（Bollard et al. 2004）。这一治疗方法用在 PTLD 时，取得了一些好的结果，例如，EBV 的病毒 DNA 下降 2~3 个数量级，并能稳定病毒载量（Gustafsson et al. 2000；Rooney et al. 1995）；防止 PTLD 的进一步发展（Heslop et al. 2010）；移植的 CTL 防止病毒再激活的活性维持在 9 年以上（Heslop et al. 2010）。然而，NPC 和 HL 患者的治疗结果不是很令人满意。对于 NPC，标准的化疗和放疗后，仍有 15%~19%已经转移的和局部严重的患者存活率很差。对于 NPC，我们之所以考虑免疫治疗，是因为 EBV 抗原 EBNA1、LMB1 和 LMB2 是 EBV-CTL 的靶点。令人鼓舞的免疫治疗结果主要集中在反复发作的 NPC 患者，如能完全康复（Louis et al. 2010；Straathof et al. 2005）、缺少明显的毒副作用，对于有些患者还能控制疾病进一步发展（Comoli et al. 2005）。对于反复发作的 HL 患者，也能观察到外周血中 EBV DNA 下降和疾病得到控制（Bollard et al. 2004）。目前有关免疫治疗的数据还很有限，研究的患者人数少、观察的有效时间短，因此，EBV 相关肿瘤的所有免疫治疗还需进一步研究（Merlo et al. 2011）。

基于病毒的治疗方法是将肿瘤中 EBV 病毒基因组作为靶点。该方法可分为两组。一组方法是抑制 EBV 癌蛋白的表达，诱导 EBV 游离体（episome）的丢失，在 EBV 感染的肿瘤中产生细胞毒素。另一种方法就是先诱导 EBV 裂解复制，然后再用阿昔洛韦和更昔洛韦联合治疗（Ghosh et al. 2012；Israel and Kenney 2003）。EBV 相关淋巴瘤的 I/II 临床研究发现，HDAC 抑制剂丁酸精氨酸与更昔洛韦的联合治疗在一些难以治疗的患者当中取得较好的临床反应（Faller et al. 2001；Perrine et al. 2007）。多种裂解复制诱导剂，如佛波酯、DNA 甲基转移酶抑制剂和 DNA 甲基化转移酶抑制剂都已被研发出来，并且已经在体外和动物模型内进行了评估。然而，最优化的试剂目前还没有确定。综上所述，EBV 相关恶性肿瘤的抗病毒治疗已发现了一些鼓舞人心的结果，为将来大规模的、长期的研究指明了方向。

8 人乳头瘤病毒（HPV）

在 100 多种已发现的 HPV 类型中，有 15 种高风险 HPV 类型与大约 12 种癌症有关（Bharti et al. 2009；Woodman et al. 2007）。一些研究清楚地表明，HPV-16 和 HPV-18 对宫颈癌起主要致病作用。HPV 病毒的载量通常与疾病的程度、感染持续的时间、疾病的清除和疾病的预后没有很好的相关性，这可能是由于在不同 HPV 基因型中，它们的致癌潜力有很大的差异（Josefsson et al. 2000）。尽管如此，对于最高风险的 HPV-16 基因型，其病毒载量与流行的宫颈癌前兆相关，可能用于预测刚被诊断的疾病的发展和持续性感染（Gravitt et al. 2007；Josefsson et al. 2000；Xi et al. 2011）。

几个用于处理 HPV 感染和 HPV 诱导宫颈癌的抗病毒策略正在研发中，其中治疗性 HPV 疫苗和基于 RNA 干扰的治疗是两个可能的方法。此外，最近的一个体外研究表明，两个合成的聚醯胺纤维能引起 HPV 失去游离体的 DNA，其效果正在评价之中（Edwards et al. 2011）。

HPV-16 和 HPV-18 的治疗性疫苗正在实验之中，包括蛋白质/多肽疫苗和 DNA 疫苗（Bermúdez- Humarán and Langella 2010；Bharti et al. 2009）。在动物模型中，HPV 早期蛋白 E6 和 E7 的疫苗能抑制疾病的进程（Gomez-Gutierrez et al. 2007；Zwaveling et al. 2002）。在 I/II 期临床实验中，一些（但不是所有）有早期和严重病变的患者表现出抗 HPV 的 CTL 反应和 HPV 的清除（Bharti et al. 2009；Brinkman et al. 2007）。HPV 抗原刺激的自身树突状细胞疫苗也能观察到类似的

结果。在一个有127例患者的II期临床研究中，尽管有些患者出现了部分甚至完全复发，DNA疫苗在有高度病变的妇女中能诱导产生持续细胞毒性T淋巴细胞免疫应答（Brinkman et al. 2007）。这些令人鼓舞的结果表明了治疗性HPV疫苗的潜力。

RNA干扰治疗是利用反义寡核苷酸、核酶和小干扰RNA（siRNA）在转录后水平抑制HPV病毒E6和E7基因的表达。子宫癌细胞和小鼠模型的几个研究证明，RNAi治疗诱导细胞凋亡、细胞生长速率下降和细胞死亡。该方法还能使癌细胞对一些化疗（如顺铂）的敏感性升高。尽管如此，这些好的结果都只是来自临床前研究和I期临床研究，因此，其实际影响和作为长期治疗的潜力还不是很清楚。而且，用反义分子或核酶还存在一些问题，如靶向选择、释放效率和短期维持，这些问题仍然需要克服。

9　梅克尔细胞多瘤病毒

梅克尔细胞多瘤病毒（Merkel cell polyomavirus，MCV）是一种于2008年新发现的多瘤病毒（Feng et al. 2008）。25%~64%的健康人群中能检测到MCV（Carter et al. 2009；Kean et al. 2009；Tolstov et al. 2009）。许多正常的组织中也能发现MCV，如食道、肝、结肠、肺和膀胱（Loyo et al. 2010）。MCV是梅克尔细胞癌（Merkel cell carcinoma，MCC）的致病因素。MCC是一种稀少而具有侵袭性和致命的神经内分泌皮肤癌（Feng et al. 2008）。MCC的MCV病毒载量比其他组织明显地高（Loyo et al. 2010）。MCV与MCC之间的高度相关性表明，除了目前的外科切除、淋巴结手术、放射治疗和化疗外，抗病毒治疗可能是治疗MCC的一种新方法（Schrama et al. 2012）。

有关MCC的抗MCV病毒治疗的研究仍然还有限。一个体外研究表明，α干扰素对MCC可能有抗肿瘤效果（Krasagakis et al. 2008）。α干扰素已用于治疗了2个MCV阳性MCC患者，没有临床反应（Biver-Dalle et al. 2011）。然而，据报道一个62岁MCV阳性患MCC的妇女，在每天使用3 000 000IU的α干扰素治疗后，出现了好的反应（Nakajima et al. 2009）。体外和体内研究数据也表明，α干扰素和β干扰素对MCC可能有较强的抗肿瘤作用，尤其是对MCV阳性的MCC（Willmes et al. 2012）。由于数据有限，因此需要更多的研究进一步评价抗病毒治疗对MCC的效果。

10　结论与展望

致瘤病毒的抗病毒治疗方面的巨大进步是癌症预防概念和实践上的一场革命。

在慢性 HBV 和/或 HCV 感染的患者中，进行 HCC 的一级预防是目前一个现实的目标，能明显节约金钱和挽救生命（Kim et al. 2007；Toy et al. 2008）。HAART 的广泛使用也显著地降低了 HIV 感染患者的 KS 发生率。对于其他的致瘤病毒，仍然缺少方便、有效的抗病毒药物用于一级预防。尽管如此，对于一些类型 HTLV-1 诱导的 ATL，抗病毒治疗能有效地延长患者的存活时间，成为治疗的一个选择。在 EBV、HPV 和 MCV 相关的恶性肿瘤的辅助治疗方面，实验性抗病毒治疗和技术的深入研究可能会产生一些可喜的结果。

为促进新的预防或治疗方法及试剂的发展，需要进行进一步的研究，以继续提高我们对病毒相关的致癌机制的认识，以及我们对病毒动态和疾病自然史之间关系的认识。这些能增加我们对抗这些病毒的力量，并在将来产生更有利的/满意的临床结果。

（刘红旗，陶玉芬 译）

参 考 文 献

Bazarbachi A, Plumelle Y, Carlos Ramos J, Tortevoye P, Otrock Z, Taylor G, Gessain A, Harrington W, Panelatti G, Hermine O (2010) Meta-analysis on the use of zidovudine and interferon-alfa in adult T-cell leukemia/lymphoma showing improved survival in the leukemic subtypes. J Clin Oncol 28:4177–4183

Benitez-Hess ML, Reyes-Gutierrez P, Alvarez-Salas LM (2011) Inhibition of human papillo- mavirus expression using DNAzymes. Methods Mol Biol 764:317–335

Bermúdez-Humarán LG, Langella P (2010) Perspectives for the development of human papillomavirus vaccines and immunotherapy. Expert Rev Vaccines 9:35–44

Besson C, Panelatti G, Delaunay C, Gonin C, Brebion A, Hermine O, Plumelle Y (2002) Treatment of adult T-cell leukemia-lymphoma by CHOP followed by therapy with antinucleosides, alpha interferon and oral etoposide. Leuk Lymphoma 43:2275–2279

Bharti AC, Shukla S, Mahata S, Hedau S, Das BC (2009) Anti-human papillomavirus therapeutics: facts & future. Indian J Med Res 130:296–310

Biver-Dalle C, Nguyen T, Touze A, Saccomani C, Penz S, Cunat-Peultier S, Riou-Gotta MO, Humbert P, Coursaget P, Aubin F (2011) Use of interferon-alpha in two patients with Merkel cell carcinoma positive for Merkel cell polyomavirus. Acta Oncol 50:479–480

Bollard CM, Aguilar L, Straathof KC, Gahn B, Huls MH, Rousseau A, Sixbey J, Gresik MV, Carrum G, Hudson M, Dilloo D, Gee A, Brenner MK, Rooney CM, Heslop HE (2004) Cytotoxic T lymphocyte therapy for Epstein-Barr virus+ Hodgkin's disease. J Exp Med 200:1623–1633

Boulet GA, Horvath CA, Berghmans S, Bogers J (2008) Human papillomavirus in cervical cancer screening: important role as biomarker. Cancer Epidemiol Biomarkers Prev 17:810–817

Bourboulia D, Aldam D, Lagos D, Allen E, Williams I, Cornforth D, Copas A (2004) Short- and long-term effects of highly active antiretroviral therapy on Kaposi sarcoma-associated herpesvirus immune responses and viraemia. AIDS 18:485–493

Bower M, Palmieri C, Dhillon T (2006) AIDS-related malignancies: changing epidemiology and the impact of highly active antiretroviral therapy. Curr Opin Infect Dis 19:14–19

Brinkman JA, Hughes SH, Stone P, Caffrey AS, Muderspach LI, Roman LD, Weber JS, Kast WM (2007) Therapeutic vaccination for HPV induced cervical cancers. Dis Markers 23:337–352

Buster EH, Flink HJ, Cakaloglu Y, Simon K, Trojan J, Tabak F, So TM, Feinman SV, Mach T, Akarca US, Schutten M, Tielemans W, van Vuuren AJ, Hansen BE, Janssen HL (2008) Sustained HBeAg and HBsAg loss after long-term follow-up of HBeAg-positive patients treated with peginterferon alpha-2b. Gastroenterology 135:459–467

Cammá C, Giunta M, Andreone P, Craxi A (2001) Interferon and prevention of hepatocellular carcinoma in viral cirrhosis: an evidence-based approach. J Hepatol 34:593–602

Carter JJ, Paulson KG, Wipf GC, Miranda D, Madeleine MM, Johnson LG, Lemos BD, Lee S, Warcola AH, Iyer JG, Nghiem P, Galloway DA (2009) Association of Merkel cell polyomavirus-specific antibodies with Merkel cell carcinoma. J Natl Cancer Inst 101:1510–1522

Casper C (2011) The increasing burden of HIV-associated malignancies in resource-limited regions. Annu Rev Med 62:157–170

Chang TT, Gish RG, de Man R, Gadano A, Sollano J, Chao YC, Lok AS, Hamn KH, Goodman Z, Zho J, Cross A, DeHertogh D, Wilber R, Colonno R, Apelian D, Group tBAS (2006) A comparison of entecavir and lamivudine for HBeAg-positive chronic hepatitis B. N Engl J Med 354: 1001–1010

Chang MH, You SL, Chen CJ, Liu CJ, Lee CM, Lin SM, Chu HC, Wu TC, Yang SS, Kuo HS, Chen DS (2009) Decreased incidence of hepatocellular carcinoma in hepatitis B vaccinees: a 20-year follow-up study. J Natl Cancer Inst 101:1348–1355

Chen CJ, Yang HI, Iloeje UH (2009) Hepatitis B virus DNA levels and outcomes in chronic hepatitis B. Hepatology 49:S72–S84

Chua D, Huang J, Zheng B, Lau SY, Luk W, Kwong DL, Sham JS, Moss D, Yuen KY, Im SW, Ng MH (2001) Adoptive transfer of autologous Epstein-Barr virus-specific cytotoxic T cells for nasopharyngeal carcinoma. Int J Cancer 94:73–80

Comoli P, Pedrazzoli P, Maccario R, Basso S, Carminati O, Labirio M, Schiavo R, Secondino S, Frasson C, Perotti C, Moroni M, Locatelli F, Siena S (2005) Cell therapy of stage IV nasopharyngeal carcinoma with autologous Epstein-Barr virus-targeted cytotoxic T lympho- cytes. J Clin Oncol 23:8942–8949

De Paoli P, Pratesi C, Bortolin MT (2007) The Epstein Barr virus DNA levels as a tumor marker in EBV-associated cancers. J Cancer Res Clin Oncol 133:809–815

Di Marco V, Marzano A, Lampertico P, Andreone P, Santantonio T, Almasio PL, Rizzetto M, Craxi A

(2004) Clinical outcome of HBeAg-negative chronic hepatitis B in relation to virological response to lamivudine. Hepatology 40:883–891

Dienstag JL (2009) Benefits and risks of nucleoside analog therapy for hepatitis B. Hepatology 49:S112–S121

Edwards TG, Koeller KJ, Slomczynska U, Fok K, Helmus M, Bashkin JK, Fisher C (2011) HPV episome levels are potently decreased by pyrrole-imidazole polyamides. Antiviral Res 91:177–186

El-Serag HB (2012) Epidemiology of viral hepatitis and hepatocellular carcinoma. Gastroenterology 142:1264–1273.e1

Etoh KI, Yamaguchi K, Tokudome S, Watanabe T, Okayama A, Stuver S, Mueller N, Takatsuki K, Matsuoka M (1999) Rapid quantification of HTLV-1 provirus load: detection of monoclonal proliferation of HTLV-1-infected cells among blood donors. Int J Cancer 81:859–864

Faller DV, Mentzer SJ, Perrine SP (2001) Induction of the Epstein-Barr virus thymidine kinase gene with concomitant nucleoside antivirals as a therapeutic strategy for Epstein-Barr virus- associated malignancies. Curr Opin Oncol 13:360–367

Fang CT, Chen PJ, Chen MY, Hung CC, Chang SC, Chang AL, Chen DS (2003) Dynamics of plasma hepatitis B virus levels after highly active antiretroviral therapy in patients with HIV infection. J Hepatol 39:1028–1035

Feld JJ, Wong DK, Heathcote EJ (2009) Endpoints of therapy in chronic hepatitis B. Hepatology 49:S96–S102

Feng H, Shuda M, Chang Y, Moore PS (2008) Clonal integration of a polyomavirus in human Merkel cell carcinoma. Science 319:1096–1100

Gantt S, Casper C (2011) Human herpesvirus 8-associated neoplasms: the roles of viral replication and antiviral treatment. Curr Opin Infect Dis 24:295–301

Ghosh SK, Perrine SP, Faller DV (2012) Advances in virus-directed therapeutics against Epstein- Barr virus-associated malignancies. Adv Virol 2012:509296

Gill PS, Harrington W Jr, Kaplan MH, Ribeiro RC, Bennett JM, Liebman HA, Bernstein-Singer M, Espina BM, Cabral L, Allen S, Kornblau S, Pike MC, Levine AM (1995) Treatment of adult T-cell leukemia-lymphoma with a combination of interferon alfa and zidovudine. N Engl J Med 332:1744–1748

Gomez-Gutierrez JG, Elpek KG, Montes de Oca-Luna R, Shirwan H, Sam Zhou H, McMasters KM (2007) Vaccination with an adenoviral vector expressing calreticulin-human papilloma- virus 16 E7 fusion protein eradicates E7 expressing established tumors in mice. Cancer Immunol Immunother 56:997–1007

Goncalves DU, Proietti FA, Ribas JG, Araujo MG, Pinheiro SR, Guedes AC, Carneiro-Proietti AB (2010) Epidemiology, treatment, and prevention of human T-cell leukemia virus type 1-

associated diseases. Clin Microbiol Rev 23:577–589

Gravitt PE, Kovacic MB, Herrero R, Schiffman M, Bratti C, Hildesheim A, Morales J, Alfaro M, Sherman ME, Wacholder S, Rodriguez AC, Burk RD (2007) High load for most high risk human papillomavirus genotypes is associated with prevalent cervical cancer precursors but only HPV 16 load predicts the development of incident disease. Int J Cancer 121:2787–2793

Gustafsson Å, Levitsky V, Zou JZ, Frisan T, Dalianis T, Ljungman P, Ringden O, Winiarski J, Ernberg I, Masucci MG (2000) Epstein-Barr virus (EBV) load in bone marrow transplant recipients at risk to develop posttransplant lymphoproliferative disease: prophylactic infusion of EBV-specific cytotoxic T cells. Blood 95:807–814

Hermine O, Bouscary D, Gessain A, Turlure P, Leblond V, Franck N, Buzyn-Veil A, Rio B, Macintyre E, Dreyfus F, Bazarbachi A (1995) Treatment of adult T-cell leukemia-lymphoma with zidovudine and interferon alfa. N Engl J Med 332:1749–1751

Hermine O, Allard I, Lévy V, Arnulf B, Gessain A, Bazarbachi A (2002) A prospective phase II clinical trial with the use of zidovudine and interferon-alpha in the acute and lymphoma forms of adult T-cell leukemia/lymphoma. Hematol J 3:276–282

Hermine O, Dombret H, Poupon J, Arnulf B, Lefrere F, Rousselot P, Damaj G, Delarue R, Fermand JP, Brouet JC, Degos L, Varet B, de The H, Bazarbachi A (2004) Phase II trial of arsenic trioxide and alpha interferon in patients with relapsed/refractory adult T-cell leukemia/lymphoma. Hematol J 5:130–134

Heslop HE, Slobod KS, Pule MA, Hale GA, Rousseau A, Smith CA, Bollard CM, Liu H, Wu MF, Rochester RJ, Amrolia PJ, Hurwitz JL, Brenner MK, Rooney CM (2010) Long-term outcome of EBV-specific T-cell infusions to prevent or treat EBV-related lymphoproliferative disease in transplant recipients. Blood 115:925–935

Hofmann WP, Zeuzem S (2011) A new standard of care for the treatment of chronic HCV infection. Nat Rev Gastroenterol Hepatol 8:257–264

Ingiliz P, Rockstroh JK (2012) HIV-HCV co-infection facing HCV protease inhibitor licensing: implications for clinicians. Liver Int 32:1194–1199

Israel BF, Kenney SC (2003) Virally targeted therapies for EBV-associated malignancies. Oncogene 22:5122–5130

Iwanaga M, Watanabe T, Utsunomiya A, Okayama A, Uchimaru K, Koh KR, Ogata M, Kikuchi H, Sagara Y, Uozumi K, Mochizuki M, Tsukasaki K, Saburi Y, Yamamura M, Tanaka J, Moriuchi Y, Hino S, Kamihira S, Yamaguchi K (2010) Human T-cell leukemia virus type I (HTLV-1) proviral load and disease progression in asymptomatic HTLV-1 carriers: a nationwide prospective study in Japan. Blood 116:1211–1219

Janssen HLA, van Zonneveld M, Senturk H, Zeuzem S, Akarca US, Cakaloglu Y, Simon C, So TMK, Gerken G, de Man RA, Niesters HGM, Zondervan P, Hansen B, Schalm SW (2005) Pegylated interferon alfa-2b alone or in combination with lamivudine for HBeAg-positive chronic hepatitis B: a randomised trial. Lancet 365:123–129

Jones M, Nunez M (2011) HIV and hepatitis C co-infection: the role of HAART in HIV/hepatitis C virus management. Curr Opin HIV AIDS 6:546–552

Jonson AL, Rogers LM, Ramakrishnan S, Downs LS Jr (2008) Gene silencing with siRNA targeting E6/E7 as a therapeutic intervention in a mouse model of cervical cancer. Gynecol Oncol 111:356–364

Josefsson AM, Magnusson PKE, Ylitalo N, Sørensen P, Qwarforth-Tubbin P, Andersen PK, Melbye M, Adami H-O, Gyllensten UB (2000) Viral load of human papilloma virus 16 as a determinant for development of cervical carcinoma in situ: a nested case-control study. Lancet 355:2189–2193

Kchour G, Makhoul NJ, Mahmoudi M, Kooshyar MM, Shirdel A, Rastin M, Rafatpanah H, Tarhini M, Zalloua PA, Hermine O, Farid R, Bazarbachi A (2007) Zidovudine and interferon- alpha treatment induces a high response rate and reduces HTLV-1 proviral load and VEGF plasma levels in patients with adult T-cell leukemia from North East Iran. Leuk Lymphoma 48:330–336

Kchour G, Tarhini M, Kooshyar MM, El Hajj H, Wattel E, Mahmoudi M, Hatoum H, Rahimi H, Maleki M, Rafatpanah H, Rezaee SA, Yazdi MT, Shirdel A, de The H, Hermine O, Farid R, Bazarbachi A (2009) Phase 2 study of the efficacy and safety of the combination of arsenic trioxide, interferon alpha, and zidovudine in newly diagnosed chronic adult T-cell leukemia/ lymphoma (ATL). Blood 113:6528–6532

Kean JM, Rao S, Wang M, Garcea RL (2009) Seroepidemiology of human polyomaviruses. PLoS Pathog 5:e1000363

Kim WR, Benson JT, Hindman A, Brosgart C, Fortner-Burton C (2007) Decline in the need for liver transplantation for end stage liver disease secondary to hepatitis B in the US [Abstract]. Hepatology 46(Suppl):238A

Kimura H, Ito Y, Suzuki R, Nishiyama Y (2008) Measuring Epstein-Barr virus (EBV) load: the significance and application for each EBV-associated disease. Rev Med Virol 18:305–319

Koivusalo R, Krausz E, Helenius H, Hietanen S (2005) Chemotherapy compounds in cervical cancer cells primed by reconstitution of p53 function after short interfering RNA-mediated degradation of human papillomavirus 18 E6 mRNA: opposite effect of siRNA in combination with different drugs. Mol Pharmacol 68:372–382

Krasagakis K, Kruger-Krasagakis S, Tzanakakis GN, Darivianaki K, Stathopoulos EN, Tosca AD (2008) Interferon-alpha inhibits proliferation and induces apoptosis of merkel cell carcinoma in vitro. Cancer Invest 26:562–568

Kutok JL, Wang F (2006) Spectrum of Epstein-Barr virus-associated diseases. Annu Rev Pathol Mech Dis 1:375–404

Lacombe K, Rockstroh J (2012) HIV and viral hepatitis coinfections: advances and challenges. Gut

61(Suppl 1):i47–i58

Lai CL, Shouval D, Lok AS, Chang TT, Cheinquer H, Goodman Z, DeHertogh D, Wilber R, Zink RC, Cross A, Colonno R, Fernandes L, Group tBAS (2006) Entecavir versus lamivudine for patients with HBeAg-negative chronic hepatitis B. N Engl J Med 354:1011–1020

Lai CL, Gane E, Liaw YF, Hsu CW, Thongsawat S, Wang Y, Chen Y, Heathcote EJ, Rasenack J, Bzowej B, Naoumov NV, Di Bisceglie AM, Zeuzem S, Moon YM, Goodman Z, Chao G, Constance BF, Brown NA, Group tGS (2007) Telbivudine versus lamivudine in patients with chronic hepatitis B. N Engl J Med 357:2576–2588

Lau GKK, Piratvisuth T, Luo KX, Marcellin P, Thongsawat S, Cooksley G, Gane E, Fried MW, Chow WC, Paik SW, Chang WY, Berg T, Flisiak R, McCloud P, Pluck N, Group tPA-aH- PCHBS (2005) Peginterferon alfa-2a, lamivudine, and combination for HBeAg-positive chronic hepatitis B. N Engl J Med 352:2682–2695

Liaw YF (2006) Hepatitis B virus replication and liver disease progression: the impact of antiviral therapy. Antivir Ther 11:669–679

Liaw YF, Sung JJ, Chow WC, Farrell G, Lee CZ, Yuen H, Tanwandee T, Tao QM, Shue K, Keene ON, Dixon JS, Gray DF, Sabbat J, Group CALMS (2004) Lamivudine for patients with chronic hepatitis B and advanced liver disease. N Engl J Med 351:1521–1531

Liu CJ, Chuang WL, Lee CM, Yu ML, Lu SN, Wu SS, Liao LY, Chen CL, Kuo HT, Chao YC, Tung SY, Yang SS, Kao JH, Liu CH, Su WW, Lin CL, Jeng YM, Chen PJ, Chen DS (2009) Peginterferon alfa-2a plus ribavirin for the treatment of dual chronic infection with hepatitis B and C viruses. Gastroenterology 136:496–504.e3

Louis CU, Straathof K, Bollard CM, Ennamuri S, Gerken C, Lopez TT, Huls MH, Sheehan A, Wu MF, Liu H, Gee A, Brenner MK, Rooney CM, Heslop HE, Gottschalk S (2010) Adoptive transfer of EBV-specific T cells results in sustained clinical responses in patients with locoregional nasopharyngeal carcinoma. J Immunother 33:983–990

Loyo M, Guerrero-Preston R, Brait M, Hoque MO, Chuang A, Kim MS, Sharma R, Liegeois NJ, Koch WM, Califano JA, Westra WH, Sidransky D (2010) Quantitative detection of Merkel cell virus in human tissues and possible mode of transmission. Int J Cancer 126:2991–2996

Manns A, Miley WJ, Wilks RJ, Morgan OSC, Hanchard B, Wharfe G, Caranston B, Maloney W, Welles SL, Blattner WA, Waters D (1999) Quantitative proviral DNA and antibody levels in the natural history of HTLV-1 infection. J Infect Dis 180:1487–1493

Marcellin P, Lau GKK, Bonino F, Farci P, Hadziyannis S, Jin R, Lu ZM, Piratvisuth T, Germanidis G, Yurdaydin C, Diago M, Gurel S, Lai MY, Button P, Pluck N, Group tPA-aH- NCHBS (2004) Peginterferon alfa-2a alone, lamivudine alone, and the two in combination in patients with HBeAg-negative chronic hepatitis B. N Engl J Med 351:1206–1217

Marcellin P, Heathcote EJ, Buti M, Gane E, de Man RA, Krastev Z, Germanidis G, Lee SS, Flisiak R,

Kaita K, Manns M, Kotzev I, Tchernev K, Buggisch P, Weilert F, Kurdas OO, Shiffman ML, Trinh H, Washington MK, Sorbel J, Anderson J, Snow-Lampart A, Mondou E, Quinn J, Rousseau F (2008) Tenofovir disoproxil fumarate versus adefovir dipivoxil for chronic hepatitis B. N Engl J Med 359:2442–2455

Marcellin P, Bonino F, Lau GK, Farci P, Yurdaydin C, Piratvisuth T, Jin R, Gurel S, Lu ZM, Wu J, Popescu M, Hadziyannis S (2009) Sustained response of hepatitis B e antigen-negative patients 3 years after treatment with peginterferon alpha-2a. Gastroenterology 136:2169–2179.e1–4

Masarone M, Persico M (2011) Antiviral therapy: why does it fail in HCV-related chronic hepatitis? Expert Rev Anti Infect 9:535–543

Masuzaki R, Yoshida H, Omata M (2010) Interferon reduces the risk of hepatocellular carcinoma in hepatitis C virus-related chronic hepatitis/liver cirrhosis. Oncology 78(Suppl 1):17–23 Matutes E, Taylor GP, Cavenagh J, Pagliuca A, Bareford D, Domingo A, Hamblin M, Kelsey S,

Mir N, Reilly JT (2001) Interferon *a* and zidovudine therapy in adult T-cell leukaemia lymphoma: response and outcome in 15 patients. Br J Haematol 113:779–784

Merlo A, Turrini R, Dolcetti R, Zanovello P, Rosato A (2011) Immunotherapy for EBV- associated malignancies. Int J Hematol 93:281–293

Mesri EA, Cesarman E, Boshoff C (2010) Kaposi's sarcoma and its associated herpesvirus. Nat Rev Cancer 10:707–719

Mommeja-Marin H, Mondou E, Blum MR, Rousseau F (2003) Serum HBV DNA as a marker of efficacy during therapy for chronic HBV infection: analysis and review of the literature. Hepatology 37:1309–1319

Monini P, Sgadari C, Garosso MG, Bellino S, Biagio AD, Toschi E, Bacigalupo S, Sabbatucci M, Cencioni G, Salvi E, Leone P, Ensoli B, Sarcoma tCAoKs (2009) Clinical course of classic Kaposi's sarcoma in HIV-negative patients treated with the HIV protease inhibitor indinavir. AIDS 23:534–538

Moore PS, Chang Y (2010) Why do viruses cause cancer? Highlights of the first century of human tumour virology. Nat Rev Cancer 10:878–889

Munir S, Saleem S, Idrees M, Tariq A, Butt S, Rauff B, Hussain A, Badar S, Naudhani M, Fatima Z, Ali M, Ali L, Akram M, Aftab M, Khubaib B, Awan Z (2010) Hepatitis C treatment: current and future perspectives. Virol J 7:296

Nakajima H, Takaishi M, Yamamoto M, Kamijima R, Kodama H, Tarutani M, Sano S (2009) Screening of the specific polyoma virus as diagnostic and prognostic tools for Merkel cell carcinoma. J Dermatol Sci 56:211–213

Nguyen HQ, Magaret AS, Kitahata MM, van Rompaey SE, Wald A, Casper C (2008) Persistent Kaposi sarcoma in era of highly active antiretroviral therapy: characterizing the predictors of clinical response. AIDS 22:937–945

Niederau C, Heintges T, Lange S, Goldmann G, Niederau CM, Mohr L, Häussinger D (1996) Long-term follow-up of HBeAg-positive patients treated with interferon alfa for chronic hepatitis B. N Engl J Med 334:1422–1427

Okayama A, Stuver S, Matsuoka M, Ishizaki J, Tanaka G, Kubuki Y, Mueller N, Hsieh CC, Tachibana N, Tsubouchi H (2004) Role of HTLV-1 proviral DNA load and clonality in the development of adult T-cell leukemia/lymphoma in asymptomatic carriers. Int J Cancer 110:621–625

Papatheodoridis GV, Papatheodoridis VC, Hadziyannis SJ (2001) Effect of interferon therapy on the development of hepatocellular carcinoma in patients with hepatitis C virus-related cirrhosis: a meta-analysis. Aliment Pharmacol Ther 15:689–698

Papatheodoridis GV, Manolakopoulos S, Dusheiko G, Archimandritis AJ (2008) Therapeutic strategies in the management of patients with chronic hepatitis B virus infection. Lancet Infect Dis 8:167–178

Papatheodoridis GV, Lampertico P, Manolakopoulos S, Lok A (2010) Incidence of hepatocellular carcinoma in chronic hepatitis B patients receiving nucleos(t)ide therapy: a systematic review. J Hepatol 53:348–356

Perrine SP, Hermine O, Small T, Suarez F, O'Reilly R, Boulad F, Fingeroth J, Askin M, Levy A, Mentzer SJ, Di Nicola M, Gianni AM, Klein C, Horwitz S, Faller DV (2007) A phase 1/2 trial of arginine butyrate and ganciclovir in patients with Epstein-Barr virus-associated lymphoid malignancies. Blood 109:2571–2578

Poiesz BJ, Ruscetti FW, Gazdar AF, Bunn PA, Minna JD, Gallo RC (1980) Detection and isolation of type C retrovirus particles from fresh and cultured lymphocytes of a patient with cutaneous T-cell lymphoma. Proc Natl Acad Sci U S A 77:7514–7519

Potthoff A, Manns MP, Wedemeyer H (2010) Treatment of HBV/HCV coinfection. Expert Opin Pharmacother 11:919–928

Proietti FA, Carneiro-Proietti AB, Catalan-Soares BC, Murphy EL (2005) Global epidemiology of HTLV-I infection and associated diseases. Oncogene 24:6058–6068

Putral LN, Bywater MJ, Gu W, Saunders NA, Gabrielli BG, Leggatt GR, McMillan NA (2005) RNA interference against human papillomavirus oncogenes in cervical cancer cells results in increased sensitivity to cisplatin. Mol Pharmacol 68:1311–1319

Qu LS, Chen H, Kuai XL, Xu ZF, Jin F, Zhou GX (2012) Effects of interferon therapy on development of hepatocellular carcinoma in patients with hepatitis C-related cirrhosis: A meta-analysis of randomized controlled trials. Hepatol Res 42:782–789

Ratner L, Harrington W, Feng X, Grant C, Jacobson S, Noy A, Sparano J, Lee J, Ambinder R, Campbell N, Lairmore M (2009) Human T cell leukemia virus reactivation with progression of adult T-cell leukemia-lymphoma. PLoS ONE 4:e4420

Rooney CM, Smith CA, Ng CYC, Loftin S, Li C, Krance RA, Brenner MK, Heslop HE (1995) Use of gene-modified virus-specific T lymphocytes to control Epstein-Barr-virus-related lymphoproliferation. Lancet 345:9–13

Schrama D, Ugurel S, Becker JC (2012) Merkel cell carcinoma: recent insights and new treatment options. Curr Opin Oncol 24:141–149

Sima N, Wang S, Wang W, Kong D, Xu Q, Tian X, Luo A, Zhou J, Xu G, Meng L, Lu Y, Ma D (2007) Antisense targeting human papillomavirus type 16 E6 and E7 genes contributes to apoptosis and senescence in SiHa cervical carcinoma cells. Gynecol Oncol 106:299–304

Singal AK, Singh A, Jaganmohan S, Guturu P, Mummadi R, Kuo YF, Sood GK (2010) Antiviral therapy reduces risk of hepatocellular carcinoma in patients with hepatitis C virus-related cirrhosis. Clin Gastroenterol Hepatol 8:192–199

Soriano V, Vispo E, Labarga P, Medrano J, Barreiro P (2010) Viral hepatitis and HIV co- infection. Antiviral Res 85:303–315

Straathof KCM, Bollard CM, Popat U, Huls MH, Lopez T, Morriss MC, Gresik MV, Gee AP, Russell HV, Brenner MK, Rooney CM, Heslop HE (2005) Treatment of nasopharyngeal carcinoma with Epstein-Barr virus-specific T lymphocytes. Blood 105:1898–1904

Sung JJ, Tsoi KK, Wong VW, Li KC, Chan HL (2008) Meta-analysis: treatment of hepatitis B infection reduces risk of hepatocellular carcinoma. Aliment Pharmacol Ther 28:1067–1077

Sunil M, Reid E, Lechowicz MJ (2010) Update on HHV-8-associated malignancies. Curr Infect Dis Rep 12:147–154

Tolstov YL, Pastrana DV, Feng H, Becker JC, Jenkins FJ, Moschos S, Chang Y, Buck CB, Moore PS (2009) Human Merkel cell polyomavirus infection II. MCV is a common human infection that can be detected by conformational capsid epitope immunoassays. Int J Cancer 125:1250–1256

Toy M, Veldhuijzen IK, De Man RA, Richardus J, Schalm SW (2008) The potential impact of long-term nucleoside therapy on the mortality and morbidity of high viremic chronic hepatitis B [Abstract]. Hepatology 48(Suppl):717A

Tsukasaki K, Hermine O, Bazarbachi A, Ratner L, Ramos JC, Harrington W Jr, O'Mahony D, Janik JE, Bittencourt AL, Taylor GP, Yamaguchi K, Utsunomiya A, Tobinai K, Watanabe T (2009) Definition, prognostic factors, treatment, and response criteria of adult T-cell leukemia-lymphoma: a proposal from an international consensus meeting. J Clin Oncol 27:453–459

van Zonneveld M, Honkoop P, Hansen BE, Niesters HG, Darwish Murad S, de Man RA, Schalm SW, Janssen HL (2004) Long-term follow-up of alpha-interferon treatment of patients with chronic hepatitis B. Hepatology 39:804–810

Willmes C, Adam C, Alb M, Volkert L, Houben R, Becker JC, Schrama D (2012) Type I and II IFNs inhibit Merkel cell carcinoma via modulation of the Merkel cell polyomavirus T antigens. Cancer Res 72:2120–2128

Wong GL, Yiu KK, Wong VW, Tsoi KK, Chan HL (2010) Meta-analysis: reduction in hepatic events following interferon-alfa therapy of chronic hepatitis B. Aliment Pharmacol Ther 32:1059–1068

Woodman CB, Collins SI, Young LS (2007) The natural history of cervical HPV infection: unresolved issues. Nat Rev Cancer 7:11–22

Xi LF, Hughes JP, Castle PE, Edelstein ZR, Wang C, Galloway DA, Koutsky LA, Kiviat NB, Schiffman M (2011) Viral load in the natural history of human papillomavirus type 16 infection: a nested case-control study. J Infect Dis 203:1425–1433

Yang YF, Zhao W, Zhong YD, Xia HM, Shen L, Zhang N (2009) Interferon therapy in chronic hepatitis B reduces progression to cirrhosis and hepatocellular carcinoma: a meta-analysis. J Viral Hepat 16:265–271

Yeh ML, Hung CH, Huang JF, Liu CJ, Lee CM, Dai CY, Wang JH, Lin ZY, Lu SN, Hu TH, Yu ML, Kao JH, Chuang WL, Chen PJ, Chen DS (2011) Long-term effect of interferon plus ribavirin on hepatitis B surface antigen seroclearance in patients dually infected with hepatitis B and C viruses. PLoS ONE 6:e20752

Zhang CH, Xu GL, Jia WD, Li JS, Ma JL, Ge YS (2011) Effects of interferon treatment on development and progression of hepatocellular carcinoma in patients with chronic virus infection: a meta-analysis of randomized controlled trials. Int J Cancer 129:1254–1264

Zhou J, Peng C, Li B, Wang F, Zhou C, Hong D, Ye F, Cheng X, Lu W, Xie X (2012) Transcriptional gene silencing of HPV16 E6/E7 induces growth inhibition via apoptosis in vitro and in vivo. Gynecol Oncol 124:296–302

Zwaveling S, Ferreira Mota SC, Nouta J, Johnson M, Lipford GB, Offringa R, van der Burg SH, Melief CJM (2002) Established human papillomavirus type 16-expressing tumors are effectively eradicated following vaccination with long peptides. J Immunol 169:350–358